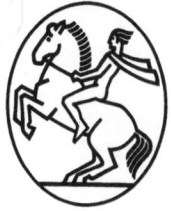

Advanced Intraoperative Technologies in Neurosurgery

Edited by V. A. Fasano

Authors:

R. E. Anderson
J. E. Boggan
L. J. Cerullo
M. C. Chan
G. J. Dohrmann
M. S. B. Edwards
V. A. Fasano
J. M. Gilsbach

A. Harders
R. M. Ikeda
P. J. Kelly
E. R. Laws, Jr.
G. Lee
T. Letardi
D. T. Mason
C. R. Neblett

R. W. Rand
A. Renieri
I. L. Richmond
J. M. Rubin
A. W. Silberman
R. Urciuoli
R. E. Wharen, Jr.

Springer-Verlag Wien New York

Professor VICTOR ALDO FASANO
Director of the Institute of Neurosurgery,
University of Turin, Italy

With 124 partly colored Figures

Library of Congress Cataloging-in-Publication Data. Main entry under title: Advanced intraoperative technologies in neurosurgery. 1. Nervous system—Surgery. 2. Lasers in surgery. 3. Ultrasonics in surgery. I. Fasano, V. A. (Vittorio Aldo), 1920– . [DNLM: 1. Neurosurgery—methods. WL 368 A244] RD593.A38 1986. 617'.48. 85-17327.

ISBN 978-3-7091-8812-5   ISBN 978-3-7091-8810-1 (eBook)
DOI 10.1007/978-3-7091-8810-1

Preface

Since the introduction of electrosurgery the techniques of surgery on the nervous system have passed through further improvements (bipolar coagulation, microscope), even if the procedure was not substantially modified. Today, laser represents a new "discipline", as it offers a new way of performing all basic maneuvers (dissection, demolition, hemostasis, vessel sutures). Furthermore, laser offers the possibility of a special maneuver, namely reduction of the volume of a tumoral mass through vaporization. Its application is not restricted to traditional neurosurgery but extends also to stereotactic and vascular neurosurgery. Laser surgery has also influenced the anesthesiologic techniques.

At the same time new instrumentation has been introduced: CUSA ultrasonic aspiration, echotomography, and Doppler flowmeter. I have had the chance to utilize these new technologies all at a time and have come to the conclusion that we are facing the dawn of a new methodology which has already shown its validity and lack of inconveniences, and whose object is to increase the precision of neurological surgery.

The technological development is still going on, and some improvements are to be foreseen. Laser scalpel is splitting the initial laser surgery into NO-TOUCH and TOUCH surgery with laser. As new instrumentarium will be developed, a variable and tunable beam will become available. For example, in a few years Free Electron Laser will further add to the progress in this field.

We have also included a chapter on local hyperthermia, as we think that its development will raise renewed interest in malignant tumors and give neurosurgeons and patients a glimmer of hope.

We may certainly say that all these new technologies have already improved the traditional procedures; it may well be that they will eventually substitute them. New solutions in all fields of neurosurgery will be the consequence.

All neurosurgeons are interested in keeping pace with these rapid developments. Their consistent presentation is the principal goal of this volume.

I am very grateful to all my colleagues, whose knowledge of the subject is based on vast surgical experience, for their enthusiastic contributions.

My very grateful thanks are due to all my assistants of the Department of Neurosurgery of the University of Torino, who have always collaborated with me in the development of the use of new technologies.

I should like to thank the following for their valuable contributions:

The Administration of the Ospedale Maggiore di S. Giovanni Battista e della Città di Torino.

The Cassa di Risparmio di Torino; the Istituto Bancario S. Paolo di Torino; G. S. G. Laser, Torino; Biomatic, Milano; Stern, Bolzano; Sharplan, Tel Aviv; Medilas, München; Cooper, Santa Clara, California; Prof. Nozio Daikuzono, President of the Surgical Laser Technologies, Japan Co. Ltd., Japan.

My sincere appreciation is due to Dr. Saverio M. Peirone (Professore Associato di Zoologia, Facoltà di Veterinaria, Università di Torino) to whom I owe the histological studies.

I must acknowledge the competence and dedication of my assistant Dr. Roberto M. Ponzio, who showed admirable patience in helping me write my text.

I am also grateful to Dr. Michael Mostert (lettore di lingua inglese, Facoltà di Medicina, Università di Torino) for his kind supervision of my English manuscript.

For the interest shown in our common research, the considerable effort and constant Editorial Assistance in assembling this volume we are deeply indebted to Springer-Verlag Wien.

For the secretarial work and general supervision I thank particularly Miss Elisabeth Lainer of the Editorial Department of Springer-Verlag and my collaborator Dr. Merita Ferrero.

Torino, September 1985   V. A. FASANO

Contents

List of Contributors IX

1. Intraoperative Ultrasound

Intraoperative Real-Time Ultrasonography: Localization, Characterization
and Instrumentation of Lesions of Brain and Spinal Cord. By G. J.
DOHRMANN and J. M. RUBIN 3
Intraoperative A-Mode Echoencephalography in Neurosurgery. By V. A.
FASANO 20
Intraoperative Dopplersonography. By J. M. GILSBACH and A. HARDERS . 27

2. Laser Neurosurgery

Historical Introduction. By V. A. FASANO 51
Laser Physic. By V. A. FASANO 53
Laser Effect on Normal Nervous Tissue (CO_2-Nd: YAG). Histological Data.
By V. A. FASANO 72
Laser Effect on Normal Vessels (CO_2-Nd: YAG-Argon). Histological Data.
By V. A. FASANO 85
Laser. A Progress of the Traditional Surgical Procedure. By V. A. FASANO 93
Principles of Laser Surgery. By V. A. FASANO 97
Laser Safety. By V. A. FASANO 103
Laser Neurosurgical Techniques. By V. A. FASANO 107
Contact Laser. By V. A. FASANO 140
The Argon Laser and Its Application in Neurological Surgery. By M. S. B.
EDWARDS and J. E. BOGGAN 145
Laser in the Removal of Extraaxial Tumors of the Brain and Spinal Cord. By
L. J. CERULLO 154
The Stereotactic CO_2 Laser: Instrumentation, Methodology and Clinical
Results. By P. J. KELLY 162
The Use of Lasers in Nerve Repair. By I. L. RICHMOND 175
Laser Vascular Application: Reconstructive and Reparative. By C. R.
NEBLETT 184
Application of Laser for Vaporization of Atherosclerotic Disease. By G. LEE,
M. C. CHAN, R. M. IKEDA, and D. T. MASON 195

Contents

Photoradiation Therapy with Hematoporphyrin Derivative in the Management of Brain Tumors. By R. E. WHAREN, JR., R. E. ANDERSON, E. R. LAWS, JR. 211
Anesthesiological Techniques in Laser Neurosurgery. By R. URCIUOLI . . 228
The Light for the Future: Excimer and Free-Electron Lasers. By T. LETARDI and A. RENIERI 236
The Role of Laser in Neurosurgery. Conclusions. By V. A. FASANO. . . 251

3. Ultrasonic Aspiration in Neurosurgery

Ultrasonic Aspiration in Neurosurgery. By V. A. FASANO 257

4. Localized Hyperthermia for the Treatment of Cerebral Tumors

Localized Hyperthermia for the Treatment of Cerebral Tumors. By A. W. SILBERMAN and R. W. RAND 277

Subject Index 305

List of Contributors

ANDERSON, R. E., Department of Neurologic Surgery, Mayo Clinic, Mayo Medical School, Rochester, MN 55905, U.S.A.

BOGGAN, J. E., The Department of Neurosurgery, University of California, Davis, California, U.S.A.

CERULLO, L. J., University Neurosurgeons, S.C., 676 N. St. Clair, Suite 1950, Chicago, IL 60611, U.S.A.

CHAN, M. C., Western Heart Institute, St. Mary's Hospital and Medical Center, 450 Stanyan Street, San Francisco, CA 94117, U.S.A.

DOHRMANN, G. J., Associate Professor of Neurosurgery, Section of Neurosurgery, H.B. 405, University of Chicago Medical Center, 5841 South Maryland Avenue, Chicago, IL 60637, U.S.A.

EDWARDS, M. S. B., Associate Professor of Neurosurgery and Pediatrics, Department of Neurological Surgery, University of California, 1360 Ninth Avenue, Suite 210, San Francisco, CA 94122, U.S.A.

FASANO, V. A., Professor, Direttore dell'Istituto di Neurochirurgia, Università di Torino, Via Cherasco 15, I-10126 Torino, Italy.

GILSBACH, J. M., Professor, Abteilung Allgemeine Neurochirurgie, Neurochirurgische Universitätsklinik, Klinikum der Albert-Ludwigs-Universität, Hugstetterstrasse 55, D-7800 Freiburg i. Br., Federal Republic of Germany.

IKEDA, R. M., Western Heart Institute, St. Mary's Hospital and Medical Center, 450 Stanyan Street, San Francisco, CA 94117, U.S.A.

HARDERS, A., Abteilung Allgemeine Neurochirurgie, Neurochirurgische Universitätsklinik, Klinikum der Albert-Ludwigs-Universität, Hugstetterstrasse 55, D-7800 Freiburg i. Br., Federal Republic of Germany.

KELLY, P. J., Associate Professor of Neurosurgery, Department of Neurologic Surgery, Mayo Clinic, Rochester, MN 55905, U.S.A.

LAWS, E. R., JR., Department of Neurologic Surgery, Mayo Clinic, Mayo Medical School, Rochester, MN 55905, U.S.A.

LEE, G., Director of Research, Western Heart Institute, St. Mary's Hospital and Medical Center, 450 Stanyan Street, San Francisco, CA 94117, U.S.A.

LETARDI, T., ENEA-Dip. TIB, Divisione Fisica Applicata, C.R.E. Frascati, C.P. 65, I-00044 Frascati (Roma), Italy.

MASON, D. T., The Western Heart Institute, St. Mary's Hospital and Medical Center, 450 Stanyan Street, San Francisco, CA 94117, U.S.A.

NEBLETT, C. R., Clinical Assistant Professor of Neurological Surgery, 1748 Scurlock Tower, 6560 Fannin Street, Houston, TX 77030, U.S.A.

RAND, R. W., Professor of Neurological Surgery, Division of Neurosurgery, Department of Surgery, UCLA School of Medicine, 760 Westwood Plaza, Los Angeles, CA 90024, U.S.A.

RENIERI, A., ENEA-Dip. TIB, Divisione Fisica Applicata, C.R.E. Frascati, C.P. 65, I-00044 Frascati (Roma), Italy.

RICHMOND, I. L., Commonwealth Neurosurgery, Ltd., 908 Medical Tower, Norfolk, VA 23507, U.S.A.

RUBIN, J. M., Associate Professor, Department of Radiology, University of Michigan Hospitals, Ann Arbor, Michigan, U.S.A.

SILBERMAN, A. W., Division of Surgical Oncology, University of California, 9th Floor Louis Factor Building, Los Angeles, CA 90024, U.S.A.

URCIUOLI, R., Istituto di Neurochirurgia, Università di Torino, Via Cherasco 15, I-10126 Torino, Italy.

WHAREN, R. E., JR., Department of Neurologic Surgery, Mayo Clinic, Mayo Medical School, Rochester, MN 55905, U.S.A.

1. Intraoperative Ultrasound

Intraoperative Real-Time Ultrasonography: Localization, Characterization and Instrumentation of Lesions of Brain and Spinal Cord

GEORGE J. DOHRMANN[1] and JONATHAN M. RUBIN[2]

[1] Section of Neurosurgery, University of Chicago Medical Center, Chicago, Ill. (U.S.A.)
[2] Department of Radiology, University of Michigan Hospitals, Ann Arbor, Mich. (U.S.A.)

Contents

I. Introduction		3
II. The Real-Time Ultrasound Scanner		4
III. Brain		6
	A. Technique	6
	B. Localization/Characterization	8
	C. Instrumentation	10
IV. Spinal Cord		14
	A. Technique	14
	B. Localization/Characterization	15
	C. Instrumentation	18
V. Carotid Endarterectomy		18
VI. Summary		18
References		18

I. Introduction

As tissue of the central nervous system is so delicate and as manipulation or exploration of the tissue could increase the morbidity of the operative procedure, precise localization of lesions within the brain or spinal cord is mandatory. Angiograms, computed tomographic (CT) scans and magnetic resonance (MR) scans demonstrate the lesion but do so from a given perspective; this perspective is often quite different from the position of the

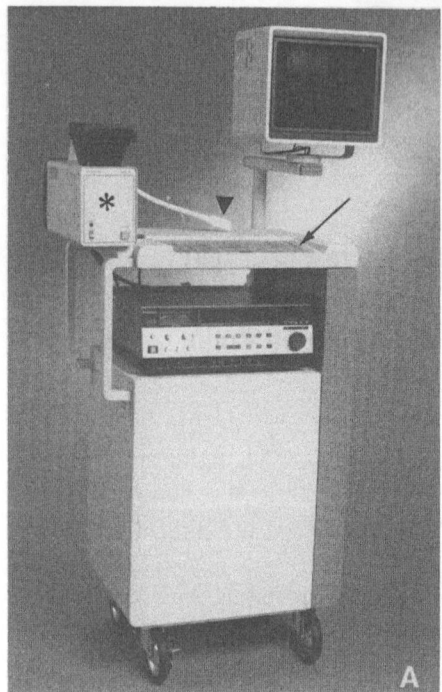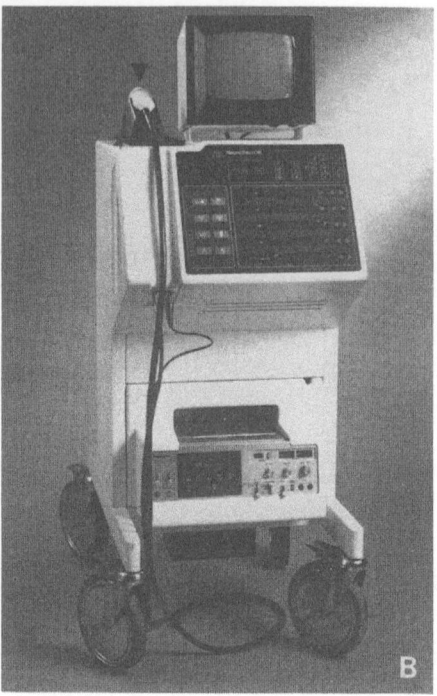

Fig. 1. Photographs of two types of real-time ultrasound scanners specifically designed for intraoperative use. A) Scanhead (arrowhead) connected by cable to scanner; videoscreen and videotape recorder are seen; Polaroid camera attachment (asterisk); pressure panel (arrow) to control scanner (Codman and Shurtleff, Inc., Randolph, MA 02368, U.S.A.). B) Cable connects scanhead (arrowhead) to scanner. Videoscreen is at top and videotape recorder is at bottom; pressure-sensitive control panel is seen at center (Advanced Technology Laboratories, Inc., Bellevue, WA 98005, U.S.A.). *Note:* Although various real-time ultrasound scanners may work for use in the operating room, the above scanners were designed to be used by the surgeon during the operative procedure and are "preset" for imaging of brain and spinal cord

patient on the operating table and there is a limited area of tissue exposure. The lesion is usually located beneath the surface of brain or spinal cord. We thought that intraoperative real-time ultrasound imaging would help with this localization and also serve to characterize the tissue (*i.e.,* solid tumor vs. necrosis vs. cyst) and we worked to develop neurosurgical real-time ultrasound imaging to aid with such problems[2-5, 9-13].

II. The Real-Time Ultrasound Scanner

Each ultrasound scanner consists of a control panel, a videotape recorder and a videoscreen (Figs. 1 A and B). The ultrasound transducers are contained within the scanheads and these scanheads are connected to the scanner by cables (Fig. 2). The transducers produce the sound waves and receive echos of the sound waves back from the tissue beneath. The reflected sound waves are interpreted by the scanner and displayed as a gray scale on the videoscreen. Greater echogenicity (as with tumors) is seen as more white and areas that transmit sound (such as CSF) are seen as black; tissue of the central nervous system is seen as shades of gray[1-15]. The scanner designed

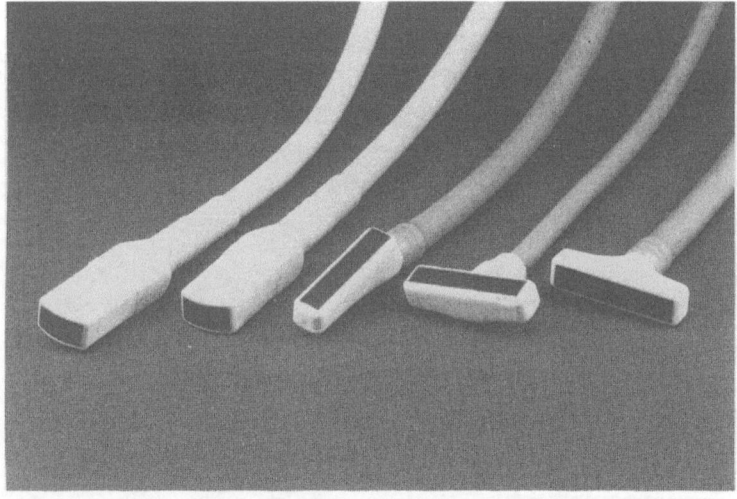

Fig. 2. Scanheads designed in various shapes and sizes for intraoperative use

for intraoperative use is controlled by a pressure sensitive panel; as such it may be covered by a transparent sterile drape and the neurosurgeon can operate the machine intraoperatively (Figs. 1 A and B). Transducers of different frequencies (3, 5, and 7.5 MHz) are within the scanheads and each has a specific use (Fig. 2). To image most of the intracranial contents, a 3 MHz transducer is used; it gives much penetration but the resolution is less. As the transducer frequency increases (5 and 7.5 MHz), the penetration decreases but the resolution becomes greater. Usually the lower frequency transducer is used to image much of brain and, thereby, to gain orientation and then a higher frequency transducer is used to better image the area of interest. A videotape recorder and/or a polaroid camera record the images. The scanner will measure the distance to the lesion and also the lesion diameter.

This type of ultrasound imaging is termed "real time" because the process is dynamic; the action (*i.e.,* pulsation of arteries, etc.) can be seen as it happens.

Scanheads are now produced in various shapes and sizes for

intraoperative use (Fig. 2). Some may be better for intracranial procedures, some for intraspinal procedures and some for procedures on the cervical carotid artery system.

Ultrasound imaging of the brain or spinal cord cannot be done preoperatively because they are encased in bone; however, the bone is removed in operative procedures and the brain and spinal cord can then be imaged very well. Because of this ultrasound imaging is the ideal method for dynamic imaging of brain and spinal cord in the operating room.

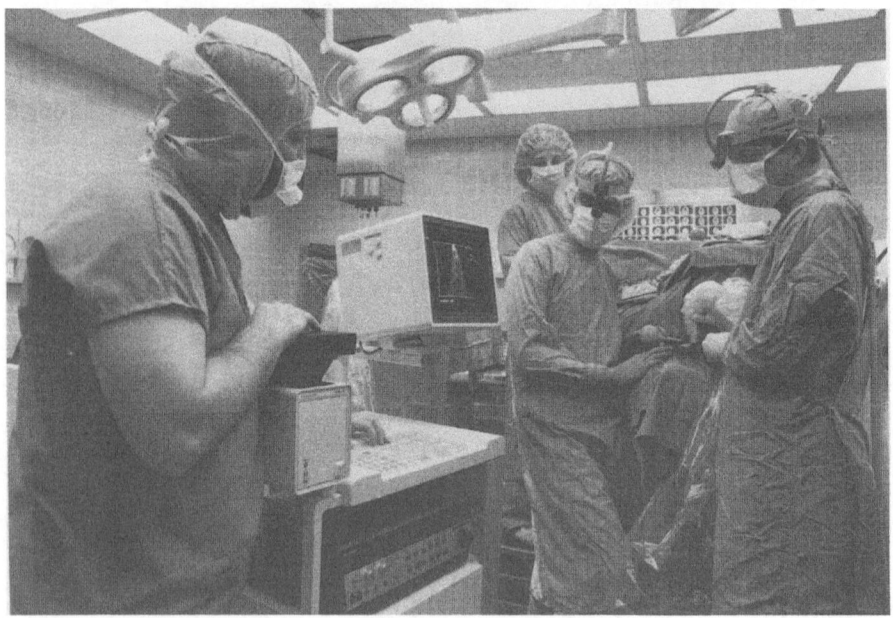

Fig. 3. Operating room arrangement for intraoperative ultrasound scanning

III. Brain

A. Technique

For intraoperative imaging the scanhead is covered with a sterile transparent plastic drape and touched to the surface of dura as exposed by craniotomy, craniectomy or large burr hole (Fig. 3). Several drops of saline are used as the coupling agent between the scanhead and the dura to maintain good contact (Fig. 4). The ultrasound is produced in a plane approximately 5 mm in thickness. If the dural exposure is lateral, then imaging in the coronal or transaxial planes can be done depending upon how the "plane of sound" is oriented. If the dural exposure is near the vertex, coronal or sagittal imaging of the brain can be obtained. It should be

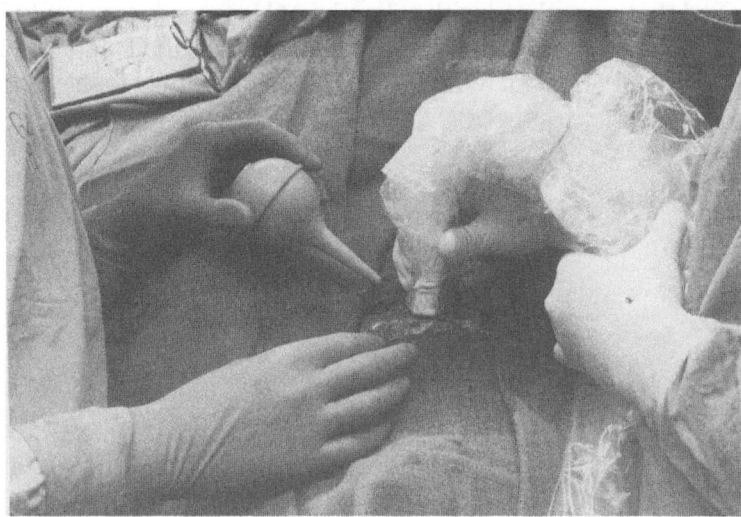

Fig. 4. Scanhead is covered with a sterile drape and touched to the surface of dura; several drops of saline are used to give good acoustic contact

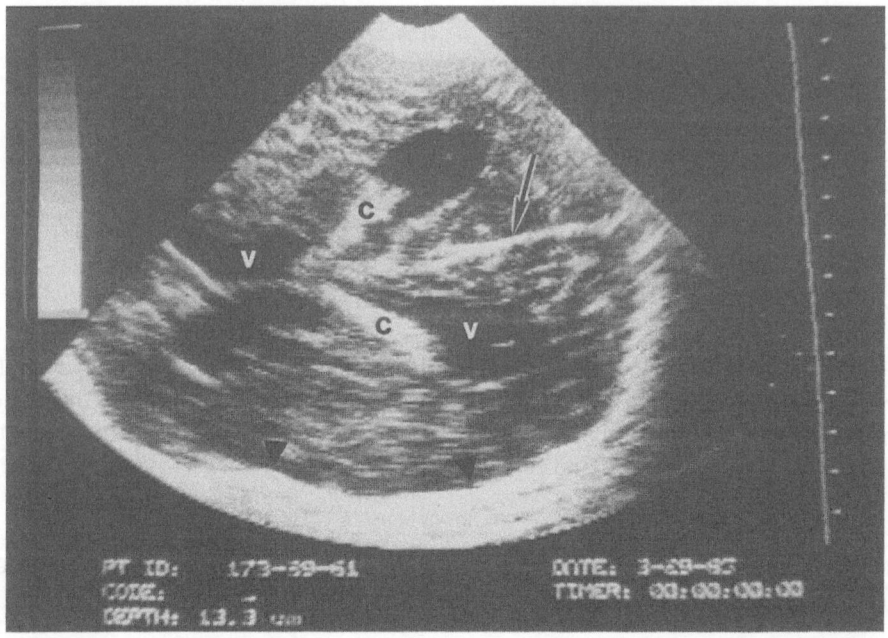

Fig. 5. Transaxial ultrasound scan of brain. Lateral ventricles (*V*); choroid plexuses (*C*); falx (arrow); skull of opposite side of head (arrowheads). (To image both sides of brain, a low frequency—3 MHz—transducer was used)

emphasized that a scanhead with a 3 or 3.5 MHz transducer should be used first; the ventricles and falx should then be identified and orientation thereby obtained (Fig. 5). When the area of interest is located, then the

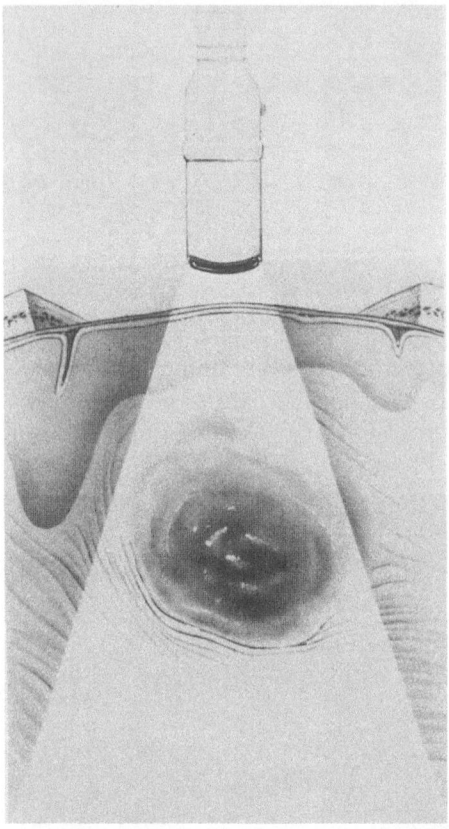

Fig. 6. Drawing showing ultrasound scanhead at top being used to image small brain tumor. Scanhead is touched to dura or to saline on surface of dura; the plane of ultrasound is seen (compare to Fig. 7). Reproduced with permission of Codman and Shurtleff, Inc., U.S.A.

scanhead with higher frequency transducers (5 and 7.5 MHz) could be used to see the area in more detail.

B. Localization/Characterization

Tumors are seen to be more echogenic than brain and the surrounding edema can be imaged as well[5, 10]. Ultrasound imaging is particularly useful in locating small metastatic tumors (Figs. 6 and 7). In addition, the ultrasound can characterize the lesions (*i.e.,* solid vs. necrotic vs. cystic

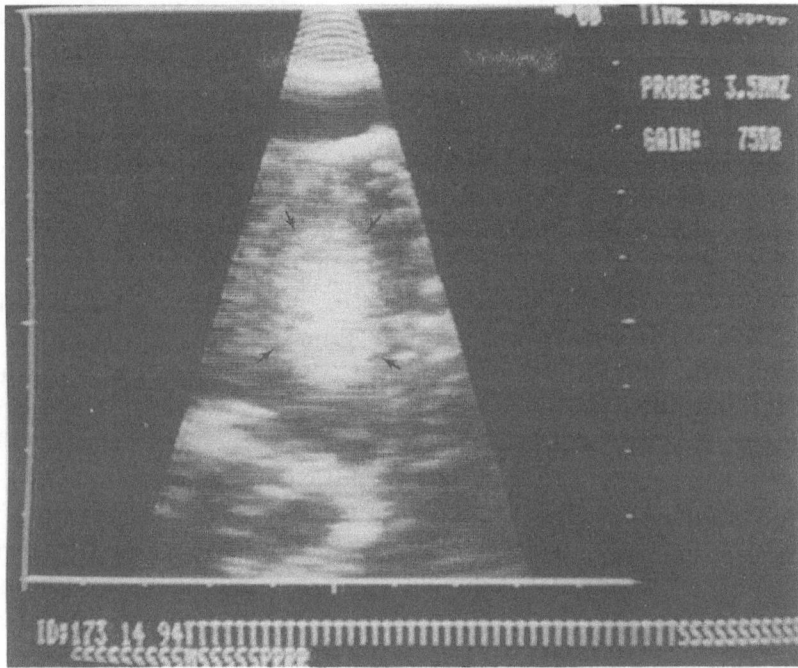

Fig. 7. Static image of intraoperative ultrasound scan showing the triangular plane of ultrasound; small metastatic tumor (arrows) within brain (compare to Fig. 6)

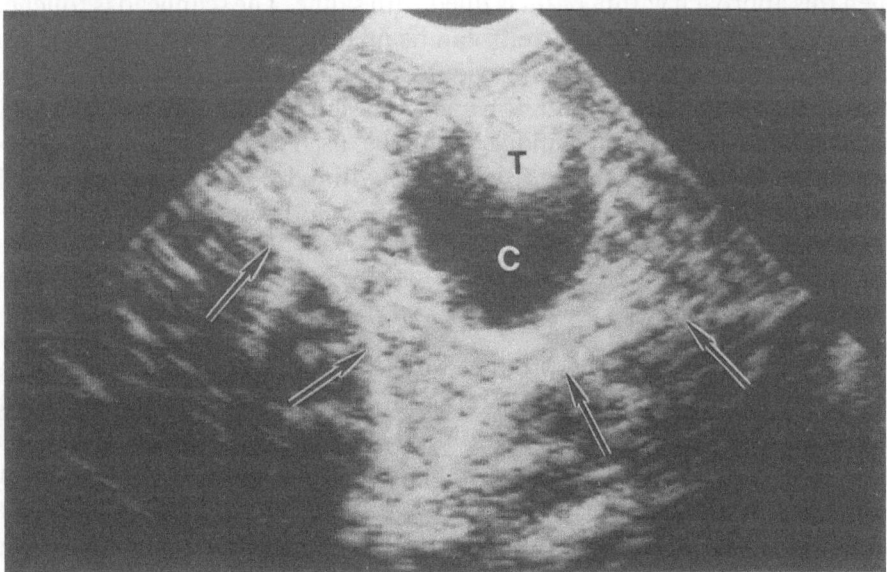

Fig. 8. Ultrasound scan showing cerebellar cyst (*C*) with mural tumor nodule (*T*); tentorium (arrows)

regions) (Fig. 8). Abscesses and cysts can be readily located using intraoperative ultrasound; "daughter abscesses" or loculated portions of abscesses or cysts can be identified and the effects of drainage procedures assessed.

Acute intracerebral hematomas can be seen as more echogenic than the surrounding brain and these can be approached and evacuated precisely. Angiomas and arteriovenous malformations may be located using ultrasound and sometimes the feeding vessel(s) can be imaged as well, thus allowing an accurate operative approach to them. Should local or distant hemorrhage occur during an operation on vascular malformations, the ultrasound can be used to identify it. In patients with penetrating head trauma, fragments of indriven bone or foreign bodies (metal, glass, wood, plastic, etc.), whether radioopaque or not, can be seen with ultrasound and these can be removed using continuous ultrasound guidance.

Giant aneurysms can be imaged with ultrasound and the region of the thickened wall can be identified. The residual lumen with blood swirling within can also be imaged. If a debulking procedure is planned, knowledge of the thickness of the wall of the aneurysm is very important. Thrombogenic needles can be placed in the region of the neck of the aneurysm and the blood in the lumen can be seen to form a thrombus. All of this can be done under intraoperative ultrasound guidance.

Small lesions deep within the brain can be approached directly and precisely using real-time ultrasound imaging in the operating room. A small topectomy is performed and dissection carried down for a short distance, then this approach within brain is filled with saline. The scanhead is touched to the saline and the "saline well" can be imaged as can the lesion, and the approach may be modified as needed. Repeating this technique can lead the neurosurgeon directly to the lesion and the lesion could be resected *en bloc* if so desired. This same technique could be used to gauge the extent of resection of a tumor. The operative cavity within brain could be filled with saline and residual tumor could be identified and resected.

C. Instrumentation

The plane of ultrasound produced by the transducers is narrow, only a matter of millimeters in width (Fig. 6). An instrument passed with ultrasound guidance must stay within that plane to be imaged. If it passes out of the plane on either side, it will no longer be seen from that point on. For this reason it is important to use an instrument guide when passing a biopsy cannula, ventricular catheter, etc. under ultrasound guidance (Fig. 9). Such a guide allows the instrument to be moved in and out within the scan plane but does not allow the instrument to move laterally out of the scan plane. Various instrument guides are available, and these can be set

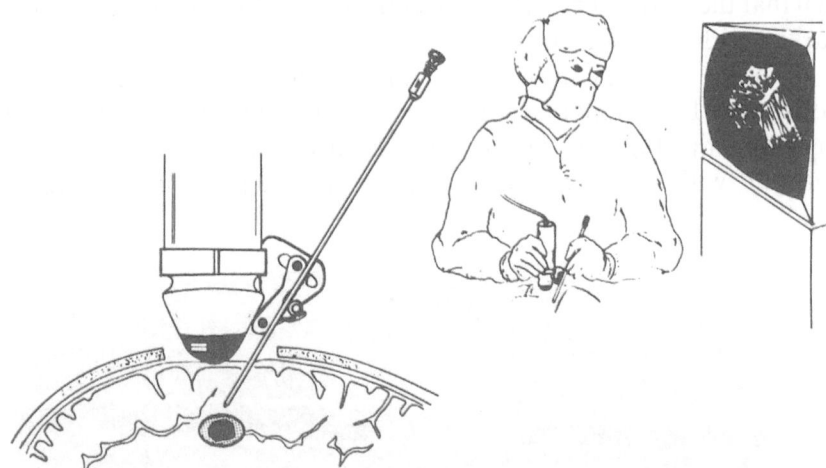

Fig. 9. Line showing the biopsy of an intracranial lesion via craniectomy using an instrument guide and a biopsy cannula (compare to Fig. 10)

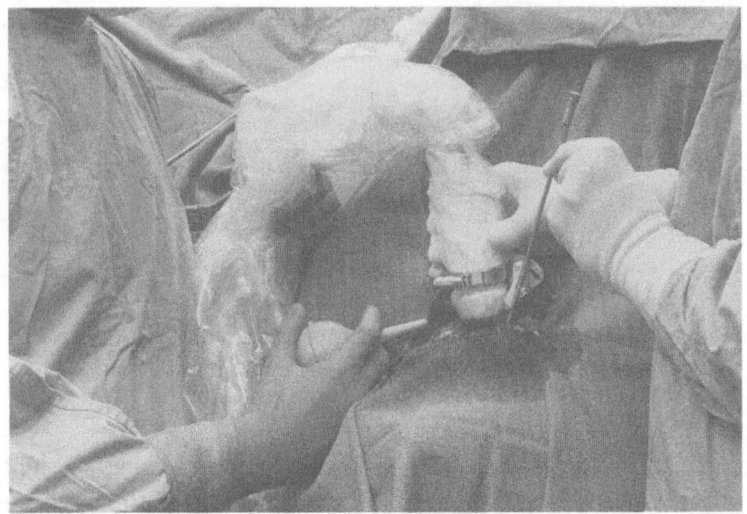

Fig. 10. Biopsy of deep brain tumor using intraoperative ultrasound guidance. Sterilely-draped scanhead is touched to dura and the target is imaged on the videoscreen. The scanner measures the depth of the lesion and the instrument guide is set for that depth and the biopsy cannula is advanced through a small dural incision down to the lesion. The biopsy is taken and the procedure is recorded on videotape. Scanning is continued for several minutes post-biopsy to watch for possible hemorrhage. Note specially designed biopsy cannula for use in ultrasound-guided biopsies of brain (American V. Mueller, McGaw Park, IL 60085, U.S.A.)

such that the instrument will intersect the target (Fig. 10). Often the target is marked with a cursor on the videoscreen.

Biopsy of deep lesions is done with a cannula* specifically designed for ultrasound. It is similar to a Dorsey cannula but longer and with etched rings at its tip (Fig. 10). The length is needed because of the "dead space" involved with the instrument guide; the etched rings increase the

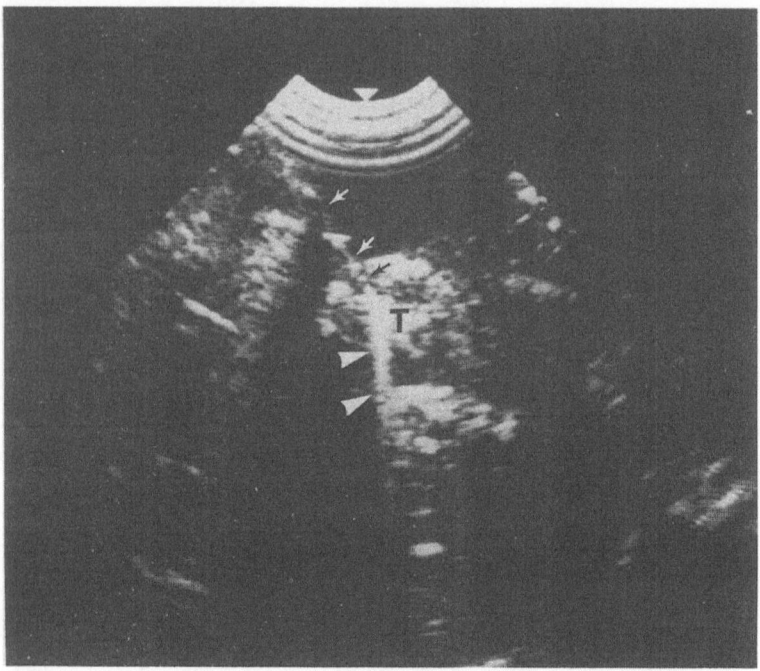

Fig. 11. Biopsy of deep brain tumor (*T*). Biopsy cannula (arrows); reverberations (arrowheads) from very echogenic tip of biopsy cannula

echogenicity of the tip and it shows up on the videoscreen as a bright dot at the tip of the cannula (Fig. 11). For this reason the tip of the instrument can always be identified. Should the tip of the instrument deviate laterally out of the scan plane for any reason, this situation can be identified immediately and corrected.

Using intraoperative ultrasound this biopsy cannula is advanced to the tumor (Fig. 11) and the stylet is then removed and the cannula is advanced into the tumor; a core of tissue is thereby obtained[2, 9]. The entire procedure can be recorded on videotape and the exact region of the lesion biopsied

_____

* Dohrmann-Rubin biopsy cannula, American V. Mueller, McGaw Park, IL 60085, U.S.A.

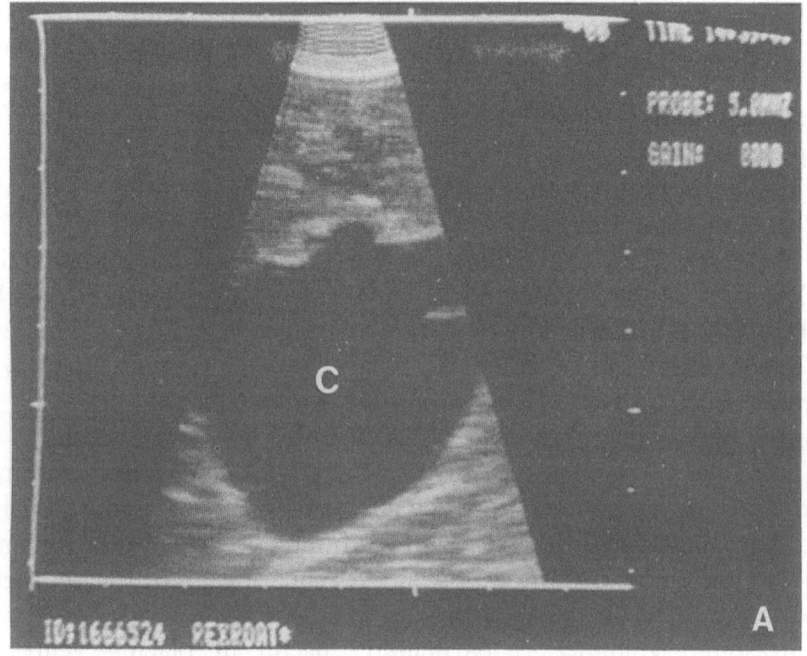

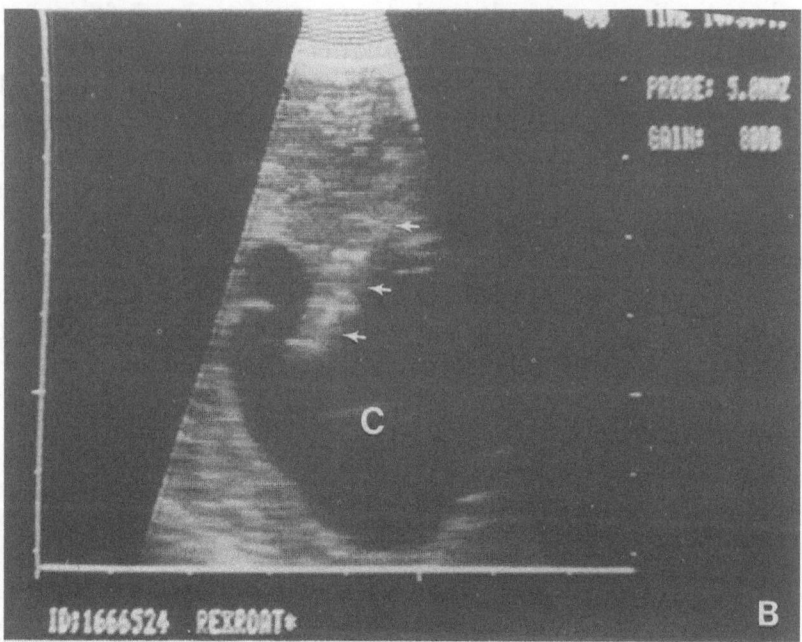

Fig. 12. Cerebellar cyst shown on ultrasound scans. A) Cyst (*C*). B) Catheter (arrows) being introduced into cyst (*C*) using continuous ultrasound guidance

could be identified. This is helpful if the neuropathologist reports "gliosis near tumor or low grade astrocytoma". The ultrasound imaging has shown that the tissue came from the tumor itself and, therefore, it is not necessary to perform another biopsy. If desired, several regions of the tumor can be sampled as well.

Drainage of cysts or abscesses can be accomplished in ultrasound-guided procedures using an instrument guide as above (Figs. 12 A and B). Cysts and abscesses often can be seen to collapse postdrainage. Sometimes loculations or daughter abscesses, not noted on CT scans, are seen and these can be drained. Multiple abscesses can be drained with little manipulation and no exploration of brain tissue. Occasionally an area of cerebritis will resemble an abscess on CT scan appearing as a contrast-enhancing ring lesion; however, ultrasound can distinguish this from an abscess.

Ventricular catheters can be advanced into various structures within the brain using intraoperative ultrasound guidance (Figs. 12 A and B). We have chosen the ventricular catheter* with the finned tip because the fins make the tip of the catheter more echogenic. As such the tip of the ventricular catheter can always be identified.

Ultrasound guidance is particularly useful in placing ventricular catheters within small or normal-sized ventricles (*i.e.,* patients with head trauma requiring ventricular catheter for intracranial pressure monitoring or patients needing a ventricular catheter/Ommaya reservoir for intrathecal chemotherapy)[5, 9]. Sometimes in the latter group of patients the CSF pressure is so low that there is no CSF drainage upon placing the catheter within the frontal horn of the lateral ventricle. Proper placement is shown by ultrasound imaging; however, to further confirm the intraventricular position, air may be injected into the catheter/Ommaya reservoir and air bubbles can be seen to go out into the ventricle. In patients with hydrocephalus, optimal positioning of the ventricular catheters may be obtained using intraoperative ultrasound guidance[14]. Ventricular catheters can be guided to drain deep cysts within the brain and, if necessary, these catheters can be left within the cysts and connected to reservoirs or converted to shunting systems.

IV. Spinal Cord

A. Technique

With the patient in a prone position, a laminectomy is performed. The wound is then filled with saline and the sterilely-draped scanhead (7.5 MHz transducer) is touched to the saline (Fig. 13). The contents of the spinal canal are then imaged on the videoscreen of the ultrasound scanner. With

---

* Cordis Corporation, Miami, FL 33152, U.S.A.

this technique it is not necessary to touch the scanhead to the dural covering of the spinal cord. Depending upon which way the scanhead is held, the plane of ultrasound can be oriented to give cross-sectional or longitudinal images of the spinal cord and associated structures. Beneath the saline the posterior aspect of the dura is seen and beneath that the subarachnoid space

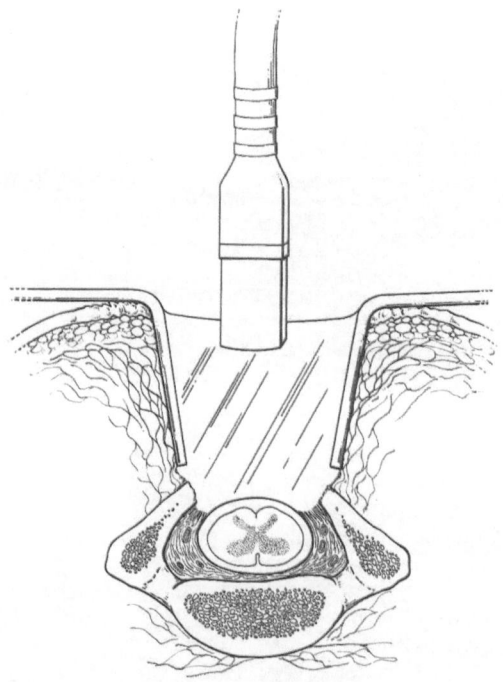

Fig. 13. Line drawing showing imaging of spinal cord and surrounding structures following laminectomy with patient in prone position. The wound is filled with saline and the sterile scanhead (7.5 MHz transducer) is touched to the saline and the contents of the spinal canal are imaged on the videoscreen

is noted. The spinal cord can be seen within the dural sac and the region of the central canal can be seen to be more echogenic than the rest of the spinal cord. Vertebral bodies are imaged as well[3, 8, 12].

B. Localization/Characterization

Intramedullary neoplasms are more echogenic (more white) than the surrounding spinal cord (Fig. 14)[3, 11]. Some neoplasms may be seen to contain cysts (Fig. 14). The location of the tumor can be determined using ultrasound as can the extent of resection (? residual tumor).

The various fluid-filled cavities of syringomyelia can be imaged and drainage of these assessed via ultrasound, and the best cavity for shunting may be chosen (Figs. 15 A and B)[3]. It is of interest that even though the widened spinal cord may collapse following shunting, sometimes not all of the fluid-filled cavities have drained. In these patients another shunting procedure is needed to drain the syrinx system that did not connect to the one that was shunted. Perhaps the suboptimal results obtained in the

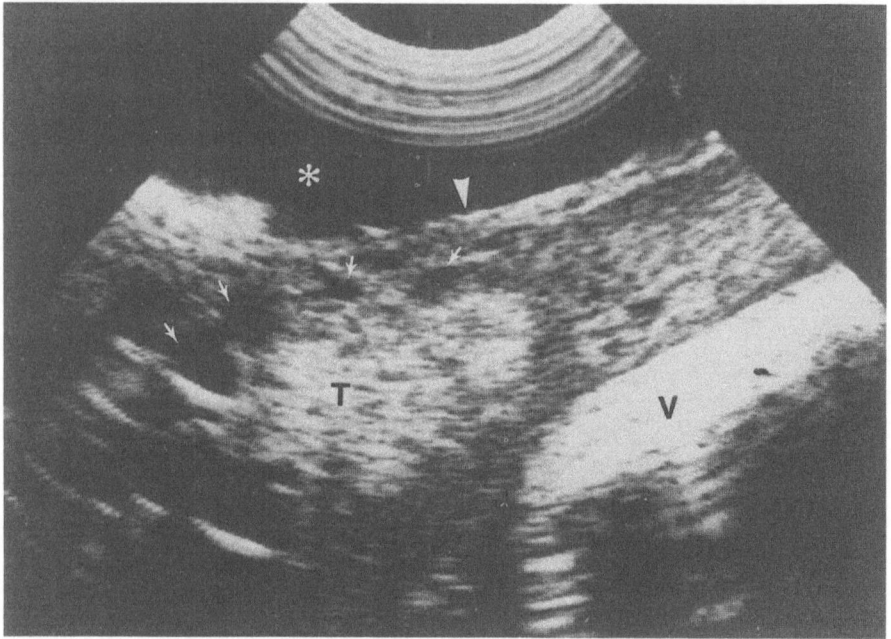

Fig. 14. Astrocytoma of spinal cord shown in longitudinal ultrasound scan. Posterior surface of dura (arrowhead) is closely juxtaposed to widened spinal cord such that no subarachnoid space is seen. Echogenic tumor tissue (*T*); cysts (arrows) within tumor; vertebral body (*V*); saline (asterisk)

treatment of patients with syringomyelia may be related to the fact that the shunting procedures may not have been complete.

Intradural extramedullary neoplasms may be identified precisely. Tumors with extradural and intradural components, such as schwannomas, can be evaluated well with ultrasound. Extradural lesions located anterior to the spinal cord or cauda equina can be identified with ultrasound. Central discs can be imaged and complete decompression of the spinal cord/cauda equina assessed with intraoperative ultrasound. Disc fragments may be located with ultrasound; this is of particular use if the fragments have migrated from the site of extrusion from the disc space[3, 5, 11, 12].

In patients with spondylosis involving anterior and posterior compression of the spinal cord or cauda equina at multiple levels, intraoperative ultrasound is helpful in assessing the extent of decompression following laminectomy. For example, in a certain patient the posterior aspect of the dura could be seen to move well with respirations

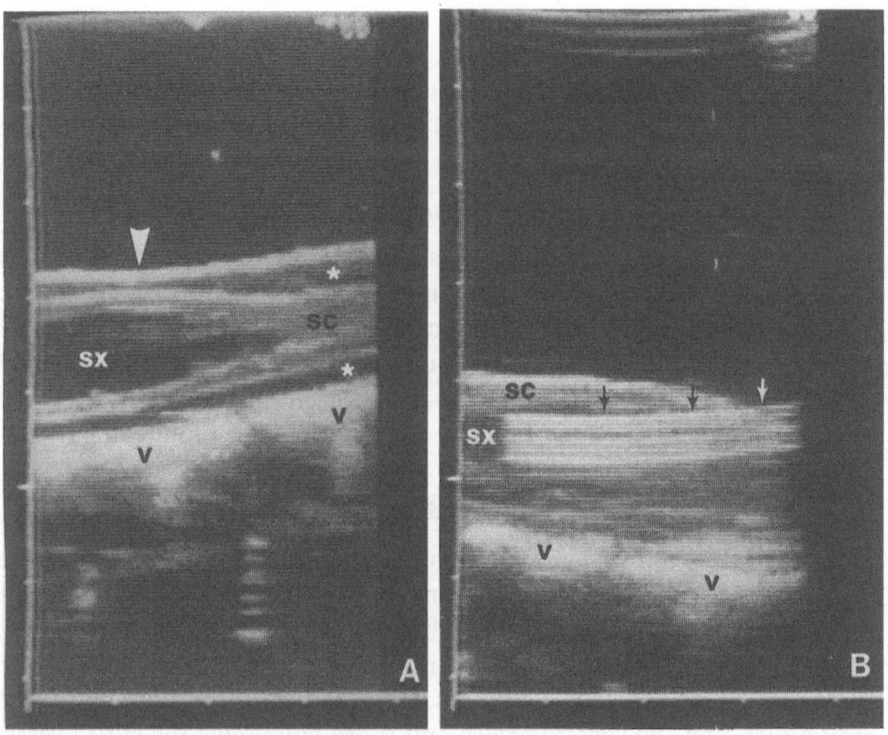

Fig. 15. Intraoperative ultrasound scans (7.5 MHz transducer) in patient with syringomyelia and one large central syrinx. A) Posterior surface of dura (arrowhead) with saline above; spinal cord (*SC*); syrinx (*SX*); subarachnoid space (asterisks); vertebral bodies (*V*). B) Shunt tube (arrows) within syrinx (*SX*); spinal cord (*SC*); vertebral bodies (*V*)

and this implied that the cervical spinal cord had been well decompressed. However, the cervical spinal cord was observed by ultrasound scanning to move rhythmically in conjunction with the heart rate; this is a sign of continuing compression of the spinal cord and transmission of the pulsations of the anterior spinal artery[6]. In this case the spinal cord was seen by ultrasound to be compressed by one of the anterior bony bars. Later, the patient had this bony bar removed via an anterior approach. Perhaps some of the suboptimal results in the treatment of cervical spondylosis are due to unsuspected continued anterior compression of the spinal cord.

Intraoperative ultrasound can assess the degree of decompression and identify immediately "pathological pulsation" of the spinal cord[6].

Intraoperative ultrasound is useful in patients with spine/spinal cord trauma. Indriven bone fragments or foreign bodies can be identified within the spinal canal. Anterior compression of the spinal cord/cauda equina by bone fragments, etc. can be identified. In some patients following the placement of Harrington or Luque rods to straighten the spine, the fractured bone anteriorly may be seen to realign and anterior decompression of the spinal cord/cauda equina accomplished. This can be monitored using intraoperative real-time ultrasound imaging in the operating room.

C. Instrumentation

Placement of catheters within cysts or syrinx cavities can be done precisely with intraoperative ultrasound guidance (Figs. 15 A and B). Following placement the positioning can be assessed and, sometimes, the catheter can be seen to have migrated superiorly and can be wedged against the wall of the cyst/syrinx. In that position it might eassily become obstructed; repositioning can be done with ultrasound monitoring.

V. Carotid Endarterectomy

Intraoperative ultrasound can be used to measure the diameter of the lumen of the cervical carotid artery. Following endarterectomy, arteriotomy closure and restoration of blood flow within the carotid system, intraoperative ultrasound imaging can be done to detect stenosis or the presence of an intimal flap. Certain scanheads have been designed to be placed directly on the carotid artery and those will image the entire vessel beneath.

VI. Summary

In summary intraoperative real-time ultrasound imaging is very useful in the neurosurgical operating room for localization, characterization and instrumentation of lesions of brain and spinal cord. The intraoperative ultrasound scanning systems described here have been designed to be used in the operating room by the neurosurgeon much as any other instrument in his surgical armamentarium.

References

1. Chandler, W. F., Knake, J. E., McGillicuddy, J. E., Lillehei, K. O., Silver, T. M., 1982: Intraoperative use of real-time ultrasonography in neurosurgery. J. Neurosurg. *57*, 157–163.
2. Dohrmann, G. J., Rubin, J. M., 1981: Use of ultrasound in neurosurgical operations: a preliminary report. Surg. Neurol. *16*, 362–366.

3. Dohrmann, G. J., Rubin, J. M., 1982: Intraoperative ultrasound imaging of the spinal cord: syringomyelia, cysts and tumors. A preliminary report. Surg. Neurol. *18*, 395–399.
4. Dohrmann, G. J., Rubin, J. M., 1985: Dynamic intraoperative imaging and instrumentation of brain and spinal cord using ultrasound. Neurol. Clin. *3*, 425–437.
5. Dohrmann, G. J., Rubin, J. M., 1985: Intraoperative diagnostic ultrasound. In: Neurosurgery (Wilkins, R. H., Rengachary, S. S., eds.), pp. 457–463. New York:. McGraw-Hill.
6. Jokich, P. M., Rubin, J. M., Dohrmann, G. J., 1984: Intraoperative ultrasonic assessment of spinal cord motion. J. Neurosurg. *60*, 707–711.
7. Masuzawa, H., Kamitani, H., Sato, J., Inoya, H., Hachiya, J., Sakai, F., 1981: Intraoperative application of sector scanning electronic ultrasound in neurosurgery. Neurol. Med. Chir. (Tokyo) *21*, 277–285.
8. Quencer, R. M., Morse, B. M., Green, B. A., Eismont, F. J., Brost, P., 1984: Intraoperative spinal sonography: adjunct to metrizamide CT in the assessment and surgical decompression of posttraumatic spinal cord cysts. A.J.R. *142*, 593–601.
9. Rubin, J. M., Dohrmann, G. J., 1982: Use of ultrasonically-guided probes and catheters in neurosurgery. Surg. Neurol. *18*, 143–148.
10. Rubin, J. M., Dohrmann, G. J., 1983: Intraoperative neurosurgical ultrasound in the localization and characterization of intracranial masses. Radiol. *148*, 519–524.
11. Rubin, J. M., Dohrmann, G. J., 1985: The spine and spinal cord during neurosurgical operations: real-time ultrasonography. Radiol. *155*, 197–200.
12. Rubin, J. M., Dohrmann, G. J., 1985: Intraoperative sonography of the spine and spinal cord. Review article. Semin. Ultrasound. CT. MR. *6*, 48–67.
13. Rubin, J. M., Mirfakhraee, M., Duda, E. E., Dohrmann, G. J., Brown, F., 1980: Intraoperative ultrasound examination of the brain. Radiol. *137*, 831–832.
14. Shkolnik, A., McLone, D. G., 1981: Intraoperative real-time ultrasonic guidance of ventricular shunt placement in infants. Radiol. *141*, 515–517.
15. Voorhies, R. M., Engel, I., Gamache, F. W., jr., Patterson, R. H., jr., Fraser, R. A. R., Lavyne, M. H., Schneider, M., 1983: Intraoperative localization of subcortical brain tumors: Further experience with B-mode real-time sector scanning. Neurosurg. *12*, 189–194.

Intraoperative A-Mode Echoencephalography in Neurosurgery

VICTOR A. FASANO

Institute of Neurosurgery, University of Turin (Italy)

Contents

1. Historical Introduction 20
2. Physical Principles.. 21
3. Surgical Applications and Results 23
References 25

1. Historical Introduction

Sound is classified by its frequency. The range of audible sound is from 16 to 18,000 cycles per second (cps). Ultrasound spans a frequency of 18,000 cps to 100,000 megacycles per second (one megacycle is one million of cycles per second or one megahertz MHz). In this discussion, ultrasound in the higher frequency ranges only is considered: from 1 to 15 MHz per second.

The first attempts to adapt ultrasound for diagnostic purposes in medicine date back to 1937. Applications were in outlining the cerebral ventricular system (Dussik, Geuttner)[1, 5]. French, Wild and Neal in 1950 demonstrated at autopsy that ultrasonic reflection or echoes were obtainable from brain tumors. In 1951 they recorded similar tumor echoes from the brain of a living patient at the time of craniotomy[3, 4]. In 1956 Leksell published a monograph that opened extensive investigation into the diagnostic applications of ultrasound. He coined the term echo encephalography to describe his technique[7, 8].

Conventionally, echo ranging has been employed to demonstrate through an intact skull the position of the structures of the midline. The thickness of the cerebral mantle can also be measured, particularly in the pediatric age group. Intraoperative transdural A-mode sonography has been used to demarcate, characterize and determine depths of such lesions.

Although the difference in ultrasonic velocities between brain and cerebral neoplasia is only slight, these differences are sufficient to provide an interface from which ultrasound can be reflected. Because of necrosis, hemorrhage, cavitation and variable cellular density within a tumor, multiple interfaces are created.

By their reflections of ultrasounds, all cerebral lesions may be divided into solid, cystic or a combination of two. When the lesion has a homogeneous consistency (metastases, fibrous meningioma) frequently uniform equal amplitude reflections of ultrasound are recorded. In contrast, a glioblastoma multiforme with its variable tissue architecture produces a tumor echo complex made up of variable-intensity ultrasonic reflections. Because of the frequent changes in consistency it is, however, difficult to classify brain tumors as to their histological type on the basis of their ultrasonic properties.

The recent innovations in echoencephalography have increased the applications in surgery. While working on methods of calibration in A-mode in order to analyze, at specific frequency and amplification, the records of a test-tube containing citrated blood (depth 2.5 cm, 4,600,000 red cells/cm^3), Ossoinig in 1970 could obtain a higher number and amplitude of peaks particularly suitable for intracranial detection. Utilizing this instrument * in several orbital tumors Ossoinig obtained a high specificity of histological diagnosis (greatest than 90%)[9]. This strict correlation between echographic pattern and pathology has been confirmed by other authors[10, 11].

2. Physical Principles

Most diagnostic conventional units employ a 2.25 MHz transducer. This sound frequency will generally penetrate 17 to 18 cm of soft tissue and return recordable echoes, attenuation depending on absorption and scattering of the acoustic energy. Absorption is the amount of energy converted into heat; scattering occurs when ultrasound travels through a medium in which tissual constituents are smaller than the wavelength used (center of scattering). Higher frequency ultrasound, having a shorter wavelength, gives better resolution of detail but poorer penetrance of tissues. For example, a 5 MHz crystal produces sound that will travel only 5 cm in soft tissue and still return meaningful echoes. Because of the high reflection, absorption and deflection properties of the skull (approximately 90% of the incident energy) transcranial detection requires a 1 MHz transducer since it has greater penetrance. Ultrasound in the megacycle range is for practical purposes not transmissible in air but is readily

---

* Kretz 7200 MA.

conducted in solids and liquids. Hence, a coupling medium that excludes air between the crystal and the structure under examination is required.

Returned echosigns are displayed on a cathode ray tube; amplitude of

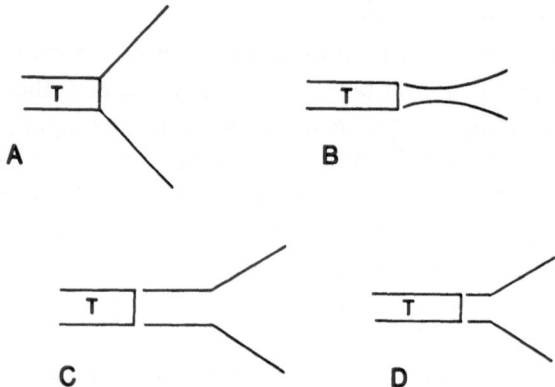

Fig. 1. Outlines of ultrasonic beams. A) Divergent beam, B) focused beam, C) collimated beam, D) slightly collimated beam (typical of the modified tissual A-mode echograph)

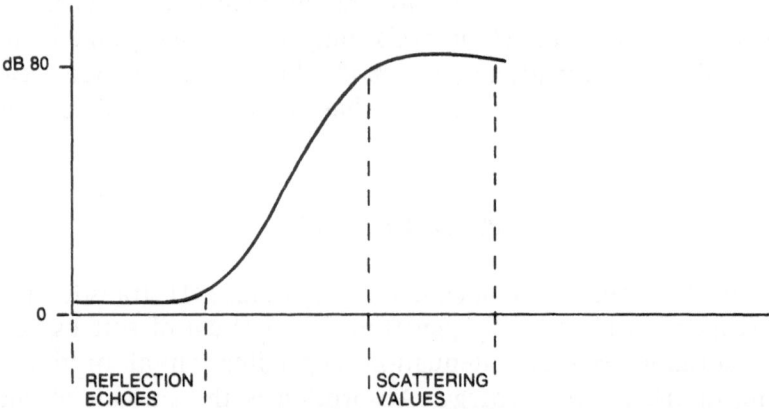

Fig. 2. Amplification of the modified A-mode used for tissual echography increasing scattering values and limiting reflected echoes

the echoes is represented on the vertical plane, depth on the horizontal plane.

The main characteristics of the modified A-mode sonograph used for tissual echography are the ultrasonic frequency of 8 MHz; the light collimation of the beam (Fig. 1); a peculiar amplification which is very high for low intensity echoes, linear for medium intensity echoes and low for high intensity echoes. This specific amplification increases scattering values limiting interference with reflected echoes (Fig. 2).

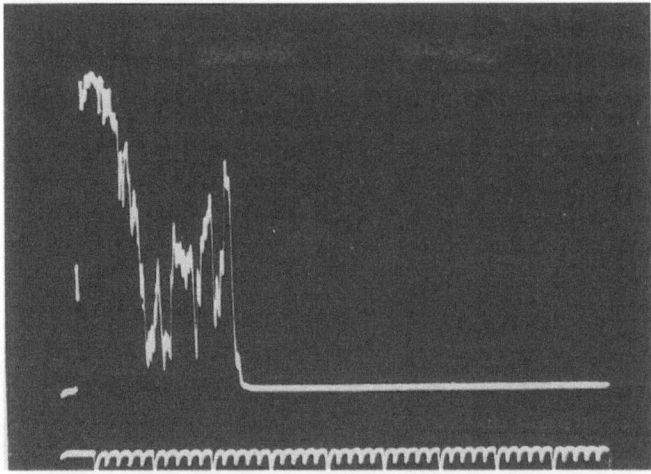

Fig. 3. Sonographic pattern (8 MHz) of a meningioma

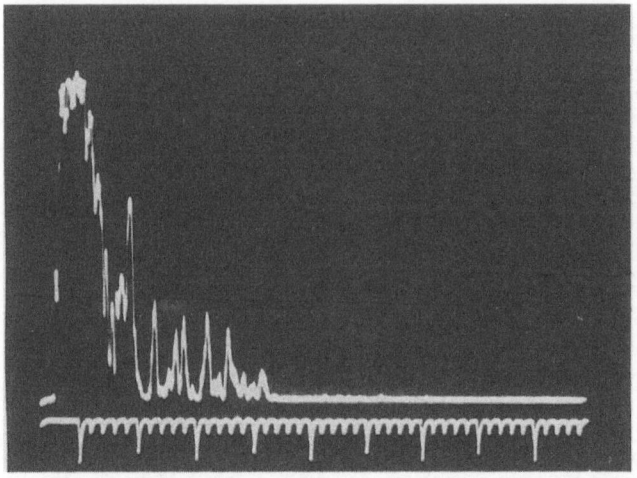

Fig. 4. Sonographic pattern (8 MHz) of an anaplastic astrocytoma

The wavelength of 190 microns at 8 MHz frequency has in fact an excellent interaction with the scattering centers. They consist in fibrous connective tissue and are present in different amount and disposition depending on the pathology of the lesion.

3. Surgical Applications and Results

On the basis of the remark of the small scattering in the nervous tissue recorded by Hill[6] in 1973, the possibility has been suggested to distinguish

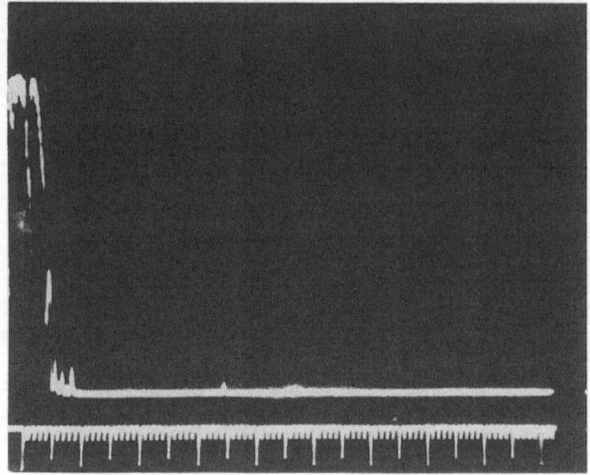

Fig. 5. Sonographic pattern (15 MHz) of normal brain

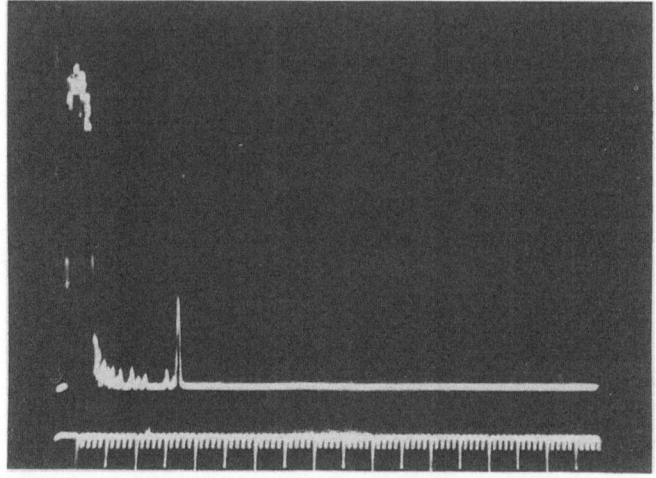

Fig. 6. Sonographic pattern (8 MHz) of edema

pathological lesions from normal brain after investigation with a modified tissual A-mode technique. Scattering in central nervous system varies with the cell or fluid infiltration and to the amount of fibrous constituents into the brain; on this basis specific tracing recorded in tumors seem to make possible an histologic identification.

Obvious differentiation exists between meningioma and glioma (Figs. 3–5). The former shows high scattering since fibrous components are consistent in tissue; peaks are considerably flattened in gliomas because of the prevalent cellular structure. Normal brain shows a flat line without scattering peaks.

The first clinical experience in neurosurgery with modified tissual A-mode is reported by Fasano in 1985[2]. The technique has been used in 15 patients. Probes were sterilized with formaline. Scanning was performed on the exposed tumor and on the walls of the surgical cavity after the removal to check the evidence of remaining neoplastic tissue. Edema and infiltrated

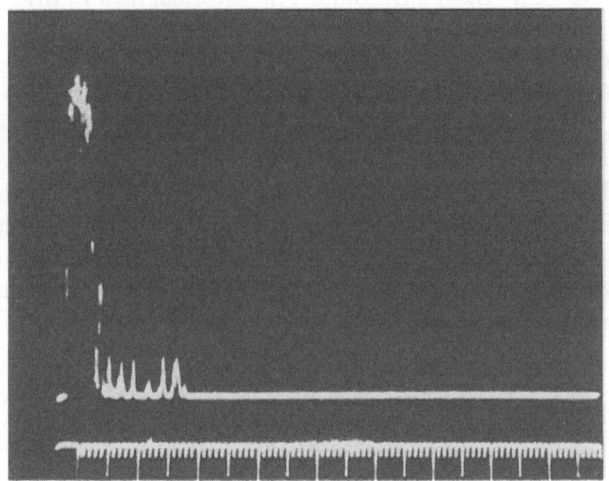

Fig. 7. Sonographic pattern (8 MHz) of gliosis

areas could be detected with an imaging capability up to 1 mm (Figs. 6 and 7). Peculiar findings could be distinguished in 6 different kinds of tumor (glioblastoma, astrocytoma, neurinoma, oligodendroglioma and metastases), pattern being closely correlated to pathology.

The advantages in comparison with intraoperative real-time sonography consist in the high specificity and sensibility in determining the outline between pathological and healthy tissues thus increasing the extent of removal. Moreover, preliminary data seem to suggest the possibility to identify the pathology of the lesion; present data are not sufficient to assess it, and an extended experience on a large number of cases is required for a definite confirmation.

References

1. Dussik, K. T., Dussik, F., Wyt, L., 1947: Auf dem Wege zur Hyperphonographie des Gehirns. Wien. Med. Wschr. 97, 425–429.
2. Fasano, V. A., Urciuoli, R., Lombard, G. F., Ponzio, R. M., Lanotte, M. M.: The use of laser and CUSA in the treatment of brain stem tumors.

International Symposium on Surgery in and around the brain stem and the third ventricle. Hannover, February 18–23, 1985. In press.

3. French, L. A., Wild, J. L., Neal, D., 1950: Detection of cerebral tumors by ultrasonic pulses: Pilot studies on postmortem material. Cancer *3*, 705–708.
4. French, L. A., Wild, J. L., Neal, D., 1951: The experimental application of ultrasonics to localization of brain tumors: Preliminary report. J. Neurosurg. *8*, 198–203.
5. Geuttner, W., Fielder, G., Paetzold, J., 1952: Über Ultraschallabbildungen am menschlichen Schädel. Acustica *2*, 148–156.
6. Hill, C. R., 1973: Medical ultrasonics: An historical review. Brit. J. Radiol. *46*, 899–905.
7. Leksell, L., 1956: Echoencephalography. 1. Detection of intracranial complications following head injury. Acta Chir. Scand. *110*, 301–315.
8. Leksell, L., 1958: Echoencephalography. 11. Midline echo from the pineal body as an index of pineal displacement. Acta Chir. Scand. *115*, 255–259.
9. Ossoinig, K. C., 1977: Echography of the eye, orbit and periorbital region. In: Orbit Roentgenology (Arger, P., ed.), p. 223. New York: J. Wiley and Sons.
10. Skalka, H. W., Callahan, M. A., Elsas, F. J., 1980: Echographic appearance of recurrent orbital retinoblastoma. J. Clin. Ultrastruct. *8*, 164–166.

Intraoperative Dopplersonography

JOACHIM M. GILSBACH and ALBRECHT HARDERS

Department of Neurosurgery, University of Freiburg Medical School,
Freiburg i. Br. (Federal Republic of Germany)

Contents

Introduction	27
Technical and Physical Background	28
Doppler Device	31
Results	33
Normal Cases	33
Anastomoses	36
Extracranial-Intracranial Bypass Procedures	37
Aneurysm Cases	40
Angioma Cases	44
Final Comments	44
References	45

Introduction

Satomura and Kaneko (1957, 1959, 1960) were the first to describe the use of an ultrasound Doppler method for investigating blood flow in the peripheral arteries and in the heart. Since then, the transcutaneous application of the method had become a standard medical procedure for noninvasive examinations of blood vessels, particularly those with stenoses and occlusions in the cervical region (Büdingen *et al.* 1982, Spencer and Reid 1981).

The method has also been used intraoperatively as an easy, atraumatic, repeatable, and reliable control of vascular and also microvascular procedures including anastomoses, endarterectomies and vascular reconstructions (van Beek *et al.* 1975, Freed *et al.* 1979). However, intraoperative applications in neurosurgery have been rare (Brawley 1969,

Friedrich *et al*. 1980, Gilsbach 1983, Hitchon *et al*. 1979, Moritake *et al*. 1980, Nornes *et al*. 1979, 1979, Nornes and Grip 1980, 1981). One reason for this is that commercially available Doppler systems were not suited for vessels with diameters of 1 millimeter and less. For some years now, prototypes and new commercially constructed systems, so-called microvascular Doppler devices, have been available (Cathignol *et al*. 1978, Eden 1984, Hartley and Cole 1974). These systems provide a high resolution, which is necessary for investigations on small vessels, and allow the use of miniaturized probes required for recordings on intracranial vessels.

Technical and Physical Background

The Doppler effect is a change in the frequency of a sound wave when the transmitter, the receiver, or the reflector move towards or away from each other. The frequency change is proportional to the velocity of the movement. When the blood flow velocity is measured according to the Doppler principle, the ultrasonic waves are emitted and received from a stationary crystal in the Doppler probe, and the erythrocytes serve as a reflector which is in motion. Thus, the difference between the emitted and received frequencies (Doppler shift) is proportional to the velocity of the red blood cells and can be expressed by the Doppler formula:

$$F = \frac{2 \cdot Fo \cdot v \cdot \cos \alpha}{c}$$

where F = the Doppler frequency (Doppler shift), Fo = the frequency of the transmitted ultrasound, v = the blood flow velocity, cos α = the angle between the transmitted ultrasound beam and the direction of the blood flow (incident angle), and c = the velocity of ultrasound in the tissue (approximately 1550 cm/second).

Theoretically, the true velocities can be calculated from the Doppler frequencies. But uncertainties due to the angle error and to an underestimation of the Doppler shift in high frequency systems (Kapp 1984) made it advisable to use only Doppler shift expressed in kHz to prevent incorrect interpretation of the results which may be possible when indicating velocity in cm per second.

Corresponding to the different flow velocities in the flowing blood the Doppler frequency consists of a frequency mixture (Doppler spectrum) (Reid 1981). This spectrum is within the audible range and can therefore be interpreted acoustically. It can also be processed and visualized by an audio spectrum analyzer, which, with the aid of a fast Fourier analysis, produces a so-called real time spectrogram. The frequencies are represented as an instantaneous function of time and the amplitude of each individual frequency is represented either in different gray shades or colors. Thus the maximum frequency, the flow pulse waveform, and the frequency distribution can be evaluated optically (Fig. 1). Further information can be obtained mathematically, *e.g.,* the time averaged maximum frequencies from the envelope, the (time averaged) mean frequencies, which correspond to the mean flow velocity across the vessel lumen, and ratios between the systolic and diastolic peak (resistance index) which indicate the peripheral resistance and compliance (Pourcelot 1974, Spencer and Reid 1981).

Reducing the Doppler spectrum to the mean frequency by a zero-crosser is easy and inexpensive but causes a loss of information, since neither the frequency distribution and the maximum frequency nor a reverse or turbulent flow can be recorded correctly. For physical reasons, an

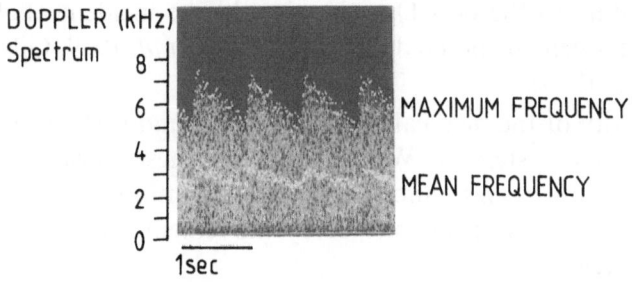

Fig. 1. Doppler frequency spectrum from a real time audio analyzer with calculated (dotted line) maximum frequencies (= envelope) and (spatial) mean frequencies. The amplitudes of the individual frequencies were characterized with different gray intensities (from Gilsbach 1983)

additional error rate of up to 20% is incurred in calculating the mean frequency (Lunt 1975, Renemann and Spencer 1974).

Medical Doppler systems have transmitted frequencies between 2 and 10 MHz depending on its application. A low frequency has a high penetration depth due to low absorption. The wave length and low reflected energy make it necessary to use large crystals. Because of the high absorption rate associated with a high frequency only superficial investigations can be done. At the same time, however, the reflection rate increases (in the 4th power with the emitted frequency), which means a high frequency is necessary for small, weakly reflecting vessels. It also compensates for the loss of energy (proportional to the area of the reflecting crystal) when miniaturized probes with small crystals are used.

For microvessels, emitted frequencies of 20 MHz proved useful (Antunes *et al.* 1983, Blair *et al.* 1981, 1981, Bandy *et al.* 1983, Cathignol *et al.* 1983, Eldridge *et al.* 1979, Freed *et al.* 1979, Pinella *et al.* 1982). These high frequencies made it possible to construct probes even with diameters below 1 millimeter.

Attempts with conventional Doppler systems failed (Friedrich *et al.* 1980) because not all microvessels could be recorded. Moritake *et al.* (1980), for example, could only obtain signals from about 70% of the recipient vessels in extra-intracranial bypass surgery.

In pulsed systems (see below), the longitudinal resolution of the sound beam depends on the electronic processing and can be increased with higher frequencies. The lateral resolution is influenced mainly by the diameter of the crystal. Therefore a high emitted frequency and a small crystal provide a high axial and lateral resolution, which is necessary for microvessels.

In clinical practice the angle dependency of the Doppler method does not have the significance which can be assumed from the cosinus function. During the operation, the probe is adjusted acoustically and under direct vision according to the best Doppler signal. The incident angle then lies constantly between 40 and 60 degrees (Eldridge *et al.* 1979, Gilsbach 1983, Kaneko *et al.* 1970).

The majority of the medical Doppler ultrasound systems are so-called continuous wave systems (CW Doppler). In these devices, one crystal continuously emits and another crystal continuously receives the ultrasound. Using this principle, every movement within the indefinite beam can be registered.

For precise recording in a definite sample volume, so-called pulsed systems were introduced. They emit the ultrasound in bursts and receive it with the same crystal (the use of one crystal makes it possible to further diminish the probe). An electronic gate enables a selective sample volume to be investigated. Its length and distance from the probe can be freely chosen (Baker 1970, 1980, Jorgensen *et al.* 1973, Peronneau *et al.* 1970).

Using a gate having the same diameter as the investigated vessel or larger, the average velocity within the entire cross-sectional area can be determined. With smaller gates, only the average velocity in the sample volume (spatial mean) can be measured. When the gates are much smaller than the vessel, so-called flow velocity profiles can be generated by moving the sample volume across the vessel diameter.

Calculations of diameter and flow volume taken from results of 20 MHz systems (Blair *et al.* 1981, Eldridge *et al.* 1979, 1984, Greene *et al.* 1980, 1981) should be interpreted very carefully because of the inaccuracy caused by relatively large gates and by the nonlinear Doppler shift measurements in high frequency systems (Kapp 1984).

The pulse repetition frequency (PRF) characterizes the time intervals between the individual sound bursts. It limits the detectable Doppler shift to one half of the PRF. If the flow velocities are higher than this half PRF, a so-called "aliasing" effect influences the interpretation of the Doppler signal (Hartley 1981).

The direction of the blood flow can be determined electronically depending on the received frequency which may be higher or lower than the emitted frequency (McLeod 1967).

Apart from providing information on the presence or absence and the direction of a blood flow, the Doppler method establishes the velocity of the red blood cells in their spatial and temporal distribution. Information can thus be obtained not only on the average velocity, but also on the distribution of the velocities within the vessel lumen. It is possible to separate the laminar flow from an irregular and turbulent flow and thus to detect localized or systemic disturbances of the blood movement. Mainly localized narrowings can be detected by the Doppler method. Recordings on the site of the lesion reveal accelerated flow velocities and changes of the flow pattern (see below), even in cases with hemodynamically noneffective stenoses. By comparing the prestenotic with the stenotic and poststenotic findings, a quantification of the degree of the narrowing can be achieved. Apart from angiography, no other method offers this possibility.

The velocity changes within the cardiac cycle, the so-called flow pulse waves, indicate local and systemic changes of resistance and compliance depending on the ratios between the systolic and diastolic flow components. Recordings made on various sites with a constant angle separate local from systemic changes by a comparison of the flow pattern.

Doppler Device

For 5 years we have been using a high frequency Doppler ultrasound system, which was originally constructed by Cathignol and co-workers (INSERM, Bron, France) (Cathignol et al. 1978). It has meanwhile undergone many modifications and is now commercially available (Eden 1984). The system is a pulsed Doppler with an emitted frequency of 20 MHz (Fig. 2, Table 1), a built in zero-crosser, an automatic gate shift, and adjustable pulse repetition frequencies and adjustable pulse durations (pulse duration = duration of the receiving period).

We exclusively use a pulse repetition frequency of 100 kHz, which offers the highest possible resolution. The theoretically possible detection of 50 kHz Doppler shift (½ of the pulse repetition frequency) has until now been limited to about 12.5 kHz by the filter arrangement. But in neurosurgical clinical practice, frequencies higher than 8–10 kHz have only been rarely found in cases of angiomas and severe vasospasms. The signal processing by the zero-crossing principle was abandoned in favor of a real time spectrum analysis, which was computed with a separate device (Angioscan I and II).

Most recordings were and can be done with a 3 mm probe, which is sufficient for superficial vessels. For the narrow conditions on the base of the brain, 1 mm and 0.6 mm probes were developed, which make it easily possible to record the individual parts of the circle of Willis (Fig. 3). The probes could be sterilized with gas for direct intraoperative investigations. By coupling the tip of the probe with a drop of saline or blood, recordings of good quality could be obtained from vessels as small as 0.2 mm. The

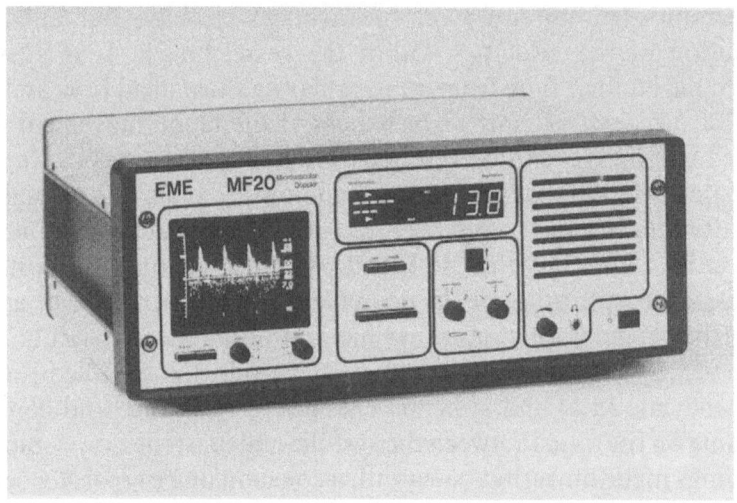

Fig. 2. The present appearance of the microvascular Doppler system with a built in spectrum analyzer (EME, Überlingen, Germany)

Table 1. *Technical Datas of the Doppler Device*

20 MHz pulsed ultrasonic Doppler Velocity Meter	
Transmitted frequency:	20 MHz
Pulse durations:	250, 450, 850, 1,500 ns
Axial resolution:	0.4, 0.7, 1.3, 2.3 mm
Lateral resolutions:	0.5, 1.1 mm
Pulse repetition frequencies:	25, 50, 100 kHz
Measuring depth:	7.5, 15, 30 mm
Maximum detectable Doppler shift:	12.5 kHz
Minimum detectable Doppler shift:	0.1 kHz

transcutaneous application was restricted to superficial vessels because of the low penetration depth (in clinical practice not more than 5 mm).

For recordings in the basal cisterns, the pulsed system helped to exclude other vessels commonly lying in the same direction in the ultrasonic beam. Because of the relatively large sample volume in comparison with vessels having diameters of 1 mm no reliable flow profiles or exact center stream measurements could be performed. We therefore used gates which were at least as large as the vessel in order to get comparable results.

Results

Normal Cases

In cases of small basal tumors or asymptomatic aneurysms, the flow pattern of normal cerebral arteries could be studied: the pulse wave forms

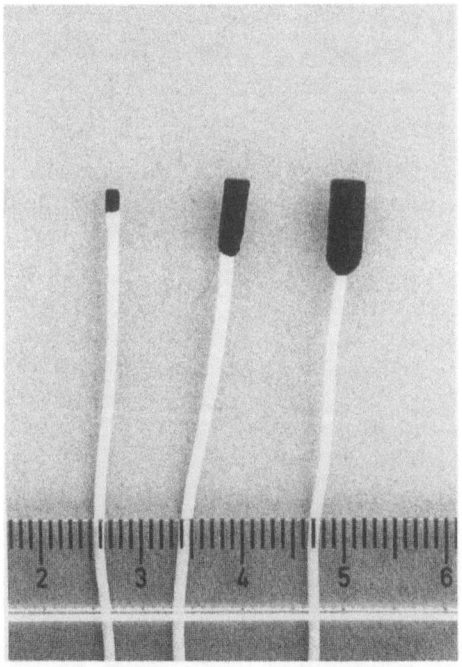

Fig. 3. Different types of sterilizable probes for intraoperative use on arteries and veins with diameters larger than 0.2 mm

corresponded to those of the internal cervical carotid artery with a high diastolic flow component as a sign of a low peripheral resistance and compliance (Figs. 4 and 5). The Doppler frequencies in the anterior part of the circle of Willis were between 1 kHz and 6 kHz (time averaged mean frequencies) in average 2.7–3.4 kHz. The resistance index varied between 0.2 and 0.7. The average value was 0.53.

The velocities in the internal carotid artery were equal to those in the trunk of the middle cerebral artery. The velocities in the anterior cerebral arteries and the branches of the middle cerebral artery were slightly slower.

The pulse wave curves and the flow velocities varied depending on the

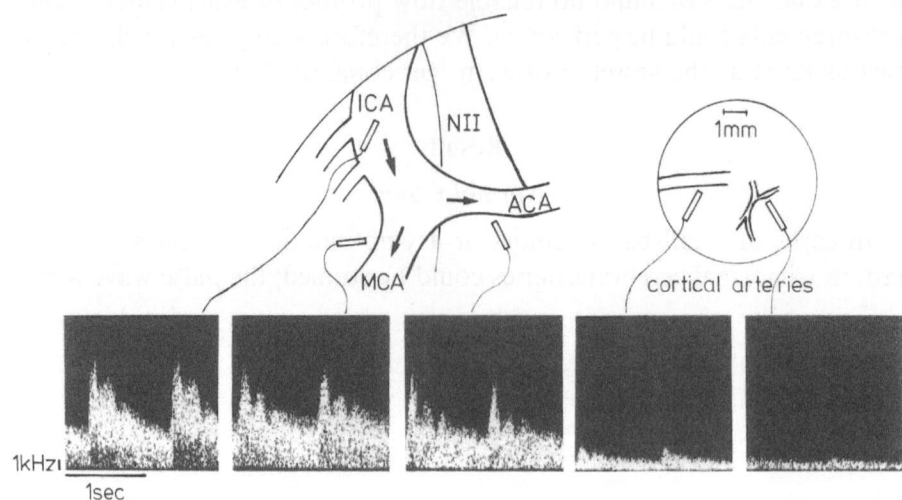

Fig. 4. Intracranial vessel tree with typical flow pattern of a normal cerebral circulation. The flow velocities decrease depending on the decrease of the vessel diameter

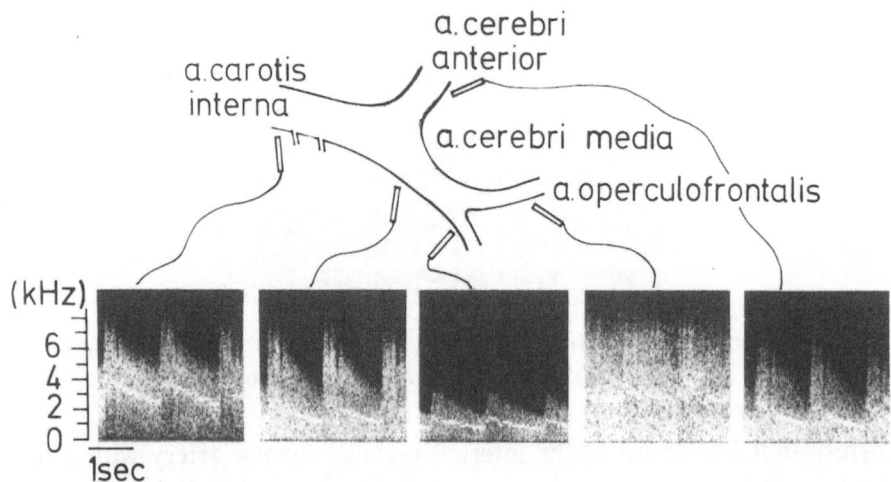

Fig. 5. Flow pattern of the intracranial internal carotid artery with its branches. In the territory of the middle cerebral artery there are accelerations with a high diastolic flow component. In this case they were a sign of a reactive hyperemia after the brain spatula pressure was released

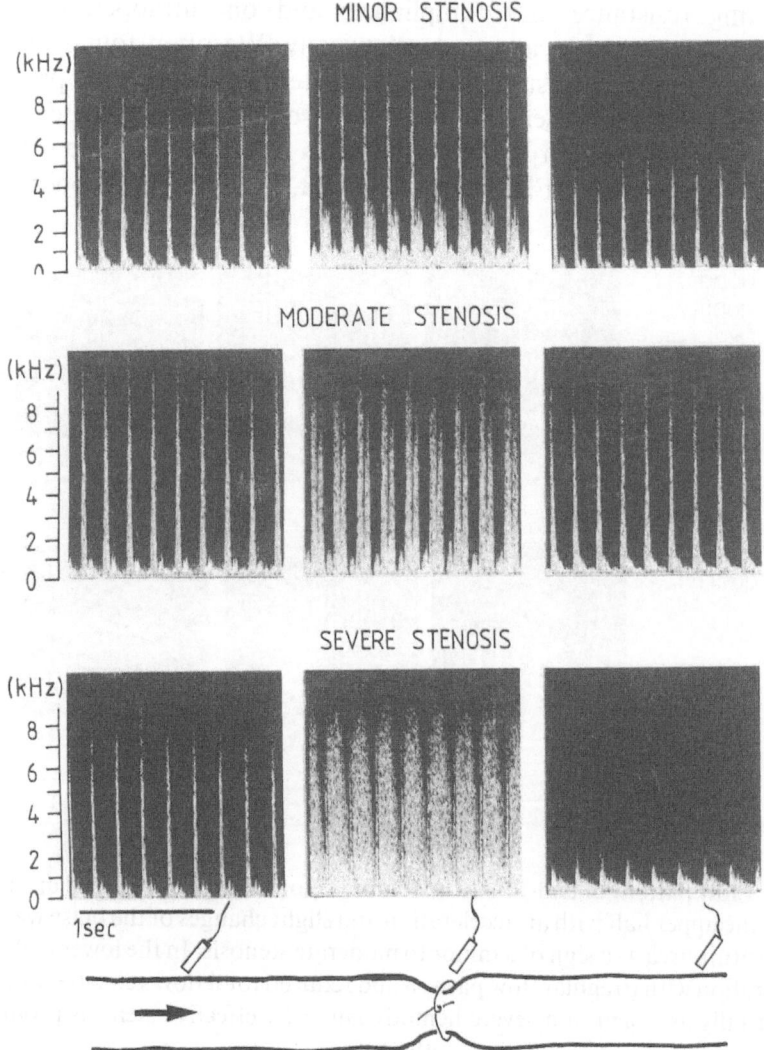

Fig. 6. Flow pattern of experimentally induced stenoses of a microvessel (common carotid artery of the rat; diameter 1 mm). Three different grades of stenoses can be distinguished according to Doppler criteria: 1. slight narrowing with a reduction below 60% of the cross sectional area with locally accelerated flow velocities; 2. moderate narrowing between 60% and 80% area reduction with locally accelerated flow velocity and changes of the flow pulse waves; 3. severe narrowing of more than 80% with a reduction of the total flow velocity, distally damped pulsations and localized accelerations and irregularities (from Gilsbach 1983)

preexisting resistance and compliance, and on intraoperative caliber changes induced chemically or mechanically. We often found high flow velocities with a high diastolic component after releasing spatula pressure or a temporary clip, or after discontinuing a sodium nitroprusside infusion. These changes were interpreted as a sign of a reactive hyperemia with a low peripheral resistance (Fig. 5). In contrast, in cases of hypocapnia or

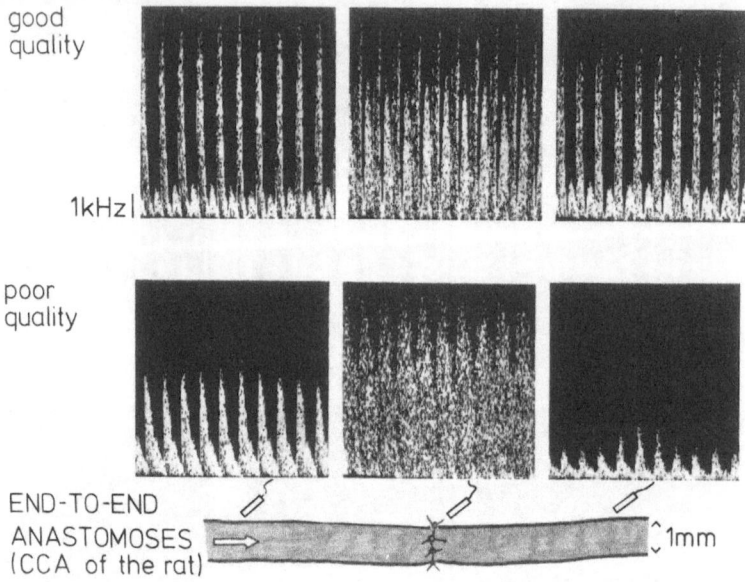

Fig. 7. Flow pattern of end-to-end anastomoses of the cerivcal carotid artery of the rat. In the upper half with an acceleration and slight changes of the pulse wave curve in the suture area as a sign of a minor to moderate stenosis. In the lower half marked acceleration with irregular flow pattern and reduced total flow velocities proximally and distally as a sign of a severe hemodynamically effective stenosis produced by the suture

arteriosclerosis there was increased resistance with a steep systolic amplitude, a low diastolic flow, and a lowered total flow velocity.

Anastomoses

In microvessels as well as in larger arteries and veins, the (un)disturbed patency of any type of anastomosis could be judged with the microvascular Doppler system. Apart from being able to immediately diagnose an open or occluded anastomosis, we were also able to check the quality of the suture by estimating the lumen narrowing and by recording irregular flow patterns in cases with wall irregularities. In minor and moderate stenoses, localized accelerations and changes in flow pattern could be observed. In cases of severe, hemodynamically effective stenoses, irregular pulse curves in the region of the narrowing and additional changes of the flow pattern in the proximal and distal segment were determined (Figs. 6 and 7). According to animal experiments (Gilsbach 1983, Freed et al. 1979) stenoses of more than 40% could be detected with the Doppler, and any necessary corrections could be made immediately and under Doppler control.

Extracranial-Intracranial Bypass Procedures

The precise and narrow beam of the microvascular Doppler system was a useful preoperative aid in mapping the course of the donor artery on the skin.

The patency of the donor artery after an anastomosis could easily be proved by a conventional Doppler or an electromagnetic flow meter. However, the patency and the flow direction of both recipient branches, the (un)disturbed flow in the region of the anastomosis area itself are also important for the success of a bypass operation and such information can only be provided by the microvascular Doppler. With this system, we are also able to detect and to immediately correct minor impairments of the anastomosis, which can become symptomatic in cases with secondary swelling or hypotension.

In cases of bypass procedures between the superficial temporal artery and a branch of the middle cerebral artery, all the recipient vessels had originally had an orthograde flow. The preexisting flow velocity was pathologically slow as in a vein in cases with bilateral internal carotid artery occlusion. In cases with unilateral occlusion, only two thirds of the patients had a pathologically slow flow velocity. In cases with stenoses of the internal cervical artery, only one half of the velocities measured were too slow.

All anastomoses were done as end-to-side sutures with a fish-mouth incision of the donor artery. In all patients, recordings could be obtained from all parts of the bypass, including the suture area itself. After the temporary clips were released, 90% of the anastomoses showed undisturbed flow pattern. They had no irregularities or marked accelerations at the site of the temporary clip or in the suture region. 97% of all recipient arteries had a bilateral flow distribution. That means that in addition to the original, mostly increased distal orthograde flow, there was a reversed flow in the proximal segment of the recipient artery. There the postanastomotic flow velocities towards the Sylvian fissure were 3–5 times higher than the original orthograde velocities. In the donor artery, the flow velocities were 3–4 times higher than before anastomosis and the flow pattern changed from the external type with a low enddiastolic flow to an internal type with a relatively high diastolic flow (Fig. 8).

About 10% of the patients had stenoses or occlusions of their anastomoses, all of which could be detected intraoperatively. The absence

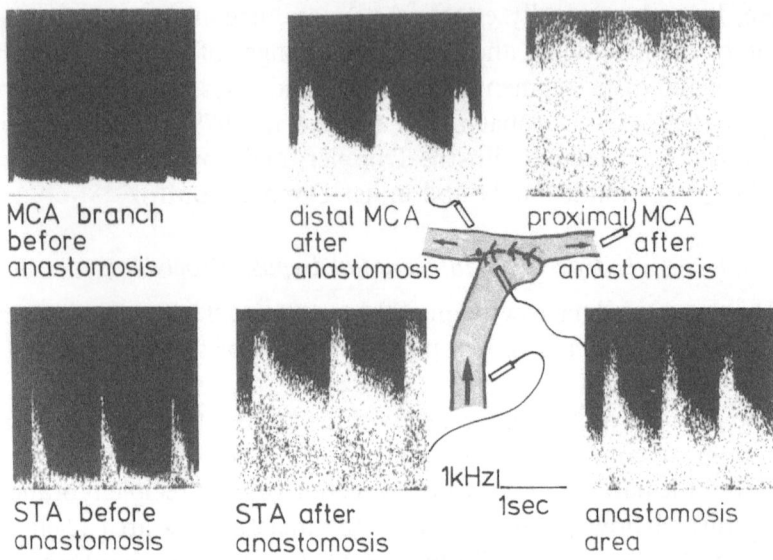

Fig. 8. Flow pattern of a well-functioning extracranial-intracranial anastomosis between the superficial temporal artery and a branch of the middle cerebral artery. Note the bidirectional flow in the recipient vessel and the increase of the velocities both in the recipient vessel and in the donor artery, in which a change from the external to internal type can be observed

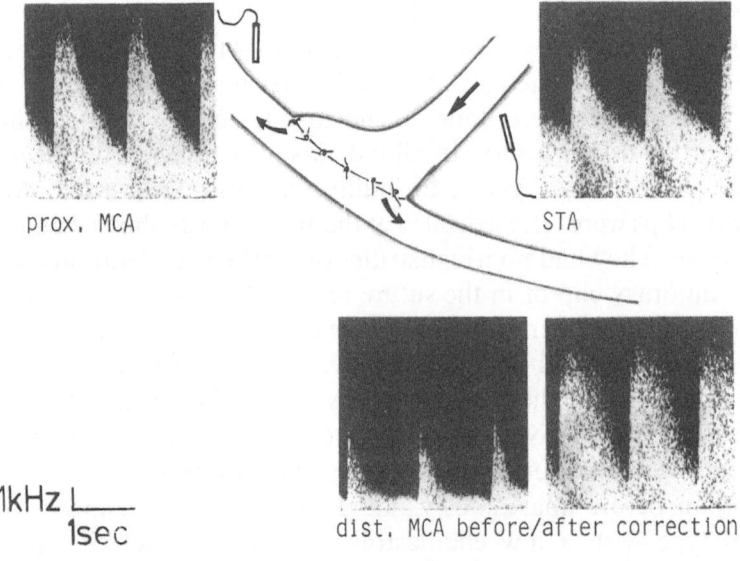

Fig. 9. Flow pattern of an anastomosis with a stenosis of the distal acute angeled part of the suture. After "milking" a normal bypass flow could be restored

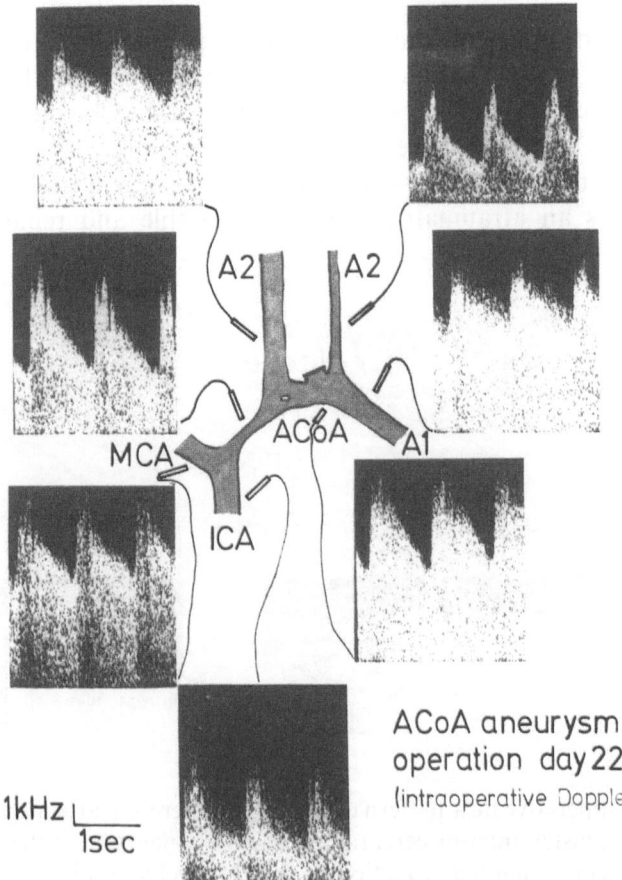

1kHz |__
     1sec

ACoA aneurysm
operation day 22
(intraoperative Dopple

Fig. 10. Intraoperative flow pattern of the dissected and visible part of the circle of Willis after clipping of an aneurysm of the anterior communicating artery. The flow in the parent arteries is undisturbed. The different flow pattern in the individual vessels depend on the individual caliber and flow variations and on narrowings produced by the hemorrhage (vasospasm) and/or mechanical irritation by the operation. (ICA: internal carotid artery, MCA: middle cerebral artery, *A1:* proximal anterior cerebral artery, *A2:* distal anterior cerebral artery, *ACoA:* anterior communicating artery)

of the Doppler signal or a "dead-end" signal indicated an occlusion, which was observed almost exclusively in the donor artery between the site of the temporary clip and the suture area. In this case, the typical bilateral flow distribution in the recipient artery did not start. In cases of a hemo-dynamically effective stenosis in the suture area or in the recipient vessel the typical increase of the flow velocities were not observed, the pulse waves were damped and the amplitudes small (Fig. 9). In all cases immediate corrections could be performed to achieve lasting patency.

Aneurysm Cases

Even under the operating microscope, there are occasionally uncertainties as to the exclusion of an aneurysm and the undisturbed patency of the parent arteries. The outer aspect may be misleading and an angiographic intraoperative control is normally not available. The microvascular Doppler now offers for the first time a tool to the surgeon which allows an atraumatic, simple, repeatable and reliable electronic

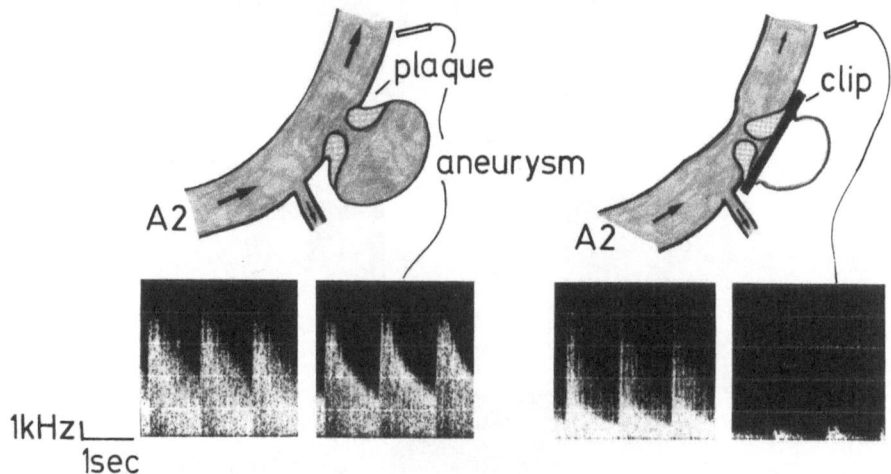

Fig. 11. Intraoperative flow pattern of the anterior cerebral artery with its branches in a case of a distal anterior cerebral artery (*A 2*) aneurysm. After an attempt to position the clip a marked reduction of the flow velocities in the distal segment occurred due to a lumen reduction by displaced calcified plaques which could not be seen from the outside. In this case a definitive exclusion was not possible

"view" into the vessel lumen (Fig. 10). We found a striking discrepancy between the outer aspect and the result of the Doppler investigation in 10% of our cases, especially in large aneurysms or aneurysms with calcified necks (Fig. 11). In the majority of the cases, a disturbed patency of a parent artery could be corrected by repositioning the clip or by neck resection and vessel wall suture.

Hemodynamically effective stenoses due to a tight clip were indicated by a markedly reduced flow velocity in comparison with the preexisting findings (Fig. 11). The detection of a localized acceleration, which is important for recognizing a minor stenosis was restricted mostly by the size of the probe, the spring of the clip, and the narrow conditions at the base of the brain.

The response of the cerebral vessels to mechanical and chemical stimuli during the operation often brought on changes in the flow pattern. This

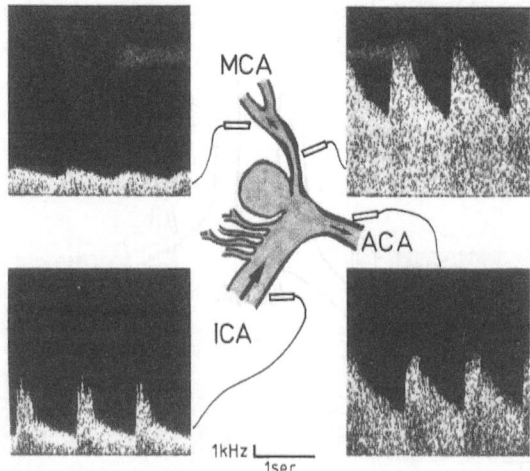

Fig. 12. Flow pattern of the internal carotid artery bifurcation with an aneurysm. Note the accelerated flow velocities in the proximal part of the middle cerebral artery (*MCA*) and the slow flow velocities with damped pulsations distally as a sign of a hemodynamically effective narrowing (vasospasm). Also slight accelerations in the anterior cerebral artery (*ACA*)

Table 2. *Comparison Between Intraoperative Doppler Findings and Direct Postoperative Angiography.* Severe means a 60–80% stenosis and moderate 30–60%

Doppler	Angiography		
	No/moderate stenosis	Severe stenosis	Occlusion
No/moderate stenosis	80%	0%	0%
Severe stenosis	12%	5%	0%
Occlusion	0%	0%	3%

restricted the significance of the absolute flow velocities, as do the anatomical properties, which in some cases make it impossible to achieve an optimum incident angle.

In patients operated on between the 4th and the 21th day after a subarachnoid hemorrhage, localized accelerations in one or more segments of the circle of Willis occurred in 65% (Fig. 12). These signs of vasospasms were also found among 9% of the patients operated on early. However, the

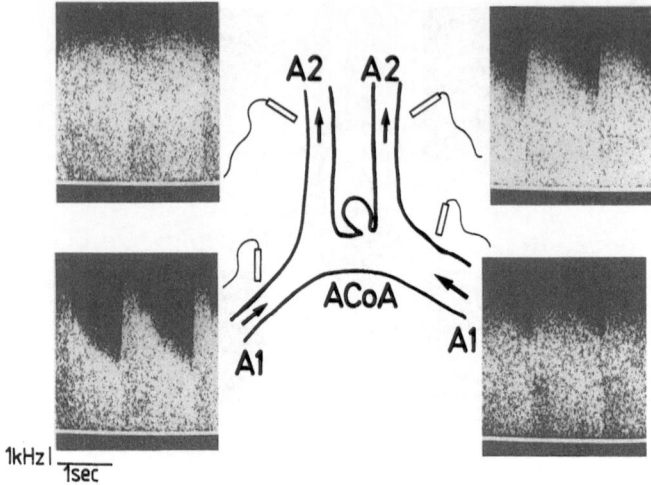

Fig. 13. Anterior communicating aneurysm with generally high and irregular flow pattern with normal vessel calibers as a sign of a reduced peripheral resistance. A common finding in acute aneurysm surgery. (The lack of pulsations in high velocities is partially due to an artefact by the filter arrangement which cuts frequencies above 12.5 kHz)

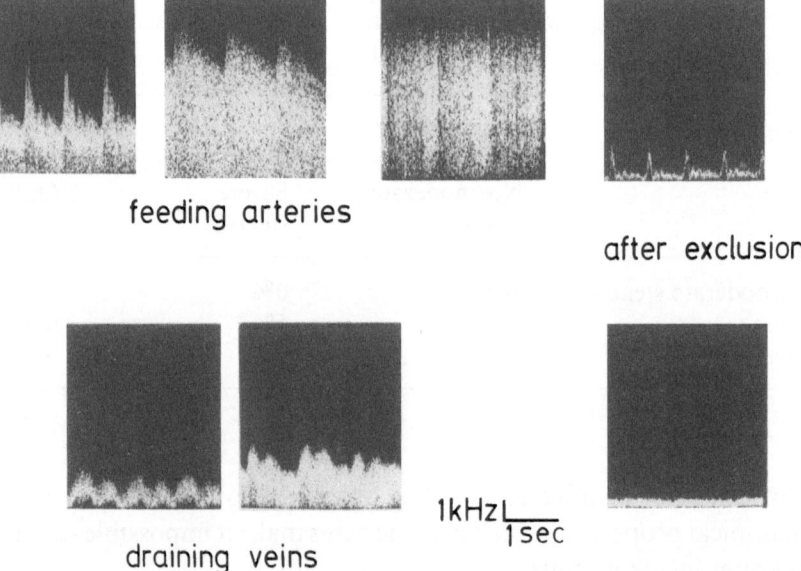

Fig. 14. Flow pattern of an intracerebral arteriovenous malformation. Depending on the diameter and flow volume in the arteries, an accelerated to irregular flow with high diastolic components is found. The veins show marked pulsations but with smooth peaks

reevaluation of their history revealed additional previous bleedings, which
were responsible for the pseudo-early development of vasospasm.

A comparison between the intraoperative Doppler findings and a
control angiography at the end of the operation in the same anesthesia

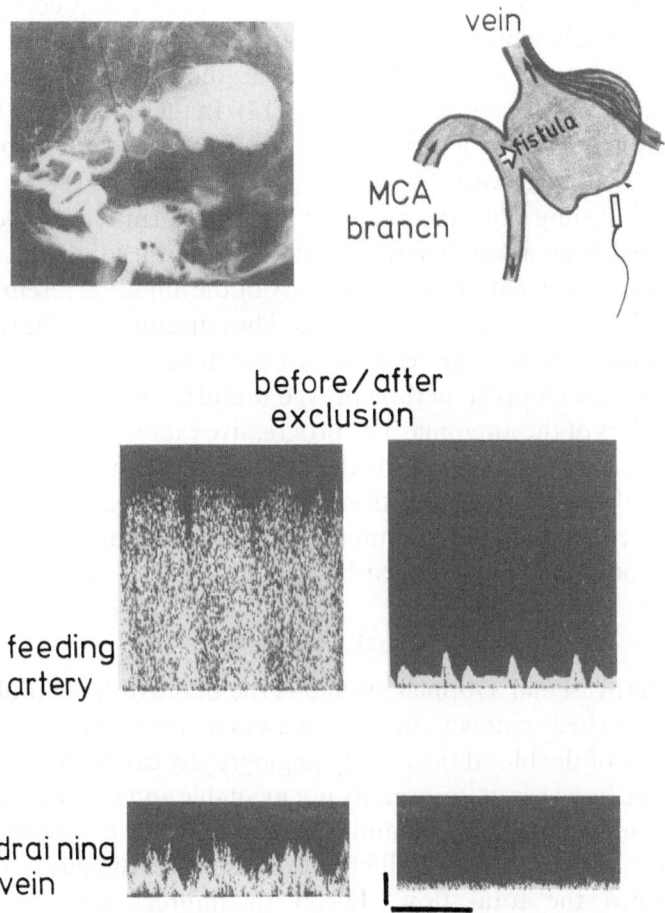

Fig. 15. Flow pattern of an intracerebral arteriovenous fistula with a large draining
vein before and after occlusion of the fistula. After exclusion of the shunt the
pulsations in the vein disappear and the velocities in the artery are reduced with
signs of a raised peripheral reduction

showed a good correlation (Table 2). In no case did the Doppler fail to
detect a severe stenosis. In 12%, the angiography showed normal vessel
calibers, despite high intraoperative velocities. In these cases the spasm had
disappeared by the end of the operation or a reduction of the peripheral
resistance caused the acceleration. The latter finding was found in 51% of
the patients with early aneurysm surgery. In these cases, the fast flow

velocities were more or less generalized and not circumscribed (Fig. 13). We interpreted this as low resistance due to the acute bleeding and/or lowered intracranial pressure during operation.

Angioma Cases

High flow velocities with a relatively high diastolic flow component were typical for vessels which feed an angioma or a fistula. Depending on the caliber of the vessel and the flow volume, the flow pattern varied from accelerated forms to irregular types (Fig. 14). In these cases, the limits of the Doppler system were reached because the velocities were higher than the device was able to record.

A vessel feeding both the angioma and the normal brain could not be distinguished from a purely pathological angioma-feeding vessel (Fig. 15).

The venous flow pattern in the vicinity of the angioma resembled that of arteries with slightly damped pulsations. They disappeared the further away from the malformation the recordings were done.

Clinically the Doppler method proved useful in detecting, localizing, and tracing feeders of the angioma. The progressive exclusion of the shunt could be recognized by the decrease of the diastolic flow in the feeding arteries (Figs. 14 and 15). Remnants of the AVM in visible areas could be detected, however, the existance of remaining non visible fistulas could not be ruled out. This could only be achieved by angiography.

Final Comments

The microvascular Doppler system is the best available tool to control the (un)disturbed patency in neurovascular operations and localized disturbances of the blood flow. Only angiography can provide comparable information, however, it is normally not available and is not ideal for vessels with diameters of about 1 mm and less. The Doppler principle enables the investigator to detect minor reductions of the vessel lumen which have not yet disturbed the total flow. Direct or indirect flow measurements (electromagnetic flowmeter, or perfusion measurements), however, are significant only in cases with marked changes of the blood flow. For example, in cases of stenoses only narrowings of more than 80% can be detected, while the Doppler system helps to recognize narrowings from 40% on. With the present technical equipment, the method is not well suited for quantitative measurements. But, theoretically, the angle dependence can be compensated for by special double crystal probes and a microprocessor, and the diameter of the vessel could perhaps be measured with very small gates and/or A-scan systems. Then we will be able to perform not only qualitative intraoperative measurements of the cerebral circulation under normal and pathological conditions—which are for the first time possible—but also quantitative ones.

Further miniaturization of the probes with diameters of less than 0.6 mm will make the microvascular Doppler system suited for an intravasal application for example on the tip of catheters.

References

1. Antunes, J. L., Muraszko, K., Stark, R., 1983: Pituitary portal blood flow in primates: a Doppler study. Neurosurgery *12*, 492–495.
2. Baker, D. W., 1970: Pulsed ultrasonic Doppler blood-flow sensing. IEEE Trans. Sonics Ultrastruct. *17*, 170–185.
3. Baker, D. W., 1980: Applications of pulsed Doppler techniques. Radiol. Clin. N. Amer. *18*, 79–103.
4. Bandyk, D. F., Zierler, R. E., Berni, G. A., Thiele, B. L., 1983: Pulsed Doppler velocity patterns produced by arterial anastomoses. Ultrasound Med. Biol. *9*, 79–87.
5. Van Beek, A. L., Link, W. J., Bennett, J. E., 1975: Ultrasound evaluation of microanastomosis. Arch. Surg. *110*, 945–949.
6. Blair, W. F., Greene, E. R., Eldridge, M., Cipoletti, R., 1981: Hemodynamics after microsurgical anastomosis: the effects of topical lidocaine. J. Microsurg. *2*, 157–164.
7. Blair, W. F., Greene, E. R., Omer, G. E., 1981: A method for the calculation of blood flow in human digital arteries. J. Hand. Surg. *6*, 90–96.
8. Bradley, E. L., Saceri, O., 1972: The velocity of ultrasound in human blood under varying physiologic parameters. J. Surg. Res. *12*, 290–297.
9. Brawley, B. W., 1969: Determination of superior sagittal sinus patency with an ultrasonic Doppler flow detector in parasagittal meningioma. J. Neurosurg. *30*, 315–316.
10. Büdingen, H. J., von Reutern, G.-M., Freund, H.-J., 1982: Doppler-Sonographie der extrakraniellen Hirnarterien. Stuttgart-New York: Thieme.
11. Cathignol, P., Chapelon, J. Y., Fourcade, C., 1978: Vélocimètre Doppler à l'usage des petits vaisseaux, le Microflo. Biosigma (Paris) 426–429.
12. Cathignol, D., Chapelon, J. Y., Mestas, J. L., *et al.,* 1983: Description et application d'un vélocimètre ultrasonore Doppler pour les petits vaisseaux. Med. Biol. Engn. *21*, 358–364.
13. Eden, A., 1984: Doppler techniques and neurosurgery. Neurosurg. Rev. 7, 193–197.
14. Eldridge, M. W., Berman, W., Greene, E. R., 1984: Femoral blood flow in term and premature infants. J. Ultrasound. Med. *3*, 53–57.
15. Eldridge, M. W., Greene, E. R., Berman, W. R., *et al.,* 1979: Ultrasonic pulsed Doppler characterization of the human neonatal peripheral circulation. Biomed. Sci. Instrum. *15*, 77–90.
16. Freed, D., Hartley, C. J., Christman, K. D., Lyman, R. C., Agrid, J., Walker, N. F., 1979: High-frequency pulsed Doppler ultrasound: a new tool for microvascular surgery. J. Microsurg. *1*, 148–153.
17. Friedrich, H., Hänsel-Friedrich, G., Seeger, W., 1980: Intraoperative Dopplersonographie an Hirngefäßen. Neurochirurgia *23*, 89–98.

18. Gilsbach, J. M., 1983: Intraoperative Doppler sonography in neurosurgery. Wien-New York: Springer.
19. Gilsbach, J. M., Schumacher, M., Hardes, A.: Intravascular application of a microvascular Doppler system. In preparation.
20. Greene, E. R., Blair, W. F., Hartley, C. J., 1980: Noninvasive pulsed Doppler velocity measurements and calculated flow in human digital arteries. Biomed. Sci. Instrum. *16*, 93–105.
21. Greene, E. R., Blair, W. F., Hartley, C., 1981: Noninvasive pulsed Doppler blood velocity measurements and calculated flow in human digital arteries. ISA Trans. *20*, 15–24.
22. Hartley, C. J., Cole, J. S., 1974: An ultrasonic pulsed Doppler system for measuring blood flow in small vessels. J. Appl. Physiol. *37*, 626–629.
23. Hartley, C. J., 1981: Resolution of frequency aliases in ultrasonic pulsed Doppler velocitimeters. IEEE Trans. Sonics Ultrastruct. *28*, 69–74.
24. Hitchon, P. W., Kassell, N. F., McDonnell, D. E., 1979: The Doppler ultrasonic flowmeter as an adjunct to operative management of cerebral arteriovenous malformations. Surg. Neurol. *11*, 345–347.
25. Jorgensen, J. E., Campau, D. J., Baker, D. W., 1973: Physical characteristics and mathematical modelling of the pulsed ultrasonic flowmeter. Med. Biol. Engng. *12*, 404–421.
26. Kaneko, Z., Shiraishi, J., Omizo, Inaoka, H., Ueshima, T., 1970: Analysis of ultrasonic blood rheogram by the sound spectrograph. Jap. Circulat. J. *34*, 1035–1045.
27. Kapp, H., 1984: personal communication.
28. McLeod, F. D., 1967: A directional Doppler flowmeter. Digest of 7th Intern. Conf. Med. Biol. Engng. (Stockholm), 213.
29. Lunt, M. J., 1975: Accuracy and limitations of the ultrasonic Doppler blood velocitymeter and zerocrossing detector. Ultrasound Med. Biol. *2*, 1–10.
30. Moritake, K., Handa, H., Yonekawa, Y., 1980: Ultrasonic Doppler assessment of hemodynamics in superficial temporal artery—middle cerebral artery anastomosis. Surg. Neurol. *13*, 249–257.
31. Nornes, H., Grip, A., Wikeby, P., 1979: Intraoperative evaluation of cerebral hemodynamics using directional Doppler technique. Part 1: Arteriovenous malformations. J. Neurosurg. *50*, 145–151.
32. Nornes, H., Grip, A., Wikeby, P., 1979: Intraoperative evaluation of cerebral hemodynamics using directional Doppler technique. Part 2: Saccular aneurysms. J. Neurosurg. *50*, 570–577.
33. Nornes, H., Grip, A., 1980: Hemodynamic aspects of cerebral arteriovenous malformations. J. Neurosurg. *53*, 456–464.
34. Nornes, H., Grip, A., 1981: Studies on hemodynamic effects of the exclusion of cerebral arterio-venous malformations. Acta Neurochir. (Wien) *56*, 134.
35. Peronneau, P., Hinglais, J., Pellet, M., Leger, F., 1970: Vélocimètre sanguin par effet Doppler à émission ultrasonore pulsée. Onde Electrique *50*, 369–384.
36. Pinella, J. W., Spira, M., Erk, Y., Freed, B., Hartley, L., 1982: Direct microvascular monitoring with implantable ultrasonic Doppler probes. J. Microsurg. *3*, 217–221.
37. Pourcelot, L., 1974: Applications cliniques de l'examen Doppler transcutane.

Les colloques de l'institut national de la Santé et de la Recherche Médicale. INSERM *34*, 213.

38. Reid, J. M., Sound and Ultrasound. In: Cerebrovascular Evaluation with Doppler Ultrasound (Spencer, M. P., Reid, J. M., eds.), pp. 23–40. Boston-London: Martinus Nijhoff.

39. Reneman, R. S., Spencer, M. P., 1974: Difficulties in processing of an analogue Doppler flow signal; with special reference to zero-crossing meters and quantification. In: Cardiovascular Applications of Ultrasound (Reneman, R. S., ed.), pp. 32–42. Amsterdam-London: North-Holland Publishing Company.

40. Satomura, S., Ultrasonic Doppler method for the inspection of cardiac function. J. Acoust. Soc. Amer. *29*, 1181.

41. Satomura, S., 1959: Study of the flow patterns in peripheral arteries by ultrasonics. J. Acoust. Soc. Jpn. *15*, 151–158.

42. Satomura, S., Kaneko, Z., 1960: Ultrasonic blood rheograph. Proc. 3rd Intern. Conf. Med. Elect. IEE, London, 254–258.

43. Spencer, M. P., Reid, J. M., 1981: Cerebrovascular Evaluation with Doppler Ultrasound. The Hague-Boston-London: Martinus Nijhoff.

2. Laser Neurosurgery

Historical Introduction

Victor A. Fasano

Institute of Neurosurgery, University of Turin (Italy)

The concept and mathematical principles underlying the Laser were set forth by Einstein in 1917[3].

During 1950's Schawflow and Townes at Columbia University and Basov and Prokhorov at the Lebeder Institute independently discovered and set forth the physical principles of microwave amplification by stimulated emission of radiation (MASER). This work revealed that wavelengths of various sizes could be made to act in accordance with Einstein's principles of stimulated emission.

The first practical laser emitting pulses of light was reported by Maiman working for the Howard Hughes Aircraft Corporation in 1960 and was a pulsed ruby laser[10].

The first gas laser, a helium-neon laser, was developed by Javan, Bennet and Herriot in 1961[7].

In the same year, Johnson and Naussau developed the Nd:YAG laser. In 1964 Patel created the CO_2 laser for Bell laboratories[12]. Argon laser was introduced around the same time.

The first clinical uses of laser were those of the argon laser for retinal detachment in 1965 by L'Esperance[3].

As a surgical instrument in neurosurgery the laser beam (Ruby Laser) was used for the first time by Rosomoff in 1965 in patients with gliomas[14].

In 1968 Bredemeier and Polany in collaboration with Yako[13] began surgical experimentation with the CO_2 laser.

Stellar in 1969, after performing animal experiments, was the first to use CO_2 laser on a patient with a brain tumor[15]. In 1970 the Nd:YAG laser was first experimentally used by Mussigang[11].

In 1972 fiberoptic technology became available for argon laser and Nd:YAG laser.

In the same year argon laser was used for the treatment of the cerebral tumors and Kamikawa[8] and Yako[6] introduced the CO_2 laser in conjunction with the microscope and the micromanipulator. The application of the laser beam in neurosurgery remained anecdotal until 1976 when Heppner and Ascher performed neurosurgical procedures with CO_2 laser in a large series of cases[1]. Around the same time Takizawa started to use CO_2 laser in Japan[16] and in 1977 Beck[2] introduced the Nd:YAG laser in neurosurgery.

In 1980 the author was the first to use the combined association of three laser sources in a patient with a cerebral glioma[4-5]. In 1980, there was renewed interest in lasers among American neurosurgeons. CO_2 laser neurosurgery workshops were established at Northwestern University of Chicago and in 1981 the first American Congress of Laser Neurosurgery was held in Chicago. In 1983 the International Association of Laser Neurosurgery was founded in Houston.

References

1. Ascher, P. W., 1977: Der CO_2-Laser in der Neurochirurgie. Wien: F. Molden Verlag.
2. Beck, O. S., 1980: The use of Neodymium:YAG and the CO_2 laser in neurosurgery. Neurosurg. Rev. *3*, 261.
3. Einstein, A., 1917: Zur Quantentheorie der Strahlung. Phys. Z. *18*, 12.
4. Fasano, V. A., Lombard, G. F., Benech, F., Tealdi, S., 1979: New technologies in neurosurgery. In: Laser Surgery III, part one (Kaplan, I., ed.), pp. 66–72. Tel Aviv: OT-PAZ.
5. Fasano, V. A., Benech, F., Ponzio, R. M., 1982: Observations on the simultaneous use of CO_2 and Nd:YAG laser in neurosurgery. Lasers Surg. Med. 155.
6. Jako, G. J., 1972: Laser surgery of the vocal cords. An experimental study with carbon dioxide laser. Laryngoscope *8*, 2204.
7. Javan, A., Bennet, W. R., jr., Herriot, D. R., 1961: Population inversion and continuous optical Maser oscillation in gas discharge containing a He-Ne misture. Phys. Rev. *6*, 106.
8. Kamikawa, K., Hayakawa, T., Ikeda, T., 1972: Argon laser treatment of brain tumors sensitized by acridine orange. Med. J. Osaka Univ. *26*, 61.
9. L'Esperance, F. A., Jr., 1965: Laser effect on retinal vasculature. Animal and clinical studies. Arch. Ophthal. *74*, 754.
10. Maiman, T. H., 1960: Stimulated optical radiation in ruby. Nature *187*, 493.
11. Mussigang, H., Rother, W., 1974: Neodymium-YAG laser as an intraoperative instrument in experimental surgery. Münch. Med. Wochenschr. *116*, 937.
12. Patel, C. K. N., 1968: High power carbon dioxide lasers. Sci. Am. *219*, 22.
13. Polany, T. G., Brademeier, C., Davis, T. W., 1970: A CO_2 laser for surgical research. Med. Biol. Eng. *8*, 541.
14. Rosomoff, H. L., Carrol, F., 1965: Effect of laser on brain and neoplasm. Surg. Forum *16*, 431.
15. Stellar, S., 1970: Experimental studies with carbon dioxide laser as a neurosurgical instrument. Med. Biol. Eng. *8*, 549.
16. Takizawa, T., 1978: Laser surgery of brain tumors. No shinkei Geka *9*, 743.

Laser Physic

Victor A. Fasano

Institute of Neurosurgery, University of Turin (Italy)

Contents

1. Generation of Laser Beams. Emission and Absorption 53
2. The Laser 55
   2.1. Active Medium, Pumping.. 55
   2.2. Optical Cavity.. 55
   2.3. Types of Lasers.. 56
3. Fundamental Characteristics of Laser Light Sources............................ 57
4. Interaction of Electromagnetic Energy with Matter.............................. 57
   4.1. Qualitative Interaction.. 57
   4.2. Quantitative Interaction 58
5. Terminology of Laser Irradiation... 60
6. Mechanisms of Tissue Effects by Laser... 61
   6.1. Thermal Effects 62
      6.1.1. Effects of Heat on Tissues 62
      6.1.2. Effects of Heat on Vessels 63
      6.1.3. Thermal Recording in Tissue.. 64
   6.2. Photochemical Reactions.. 65
   6.3. Mechanic Effects 67
   6.4. Effects Related to Electromagnetic Fields...................................... 67
   6.5. Biologic Effects... 67
References 68

Laser (Light Amplification by Stimulated Emission of Radiation) is a high intensity light source which emits a nearly parallel electromagnetic beam of given wavelength generated in a suitable atomic or molecular system by means of a quantum optical process.

1. Generation of Laser Beams. Emission and Absorption

Laser is generated in processes occurring in atoms, molecules or ions. These submicroscopic systems are called quantum systems. The basic concept of the quantum theory states that atomic or molecular systems can be in two various energy state, the first of which is their normal or basal energy state known as the ground state. The second, known as the excited state, is attained at various higher energy levels by the addition of thermal, electrical, chemical or radiation energy stimulation.

The process by which the atom initially in the lower energy level is excited to undergo the transition to an higher level absorbing some of the energy is named absorption.

An atomic or molecular system excited reverts to its own energy ground level either by radiation after some time (10^{-7}–10^{-8} seconds) (spontaneous emission), or by interaction with external incident radiation whose wavelength corresponds to the energy absorbed (stimulated emission) emitting a beam of photons.

To picture the spontaneous emission imagine that an atom is in one of its excited energy levels: Ea. After some time the atom undergo as a transition to a lower energy level: Eb. Accompanying the energy loss (Ea — Eb) light of v ab frequency appears as given by the Niels-Bohr equation

$$v\,ab = \frac{Ea - Eb}{h}$$

where:

v ab is the frequency of the photons.

Ea and Eb are two allowed energies of the atom and h is Planck's constant (6.663×10^{34} joule/second).

The atom has undergone a spontaneous transition to a lower level and in so doing has spontaneously emitted light. This light is emitted with equal probability in all directions and the frequency is not precisely v ab but is spread out over a narrow range centered at v ab. The stimulated emission occurs when an atom in the excited state (Ea) is irradiated with light. In this situation the likelihood of transition to a lower level is increased. Light from stimulated emission has precisely the frequency and direction of the stimulating light and adds constructively to it, thus increasing its intensity.

By extending the phenomena discussed so far to the case of a collection of identical atoms (medium), two special cases must be considered. The case in which most atoms in the collection are in the lower level (Eb) and light having a frequency close to v ab travels through the medium. Under this condition the atoms will absorb light and, as the light passes through the medium, its intensity will decrease. If alternatively most atoms are in the upper level (Ea) light will stimulate the atoms to emit and the results will be an increase in light intensity as it propagates. In this case the light can be said to have been amplified.

In general, whether the light intensity decreases or is amplified simply depends on the difference in densities of atoms in the two levels. The problem is to find a material in which it is possible to put more atoms in a higher energy level than in a lower one: this is termed a population inversion.

Such an atomic system, whether it be gaseous, solid or liquid, can support light amplification and can lead to a laser.

2. The Laser

2.1. Active Medium, Pumping

The laser has two basic components: an amplifying or active medium and an optical cavity. An active medium is a material consenting a population inversion. A source of energy is required to produce and maintain the population inversion by raising atoms to excited levels. This process is called pumping. The pumping of the medium by the energy source must be continued if the population inversion is to maintained, otherwise the atoms would rapidly return to their lowest energy level through the process of spontaneous emission.

2.2. Optical Cavity

The second basic components of every laser is a cavity, bound by two mirrors, forming a resonator in which the active medium is contained. Initially light is emitted in all directions spontaneously; the small fraction emitted along the axis of the cavity strikes one mirror perpendicularly at its center and is reflected to strike the second mirror similarly so being amplified as it moves through the active medium. A further consideration is needed: a standing light wave exists in the optical cavity between the two mirrors. For a standing wave to exist within the laser cavity there must be a node, or zero of intensity, at each mirror surface. This gives rise to the resonance condition that an integral number "m" of half wavelength, must equal the length of the optical cavity (L).

Because of this relationship, which must be satisfied, the optical cavity is more properly called optical resonant cavity.

$$\text{The resonance condition}: m \cdot \frac{\lambda}{2} = L$$

can be rewritten in terms of frequency of the electromagnetic wave using the formula:

$$\lambda v = C$$

where C is the velocity of light (3×10^{10} cm/second).

One than obtains:

$$Vm = \frac{mc}{2L}$$

which are the resonant frequencies of the cavity and are called the longitudinal modes of the cavity. As the cavity length increases the longitudinal modes change in frequency; therefore the resonance condition is a fundamental characteristic of lasers and the constancy of wavelength requires the optical cavity length to be kept within a small fraction of one half wavelength.

2.3. Types of Lasers

There are gas lasers, solid lasers and liquid lasers.

Gas lasers are generally pumped by producing an electrical discharge in the gas, solid lasers by powerful light sources.

The CO_2 laser has energy supplied by passing an electrical current through a mixture of helium, nitrogen and carbon dioxide contained in a cylinder with reflective surfaces. The mirrors are aligned to have a common optical axis. The optimal proportion of the gases is approximately $0.8 : 1 : 7$ and depends upon the characteristics of the laser device. The pressure of the gas mixture varies from about 10 mm Hg to a few hundred mm Hg depending upon the diameter of the tube. The discharge current is typically one or two milliampère per square millimeter of discharge. Voltage depends upon tube diameter and varies from approximately 5,000 to 15,000 V/m of discharge, the voltage per unit of length increasing as the diameter of the discharge tube decreases. This laser emits at about 106 microns in the infrared part of the spectrum; a coaxial 2 w He-Ne laser is housed within the laser head acting as a pilot light. The laser beam is directed into a beam-manipulating arm that contains a mirror in rotary joints and a focusing lens at the beam exit. This arrangement allows the surgeon to apply the focused laser beam to any point within a large area from any direction. When not in use the beam is deflected into a heat sink by a reflective shutter. This shutter is opened by a foot switch to allow the laser beam to reach the target. Flexible delivery system for CO_2 laser is in a developmental stage. For microsurgery the operating microscope is attached to both the manipulator and a specific gimballed mirror. The mirror is positioned at 45 degrees to the incident laser beam and deflects it along the viewing axis of the microscope. A lens focuses electromagnetic energy to a spot at a distance equal to the working distance of the microscope objective. By appropriate lens selection, this distance can be anything from 10 to 500 cm or more. The mirror is gimbal-mounted to permit by a joystick control steering the beam to any desired location within ± 3 degrees of the central axis of the microscope. Mechanical linkage between the joystick and the gimbal is arranged to make the motion of the beam directly proportional and in the same sense as the joystick movement with a demagnification of $7 : 1$. A new innovation is the microscan Microprocessor Controlled Micromanipulator which consents to programme automatic lasing from microprocessor memory. The surgeon traces boundries of tissue to be treated with visible He-Ne laser beam using joystick, in a second step the maneuvre is verified observing automatic retracing of selected boundries; then by depressing foot switch the lasing of tissue within selected boundries is automatically activated.

The Argon laser is an ion-gas laser. Excitation is obtained by producing an electric discharge, at very high current density, in the ionized gas. The beam is visible ranging in the blue-green part of the spectrum with a wavelength of 488–514 nm (0.48–0.51 microns). The transmission system is through fiberoptics. The beam can be directed to a hand-piece, endoscope or attachment for microscope.

The Neodymium : YAG laser is a solid state laser, made from a crystal yttrium aluminum garnet ($Y_3Al_5O_2$) with incorporated (ion doped) Nd_3^+ of certain concentration; these ions are excited by the absorption of light energy. It is accomplished by focusing the light from a discharge lamp (Kripton lamps of 1,000 watts each) on rod-like crystal by a suitable system of electrical cylindrical mirrors (optical pumps). The resonator may be arranged directly on the end surface of the cylindrical crystal or positioned away from them. The beam is emitted on a near infrared range with a wavelength of 1.06 microns. The guide beam is a coaxial 2 w He-Ne laser that is used in the laser head. Both lasers are carried over a quarts glass fiber-optic system to the handpiece, endoscope or micromanipulator attachment for the operating microscope.

Of the various types of liquid lasers, the dye laser is the most significant. This laser discovered by Sorokin in 1965 at IBM laboratories led to tunable outputs over a significant frequency range. This is in contrast to the gas and solid types, which have a very narrow wavelength profile. The active medium consists of organic dyes dissolved in solvent. When the dye is excited by external sources of a short wavelength it emits radiation at longer wavelengths or is said to fluoresce.

3. Fundamental Characteristics of Laser Light Sources

The laser beam has three essential properties:

a) Monocromaticity. All the electromagnetic waves have the same wavelength.

b) Parallelism of light rays.

c) Coherence. All the rays bear a constant relation to each other and are in phase.

As a consequence of the parallelism and coherence, all the light emitted by a laser can be concentrated in the focal spot of a lens and therefore, an extremely high energy can be obtained.

4. Interaction of Electromagnetic Energy with Matter

4.1. Qualitative Interaction

Electromagnetic radiant energy stretches over an immense range of frequencies. At the high frequency end are the γ-rays (10^{-3} A) and X-rays

$(10^{-2}$ A), then there are ultraviolet rays, visible spectrum and infrared rays; at the lower frequencies are the radio waves with wavelengths of kilometers.

The lasers most often used in surgery are all in the infrared and visible spectrum.

The diverse interactions that take place when radiant energy impinges on matter depend exclusively on the frequency of the electro-magnetic wave and tissue physical characteristics.

Electromagnetic radiant energy can be thought of a composed of photons whose individual energies E are given by the expression:

$$E = h \nu$$

where h = Planck's constant: 6.63×10^{-34} joule/second
ν = frequency (cycles per second).

The effect of electromagnetic energy on matter is a result of interactions of individual photons with individual atoms or molecules. The prevalent types of interaction of radiation with matter depend on the spectral regions. Ionization and radical formation are typical of γ-rays, X-rays and far-ultraviolet rays. Photochemical effects take place in near-ultraviolet rays and visible radiations. Thermal effects are prevalent in visible portion of the spectrum and in infrared rays.

4.2. Quantitative Interaction

The quantitative interaction of electromagnetic energy with matter is related to the concept of extinction factor (j) and follows the Lambert Beer's law:

$$I = I_{oe} - jL$$

where:
I = intensity of the beam at a certain depth in the tissue.
I_0 = initial intensity of the incident beam.
e = base of natural logarithm.

This law expresses the fact that the intensity of an incident beam in a biological tissue decreases exponentially with the depth, depending on the extinction factor.

This factor is equal to the sum of the absorption and scattering of the beam by the tissue and both are in relation to the wavelength of the incident radiation, the chemical composition and the physical state of the tissue (denser material absorbs more since there are more molecules per unit volume). Another term used is extinction length which is defined as the thickness of material that absorbs 90% of the incident energy. Therefore the absorptive properties of tissues have a fundamental role in the application of lasers to surgery: absorption characteristic of proteins, deoxyribonucleic acid (DNA), pigments, water and other intracellular molecules together determine the absorption characteristic of the tissue as a whole. Coefficient absorption (thickness of material attenuating electromagnetic radiation) of biological tissues in vivo are difficult to measure.

At the wavelength of the Nd : YAG laser the extinction length in pure water is 60 mm and that of the CO_2 laser is 0.03 mm, this means that 90% of the radiation of a Nd : YAG laser is absorbed in a 6 cm layer of water, while 0.03 mm of water are sufficient to absorb 90% of the CO_2 laser radiation.

Argon requires approximately 1 meter of water to reduce the incident energy to 90% of its original value.

Tissues, of course, are not water and variations in density, in chemical composition and structural inhomogeneities alter the coefficients of absorption. As an example, the extinction length of the Nd : YAG radiation in the stomach wall of dogs[16] and in human brain[38] have been measured experimentally and found to be about 2.3 mm and 3.5 mm respectively. The few measurements that have been made on tissue for the wavelength of the CO_2 laser confirm that tissue penetration is minimal (less than 0.2 mm) and pigment independent.

Lesion is confined totally to the irradiated surface without back scattering and forward scattering. However Nd : YAG laser has scattering both backwards and forwards so producing volume heating. Argon absorption in water is negligible, but it is color specific and has a high absorption coefficient for blood hemoglobin, melanin and cytochromes and absorption coefficient approaches that of the CO_2 laser in tissue but about 100 times as much energy is scattered laterally as is absorbed directly. The measured transmission of Argon laser into human brain is less than 0.5 mm[38]. Studies on light absorption in hemoglobin show that absorption between wavelengths of 400 and 805 nm is significantly lower in oxyhemo-globin than in hemoglobin; above 805 nm the effect is reversed, the absorption coefficient of oxyhemoglobin being higher than that of hemoglobin [37-45].

Halldorsson[17] by comparing absorbance of blood samples for He-Ne (633 nm) and Nd : YAG (1,064 nm) demonstrated that absorbance of oxygenated blood is nearly the same value for both wavelength, whereas there is a substantial difference in the absorbance of deoxygenated blood which increases almost by a factor of 2 for He-Ne laser but drops by a factor of 3.7 for the Nd : YAG laser. Since hemoglobin is totally deoxygenated during thermal denaturation[17] the dependance of the absorbance on the oxygen saturation has to be taken into account when irradiating blood vessels or tissue in sites of massive bleeding. In thermal denaturated blood an increased scattering is also assumed[17]. This causes a balancing of the reduced hemoglobin absorption of the Nd : YAG but enhances the absorption of the He-Ne laser radiation. Penetration in bleeding tissue is therefore strongly limited for wavelengths ranging between 400 and 800 nm while with Nd : YAG laser penetration depth is relatively independent of blood content.

5. Terminology of Laser Irradiation

Some of the physical parameters used to describe lasers are presented in Table 1.

The term power is related to the watts produced by the system; measurement is taken using a power meter. A rheostat controlling the voltage input to the optical cavity allows the surgeon to vary the laser output power.

Table 1. *Physical Parameters of Lasers*

TERM	SYMBOL	UNIT
POWER	P	W (WATT)
TIME	t	s (SECOND)
ENERGY	E = Pxt	Ws = J (JOULE)
AREA	A	sqcm
POWER DENSITY	I = P/A	W/sqcm
ENERGY DENSITY	L = E/A	$\frac{Ws}{sqcm} = \frac{J}{sqcm}$

Energy is the product of power and time.

Power density is expressed as watts per square centimeter. Average power density can be determined by measuring the effective spot diameter and the total power if we assume a Gaussian distribution of the intensity of the beam as it leaves the optical cavity:

$$PD = \frac{100 \times \text{power in watts}}{\text{effective beam in mm}^2}$$

Transverse electromagnetic mode (TEM) is used to describe this distribution of power over the spot area. TEMoo is the basic mode. In this mode the power is concentrated at the center of the spot (maximum intensity) diminishing towards the periphery.

Power density varies directly with power and inversely with surface area. It can be also varied by the shifts in TEMoo. Infact the transverse mode of a laser system will be affected by the shape of the mirrors (plane, spherical and so on) and by the variation of reflectivity across the surface of each mirror. In all real lasers of high-output power (greater than 5 watts) heat is generated by the pumping system, and the temperature of the resonator will change from point to point and from time to time. Changes of temperature cause expansion and/or contraction of the laser tube or rod, the mirrors, and the supporting structures. These small thermal movements in turn cause shifting of the transverse mode of the laser. Only using very elaborate structures which are often very expensive and bulky, can these thermal shifts be minimized. One simple way to minimize thermal mode shifts is to operate the laser at the desired power level for a period of 30 to 60 minutes before surgery to allow all parts of the laser to reach stable temperatures.

Many other types of intensity distribution, different from TEMoo, are possible. In $TEMo_1$ mode (or donut mode) the intensity is zero along the axis, increases as one moves away from the center and then decays to zero in a fashion similar but not equal to TEMoo mode. It is quite possible for one

Table 2. *Types of Laser Used in Surgical Applications*

LASER TYPE	WAVELENGTH (microns)	POWER / ENERGY RANGE	MODE OF OPERATION
CO_2	10.6	0.1 – 100 WATTS	CW – PULSED
Nd : YAG	1.06	5 – 120 WATTS	CW – PULSED
ARGON	0.488 – 0.516	0.001 – 20 WATTS	CW – PULSED
DYE	0.4 – 0.7	0.001 – 6 WATTS	CW – PULSED

laser to operate in several modes at the same time or to switch modes in rapid or slow succession as a consequence of thermal changes in the cavity and one mode may be more useful than another for a given application.

The energy density is a measure of the total amount of energy per unit area of tissue surface exposed, and is equal to the power density multiplied by the time of exposure.

The different temporal modes of operation of a laser are distinguished by the rate at which energy is delivered. The lasers operating in the normal pulse temporal mode have pulse durations of a few tenths of a microsecond to a few milliseconds and are often referred to as pulsed. The lasers operating continuously are termed continuous wave. In these the beam power is constant with time. Table 2 summarizes the power/energy range and modes of operation.

6. Mechanisms of Tissue Effects by Laser

Four phases of laser action at impact on tissue are described:
a) Thermal effects.
b) Photochemical reactions.
c) Development of pressure recoil and elastic shock waves.
d) Effects related to strong electromagnetic fields of the laser beam.

Bellina and coworkers[2] have divided the known effects of photon-tissue interaction in linear and not linear effects. Linear effects comprise heating, vaporization and plume phenomena. Nonlinear effects include:

a) Generation of elastic wave by: radiation pressure, electrostriction, self trapping and stimulated Brillouin.

b) Generation of ionizing radiation by: multiphoton effect, harmonic generation, stimulated Raman and electric breakdown.

6.1. Thermal Effects

Thermal action is the effect of laser beam currently utilized in surgery; it depends on the absorption of the optical energy by the tissue, with subsequent transformation into thermal energy.

Table 3. *Alterations of Tissues Due to Heat*

THERAPEUTIC RANGE	CO_2 – ARGON $\longrightarrow$ Nd : YAG $\longrightarrow$			
TEMPERATURE DEGREE	37 – 60° C	60 – 70° C	70 – 100° C	100° C
EFFECT ON TISSUE	HEATING , ENZYME DAMAGE	DENATURATION OF PROTEIN	VAPORIZATION OF TISSUE WATER	CARBONIZATION TO BURNING OF NON WATER – CONTAINING TISSUE CONSTITUENT
OPTICAL CHANGE	NONE	BLANCHING INCREASED BEAM PENETRATION, INCREASED ABSORPTION OF VISIBLE AND NEAR INFRARED RADIATION	INCREASED SCATTER AND ABSORPTION UNTIL VAPORIZATION, THEN DECREASED ABSORPTION OF INFRARED AND VISIBLE LIGHT	BLACKENING AND INCREASED ABSORPTION : SMOKE AND GAS GENERATION
MECHANICAL CHANGE	NONE	LOSS OF TISSUE STRUCTURE , DRYING	CHANGE IN TISSUE DENSITY , DRYING SEVERE SHRINKAGE	SERIOUS DAMAGE TILL ABLATION

6.1.1. Effects of Heat on Tissues

The effect of heat on tissue varies with the temperature reached from a slight pallor of the tissue to overt crater formation (Table 3). Between 37 and 60 °C simple heating occurs with a consequent speeding of temperature dependent enzyme reaction and altered water permeability characteristics. Between 60 and 70 °C denaturation of proteins occurs with loss of cell membrane integrity and alterations in the form of structural proteins. At 100 °C boiling of tissue water occurs causing cells to explode and at higher temperatures carbonization with charring is observed.

Power density, length of exposure, optical attenuation, tissue density and blood flow participate to determine the acute laser beamtissue response. If the rate of energy delivery is slow (beam defocusing or low laser power) or if absorption is decreased tissue heating is slower; conduction of heat to surrounding tissue can occur and cause more generalized but controlled heating[14], which promotes coagulation of the tissue and slow dessication. Tissue temperature ranges between 60 and 80 °C. Then, because of the lower absorbance of laser light in non-water containing tissue constituents the dehydrated tissues require much higher energy to be vaporized. As a consequence local heating and heat conduction to surrounding tissue increase and temperature higher than 100 °C are easily reached. If the rate of energy is rapid (high power density) and exceeds the capability of the tissue to dissipate heat and the sublimation threshold, there is rapid conversion of tissue water into steam. Verschueren[42] calls this vaporization process "explosive tissue evaporation", in that the vaporization of water is accompanied by a 1,000-fold increase in volume. The high energy required for the vaporization of tissue water and the sudden ejection of heated tissue and steam have a thermostatic effect (water jacket) that limits heating of surrounding non target tissue. The depth of the crater created by the laser depends on the total energy of the beam. If the energies of the beam are the same, multiple short pulses will vaporize tissue to approximately the same depth as a single long pulse. Short high-energy pulses, often used to incise tissue, produce less carbonization and lateral tissue damage because each exposure is shorter than the time needed to conduct heat away from the target and thus prevents prolonged heating of dessicated tissue, which is the cause of carbonization observed in laser lesion[11]. Less thermal diffusion from the primary lesion area to surrounding tissue was observed by Berns and coworkers for the enhanced pulsed CO_2 laser compared to the continuous wave laser[3,36]. Mihashi et al.[32] found that extension of lateral damage was greater when tissue was irradiated with a CO_2 laser at 10 watts for 0.88 seconds than when irradiated at 20 watts for 0.44 seconds. High-energy ultrashort pulses however, may cause acoustic transient, nonthermal mechanic disruption of tissue and ionization that can amplify laterally and vertically the area of laser-induced injury[13].

6.1.2. Effects of Heat on Vessels

It remains uncertain what effect is responsible for the coagulation properties of heat. It has been suggested that local compression by edema may be the main factor in occluding small vessels, and that shrinkage of the wall is probably important in producing initial instantaneous hemostasis in vessels up to 0.5–1 mm. Heat damage to vascular endothelium activating the coagulation cascade and producing secondary intravascular thrombosis seems to take the main role in coagulation of vessels up to 2–3 mm. Energy has to be calibrated to be less than what would cause charring of the wall; defocused beam and low energy are currently used.

6.1.3. Thermal Recording in Tissue

The temperature at site of impact is very high (1,500 °C in Takizawa's measurements)[39] decreasing from the center of the lesion to the external boundary following a defined range. At approximately 2 mm from the crater edge the temperature is almost equal to the primary tissue temperature[15, 35].

The conduction of heat from the laser impact area can be described by Fournier's equation:

$$P = CtA \, dt/dx$$

where:

P = power removed by thermal conduction.

Ct = thermal conductivity of the tissue.

A = Area with normal heat flow.

dt/dx = temperature gradient along path of heat flow.

Experimental studies show that thermally removed power density in living soft tissues, after CO_2 laser irradiation, is approximately 10 watts/cm^2 [32].

The vascular pattern of the tissues have a bearing on the heat dissipation. Heat of laser impact to the wall of a large artery is dissipated much faster than other tissues due to the high velocity of blood flow[44].

Various studies on heat diffusion have been made but the results are not perfectly comparable because different tissues have been used.

In a study the increase in surface temperature of irradiated normal brain tissue 2 mm from the laser spot was: 8 °C for CO_2 laser, 6 °C for argon laser, 10 °C for Nd : YAG laser. At 1 mm from the spot these values increased by 50% and at 3 mm decreased by 75%. Thermal recordings at 2 mm in depth revealed an increase in temperature of 8 °C during Nd : YAG laser irradiation; when using CO_2 and argon lasers no modifications of tissue temperature at that depth were noticed[28].

The continuous temperature recordings in cats by thermocouples positioned 5 and 10 mm below the cortical surface while applying Nd : YAG laser at various power and durations were obtained by Wharen and coworkers[47]. The magnitudes of the temperature changes at 5 and 10 mm demonstrated that, despite large increases in temperature at 5 mm, there was correspondingly very little temperature change at 10 mm. Although a 30 °C rise occurred at 5 mm after 20 watts had been applied for 8 seconds, the temperature rise at 10 mm was less than 1 °C. Similar temperature recordings were obtained for incident powers of 5–10 and 30 watts for duration of 1, 2, 4, and 8 seconds. The maximum rise in brain temperature at a depth of 5 mm for various powers and durations demonstrates a linear relationship between the brain temperature rise and the duration of the laser pulse for incident powers of 5 to 30 watts. The maximum temperature rise of the blood at a depth of 5 mm demonstrates that approximately 90% of the maximum temperature rise of the blood occurs within the first 2 to 3 seconds for incident powers of 5 to 20 watts. Prolonged duration of the pulse beyond 3 seconds results in only a small increase in blood temperature. Thus, the heating curves for brain and blood are quite distinct, since blood approaches its maximum temperature within 2 to 3 seconds while the brain temperature continues to increase at a linear rate with prolonged durations. Studies concerning thermal recordings on vessels, when using CO_2 and argon lasers are lacking.

6.2. Photochemical Reactions

Thermal effect, as described above concerns the total absorption of energy by the irradiated tissue. Photochemical effects arise instead from the selective absorption of the light by hemoglobin, melanin, pigments.

To define the participation of these reactions in determining tissue damage Yoshii et al. [49] evaluate on the dorsal spinal columns of cats the energy of laser irradiation necessary to produce marked changes in somatosensory evoked potentials when using argon laser alone and after intravenous injection of fluorescein. The amount of radiant exposure producing SEP changes was 2,699 J/cm² in the non injected group and 563 J/cm² in the fluorescein injected group; this difference represents an indirect recording of photochemical phenomena.

Sometime the absorption may be more selective and limited to some parts of the living cell; depending on their chemical structure, they can absorb one or more wavelengths of the electromagnetic spectrum. For example aminoacids present a peak of absorption at 280 nm; diphosphopyridyne nucleotides two peaks at 260 and 300 nm. Therefore we can obtain in vitro a selective destruction and/or denaturation of some cellular components, without the death of the cell. When a cell or a cellular component does not present a specific absorption peak, the latter can be artificially induced by introducing a dye into the cell or into the cellular components as a specific target.

Photoradiation therapy utilizes the photosensitizing and tumor localizing properties of certain porphyrins, in the treatment of malignant tumors.

The porphyrin most often used is a hematoporphyrin derivative (Hpd) first prepared by Schwartz and evaluated clinically for tumor localization by Lipson[25-27].

Histological evidence of experimental animal tumor damage has been described using different photosensitizers such as hematoporphyrin and white light in 1972[7] and acridine orange, and 488 nm light in 1974[41]. However, as early as 1903, Tappeneier and Jesionek described the photosensitizing effect of eosin and light on superficial tumors in man[40].

The eradication of experimental animal tumors by Hpd and light (red) was described in 1975[8] as well as the first application in treating a malignant tumor in man[21].

Hpd is currently the only photosensitizer being evaluated in man because of its now recognized superior properties of tumor localization, effective photodynamic action in vivo and its absorption in the red region of the spectrum (the most penetrating visible wavelength). The necessity of using red light to obtain penetration beyond a few mm of tissue was clear from literature[12, 38]. When tumor sites are illuminated with red light, the Hpd absorbs it producing an excited state that is then able to incite photodynamic reactions. The primary cytotoxic agent produced in this way is thought to be singlet oxygen[43] formed by energy transfer from the triplet state of excited Hpd molecules. The action of singlet oxygen is by oxidations of biological components so as to impair cell membrane function and integrity and thereby cause cell death. At the low light dosage (powers) used, there is no immediate visible change such as coagulation or necrosis. Tumor tissue death in the form of debris is noted within 24–48 hours. Normal tissues (containing little Hpd) are not irreversibly harmed.

Hyperthermia produced by the treatment light in Hpd photoradiation therapy seems to contribute to cell death and tumor necrosis in combination with the effects of the singlet oxygen. This hypothesis is particularly attractive because the various proposed mechanism of selective hyperthermia on tumor cells involve the same cellular target system as proposed for Hpd photoradiation therapy[33]. Results reported by Berns et al. who recorded a surface temperature rise up to $7\,^{\circ}C$ for a power density of $508\,mW/cm^2$ indicate that the red light employed in Hpd photoradiation therapy is sufficient to produce a rise in tissue temperature that approaches that necessary for a selective hyperthermic killing of malignant cells[4].

The distribution of Hpd in animal brain tumor models has been studied in preliminary experiences[4, 46]. Results indicate that there was minimal uptake of Hpd into normal rat brain, but significant uptake into the tumor and adjacent brain. Contrary to the rats given Hpd only or exposed to laser only a patchy pattern of coagulation necrosis in the tumors was observed in rats given Hpd and exposed to laser; significant brain edema surrounding the tumor was noticed in such cases[5].

According to experimental data[4] and preliminary clinical trials[34] photoradiation therapy did not prolong survival of treated cases[9, 48].

Recent experimental studies have shown that the activating light from the laser can be delivered directly to the tumor site by inserting the light delivery fiber through a needle placed into the tumor. Forbes[10] has used the fiber implants to advantage in cerebral tumors in man. Although results of interstitial photoradiation therapy on brain tumors remain to be assessed, this treatment apparently can be carried out safely in such cases. Similar results are reported by Laws and coworkers[24].

6.3. Mechanic Effects

Mechanic effects depend on the immediate interactions between a high power radiant energy and a biological medium. Following this interaction, acoustic and shock waves arise, due to rapidly evolving thermal gradient on the tissue. The mechanical waves push away the cells forming sometimes a crater on the tissue and the molecules can be oriented in some particular directions. Shockwaves can produce ultrasonic high frequency phenomena spreading on the surrounding space.

6.4. Effects Related to Electromagnetic Fields

According to the electromagnetic theory of light, each light photon is associated with a sinusoidal electromagnetic wave and an electric field. Damage arise from the interaction between the electromagnetic field produced by laser beam and tissues. When the electromagnetic field is quite strong the electrons movement is no longer proportional to the field itself. It means that, in this condition, some new coherent radiation can be generated at a frequency 2, 3, 4 times higher than the frequency of the field itself. For example the infrared beam of Nd:YAG can produce a green beam of 530 nm and an ultraviolet beam of 265 nm, the last one, producing ionization and free radicals with molecular damage. Besides low power laser can modify the conductivity, the dielectric constant of tissues and the polarization of cellular membranes.

6.5. Biologic Effects

The biostimulatory effects of laser beam have been reported in literature in studies on the wound healing process and on the delayed modifications occurring in lased tissues.

There is currently much interest in the use of low energy laser radiation to accelerate the healing of open wounds by selective stimulation of fibroblasts mediated functions (wound contraction, collagen synthesis and increase in tensile strength) and epithelization.

Laser stimulated fibroblast proliferation and collagen synthesis have been demonstrated in vitro with Ruby and helium-neon lasers[18, 23, 30], tissue experiments with argon revealed a similar increased proliferation of fibroblasts[20]. On the contrary a marked decrease of collagen production and DNA replication rate is reported in skin fibroblasts irradiated with Nd:YAG laser[1].

Effects on epidermal cells in vitro have not been studied.

Several authors have reported beneficial effects of laser radiation on wound healing in animal models[22, 30] as cats, dogs, mice but very few studies report researches in man or in analogous animal models. Hunter and coworkers[19] have examined the effect of helium-neon laser on the wound closure in a porcine model, an animal with a dermal structure more closely resembling that of man and concluded that the low energies used did not accelerate the healing. Concerning the study of the delayed effects occurring in lased areas after irradiation, some studies describe progressive photobiologic modifications as fibrosis consequent to inflammatory responses in tumor irradiated with Nd : YAG laser[6] and mural fibrosis and endothelial hyperplasia in vessels irradiated with argon laser[29]. Bellina[2] studied these biologic responses in irradiated tissue using a rabbit fallopian tube as model and argon laser. Results revealed delayed tissue changes associated with fibrosis which appeared to be directly related to an intravascular microcoagulation which was observed 10 days after irradiation and persisted until the 15st day. Because of the limited collateral circulation tissue necrotized and repair occurred thereafter until the 21st day of study. The second effect consisted in mucosal hyperplasia. The exact stimulus for the hyperplasia was unknown but authors suggested a photochemical reaction.

References

 1. Abergel, R. P., Meeker, C. A., Dwyer, R. M., Lasovoy, M. A., Hitto, J., 1984: Non thermal effects of Nd : YAG laser on biological functions of human skin fibroblasts in culture. Lasers Surg. Med. *3*, 279–284.
 2. Bellina, J. H., Ross, L., Holmquist, N., Voros, J. I., Moorehead, M. E., 1983: Linear and nonlinear effect of the argon laser on a fallopian tube animal model. Lasers Surg. Med. *2*, 343–356.
 3. Berns, M. W., Ishimoto, B. M., 1984: Comparison of continuous wave (CW) and superpulsed (SP) CO_2 laser effects on tissue. Lasers Surg. Med. *3*, 363.
 4. Berns, M. W., 1984: Preface: Hematoporphyrine derivative Photoradiation therapy. Lasers Surg. Med. *4*, 1–4.
 5. Boggan, J. E., Edwards, M. S. B., Berns, M. W., Walter, R. J., Bolger, C. A., 1984: Hematoporphyrin derivative photoradiation therapy of the rat 9 L gliosarcoma brain tumor model. Lasers Surg. Med. *4*, 99–105.
 6. Bown, S. G., 1983: Tumor therapy with the Nd : YAG laser. In: Neodymium-YAG laser in Medicine and Surgery (Joffe, S. N., ed.), pp. 51–58. New York-Amsterdam-Oxford: Elsevier.
 7. Diamond, I., Granelli, S., McDoangh, A. F., Nielsen, S., Wilson, C. B., Jaenicke, R., 1972: Photodynamic therapy of malignant tumors. Lancet *2*, 1175–1177.
 8. Dougherty, T. J., Grindey, G. B., Fiel, R., Weishaupt, K. R., Boyle, D. G., 1975: Photoradiation therapy II: Cure of animal tumors with hematoporphyrin and light. J. Natl. Cancer Inst. *55*, 115–119.
 9. Dougherty, T. J., Kaufman, J. E., Goldfarb, A., Weishaupt, K. R., Boyle, D. G., Mittelman, A., 1978: Photoradiation therapy for the treatment of malignant tumors. Cancer Res. *38*, 2628–2635.
10. Dougherty, T. J., Boyle, D. G., Weishaupt, K. R., Potter, W. R., Thoma, R. E., 1983: Photoradiation therapy of malignant tumors. In: New Frontiers in Laser Medicine and Surgery (Atsumi, K., ed.), pp. 161–165. Amsterdam-Oxford-Princeton: Excerpta Medica.

11. Edwards, M. S. B., Boggan, J. E., Fuller, T. A., 1983: The laser in neurological surgery. J. Neurosurg. *59*, 555–566.
12. Everett, M. A., Yearges, E., Sayre, R. M., Olson, R. L., 1983: Penetration of epidermis by ultraviolet rays. Photochem. Photobiol. *1*, 533–542.
13. Fine, S., Klein, E., Novak, W., 1965: Interaction of laser radiation with biologic systems. I: Studies on Interaction with Tissues. Fed. Proc. *24* (Suppl. 14), S 35–S 47.
14. Fox, J. L., Hayes, J. R., Stein, M. N., 1967: Experimental cranial and vascular studies of the effects of pulsed and continuous wave laser radiation. J. Neurosurg. *27*, 126–137.
15. Goldman, L., Rockwell, R. J., 1966: Laser action at cellular level. JAMA *198*, 173.
16. Halldorsson, T., Rother, W., Langehole, J., 1981: Thoretical and experimental investigations prove Nd : YAG laser treatment to be safe. Lasers Surg. Med. *1*, 253–262.
17. Halldorson, T., 1983: Alteration of optical and thermal properties of blood by Nd : YAG laser irradiation. In: New Frontiers in Laser Medicine and Surgery (Atsumi, K., ed.), pp. 98–105. Amsterdam-Oxford-Princeton: Excerpta Medica.
18. Hardy, L. B., Hardy, F. S., Fine, S., Sokal, J., 1967: Effect of ruby laser radiation on mouse fibroblast culture. Fed. Proc. *26*, 668.
19. Hunter, J., Leonard, L., Wilson, R., Snider, G., Dixon, J., 1984: Effects of low energy laser on wound healing in a porcine model. Lasers Surg. Med. *3*, 285–290.
20. Kama, J. S., Hutschenreiter, D., Waidelich, W., 1981: Effect of low-power density laser radiation on healing of open skin wounds in rats. Arch. Surg. *116*, 293–296.
21. Kelly, J. F., Snell, H. E., Berenbaum, M. C., 1975: Photodynamic destruction of human bladder carcinoma. Br. J. Cancer *31*, 237–244.
22. Kovacs, I. B., Mester, E., Garog, P., 1974: Stimulation of wound healing with laser beam in the rat. Experientia *30*, 1275.
23. Lain, T. S., Abertel, R. P., Dwyer, R. M., Uitto, J., 1983: Biological effects of laser stimulation of collagen production by low energy lasers in human skin fibroblast cultures. Lasers Surg. Med. *3*, 189.
24. Laws., E. R., Jr., Cortese, D. A., Kinsey, J. H., Eagan, R. T., Anderson, R. E., 1981: Photoradiation therapy in the treatment of malignant brain tumors: a phase I (Feasibility study). Neurosurg. *9*, 672–677.
25. Lipson, R. L., 1960: The photodynamic and fluorescent properties of a particular hematoporphyrin derivative and its use in tumor detection. Master's thesis University of Minnesota.
26. Lipson, R. L., Baldes, E. J., Olsen, A. M., 1964: A further evaluation of the use of hematoporphyrin derivative as a new aid for the endoscopic detection of malignant disease. Diseases of the Chest *46*, 676–679.
27. Lipson, R. L., Baldes, E. J., Olsen, A. M., 1961: The use of a derivative of hematoporphyrin in tumor detection. J. Nat. Cancer Inst. *26*, 1–8.

28. Lombard, G. F., Benech, F., Tealdi, S., Ponzio, R. M., 1982: Thermal effects on nervous human tissues under electro or laser surgery. J. Neurosurg. Sci. *26*, 265–271.

29. Maira, G., Mohr, G., Panisset, K., Hardy, J., 1979: Laser photocoagulation for treatment of experimental aneurysms. J. Microsurg. *1*, 137–147.

30. Mester, E., 1970: Stimulating effect of lower power laser on biological systems. Med. Biol. Eng. *8*, 430.

31. Mester, E., Spiry, T., Szende, B., Tota, J. G., 1971: Effect of laser rays on wound healing. Am. J. Surg. *122*, 532–535.

32. Mihashi, S., Hirano, M., 1979: Interaction of CO_2 laser and soft tissue. In: Laser Surgery III, part one (Kaplan, I., ed.), pp. 17–26. Tel-Aviv: OT-PAZ.

33. Overgaad, J., 1969: Effect of hyperthermia on malignant cells in vivo: A review and a hypothesis. Cancer *39*, 2637–2646.

34. Perria, C., Capuzzo, T., Cavagnaro, G., Datti, R., Francaviglia, N., Rivano, C., Trecero, V. E., 1980: First attempts at the photodynamic treatment of human gliomas. J. Neurosurg. Sci. *24*, 119–128.

35. Priebe, L. A., Welch, A. J., 1979: A dimensionless model for the calculation of temperature increase in biologic tissue exposed to non ionizing radiation. IEEE Trans Biomed. Engng. BME *26*, 244.

36. Rattner, W., Rosemberg, S., Fuller, R., 1979: Difference between continuous wave and superpulse Carbon dioxide laser in bladder surgery. Urology *13*, 265–266.

37. Sidwell, A. E., Jr., Munch, R. H., Gunzman, E., Garrow, E. S., Hogness, T. R., 1938: The salt effect of the hemoglobin-oxygen equilibrium. J. Biol. Chem. *123*, 335.

38. Svaasand, L. O., Doiron, D. R., Profio, A. E.: Light distribution in tissue during photoradiation therapy. In: Workshop on Porphirin Sensitazion. New York: Plenum Press.

39. Takizawa, T., Comparison between the laser surgical unit and the electrosurgical unit. Neurol. Med. Chir. *17*, 95–105.

40. Tappenier, H., Jesionek, A., 1903: Therapeutische Versuche mit fluoreszierenden Stoffen. Münch. Med. Wochschr. *1*, 2042–2044.

41. Tomson, S. H., Emmet, E. A., Fox, S. H., 1974: Photodestruction of mouse epithelial tumors after acridine orange and Argon laser. Cancer Res. *34*, 3124–3127.

42. Verschueren, R. C. J., Tissue reaction to the CO_2 laser in general. In: Microscopic and Endoscopic Surgery with the CO_2 Laser (Andrews, A. H., Jr., Polany, T. G., eds.), pp. 85–92. Boston-Bristol-London: John Wright-PSG.

43. Weisshaupt, K. R., Gomez, C. J., Dougherty, T. J., 1976: Identification of singlet oxygen oxygen as the cytotoxic agent in photoinactivation of a murine tumor. Cancer Res. *36*, 2326–2329.

44. Welch, A. J., Wissler, E. H., Priebe, L. A., 1980: Significance of blood flow in calculation of temperature in laser irradiated tissue. IEEE Trans Biomed. Engng. BME *27*, 164.

45. Welsch, H., Birngruber, R., Boergen, K. P., Gabel, V. P., Hillenkamp, F., 1977: The influence of scattering on the wavelength dependent light absorption in

blood. In: Proceedings of the Symposium Lasers in Medicine and Biology. Neuherberg.

46. Wharen, R. E., Jr., Anderson, R. E., Laws, E. R., Jr., 1983: Quantitation of hematoporphyrin derivative in human gliomas experimental central nervous system tumors and normal tissues. Neurosurg. *12*, 446–450.

47. Wharen, R. E., Jr., Anderson, R. E., Scheithauer, B., Sundt, T. E., Jr., 1984: The Nd : YAG laser in neurosurgery. Part 1. Laboratory investigations: dose related biological response of neural tissue. J. Neurosurg. *60*, 531–539.

48. Wile, A. G., Coffey, J., Nahabedian, M. Y., Baghdassarian, R., Mason, G. R., 1984: Laser photoradiation therapy of cancer: an update of the experience at the university of California, Irvine. Lasers Surg. Med. *4*, 5–12.

49. Yoshii, Y., Egashira, T., Maki, Y., 1984: Use of evoked responses to measure laser photoradiation tissue effects. Neurosurg. *14*, 131–134.

Laser Effect on Normal Nervous Tissue (CO_2-Nd : YAG). Histological Data

Victor A. Fasano

Institute of Neurosurgery, University of Turin (Italy)

Contents

1. Brain Tissue 72
 1.1. Morphologic Characteristics of the Acute Laser Lesion 72
 1.2. Acute Laser Effects in the Outer Periphery of the Lesion 74
 1.3. Morphologic Characteristics of the Chronic Laser Lesion 82
 1.4. Histochemical Data 82
2. Nerves 83
References 83

1. Brain Tissue

1.1. Morphologic Characteristics of the Acute Laser Lesion

The tissue changes following application of lasers to rabbit brain were studied by Beck et al. in 1979[1] using CO_2 and Nd : YAG lasers.

Focused and defocused applications were performed at power and exposure time ranging from 1 to 20 watts and ¼ to 8 seconds for CO_2 and from 22 to 45 watts and ½ to 4 seconds for Nd : YAG.

Macroscopically with defocused CO_2 laser a wide, encrusted lesion, frequently surrounded by local subarachnoid hemorrhage, is produced on the brain surface; increasing exposure time there is increasing crater formation with a well defined carbonized border zone. Focused application results in small lesions of pin-head size surrounded by a tenuous carbonized zone.

On defocused application with Nd : YAG at lower energy the lesions are frequently indetectable. At higher energy there is a paling of the brain surface, shallow pitting and sometimes accentuated hollowing with occasional sugillations in the centre of the lesions. In focused setting the

Nd:YAG laser application leaves papular or alveolate, torn and carbonized area depending upon energy. Altogether the lesions of the Nd:YAG laser are not sharply defined. At higher energy there is a relatively wide border zone with less carbonization. If the equal energy Nd:YAG laser radiation strikes a highly vascularized brain surface the lesions are more pronounced.

The nature of the tissue changes produced is identical independent of laser type. There are 4 typical zones:

a) Carbonization zone: superficial cafbonization of pia mater and adjacent brain tissue.

b) Coagulation zone with thermal honeycombing: underneath the carbonization zone, the completely coagulated tissue changes into a honeycombed, but otherwise amorphous mass. The brain surface is partly buckled or partly stripped off, resulting in craters of varying depths.

c) Zone of homogeneous coagulation: next to the coagulation zone with honeycombing, there is a zone in which the tissue coagulates but retains its original form.

d) Edema zone: all the coagulated material is surrounded mantle-like by a wide border of edema in which no recognizable tissue destruction is seen. Interstizial hemorrhage was rare and focal with Nd:YAG laser although occasional fibrin tangles were evident within vessels.

These 4 zones are found with high energy laser radiation. If the laser energy is low only limited edema appears; with increasing energy one observes homogeneous coagulation, then formation of heat honeycombing and finally carbonization. Using defocused (spot: 2 mm) CO$_2$ laser, a typical tissue lesion that extends as a half sphere into the brain tissue is produced. The size of the lesion on the surface shows no substantial relation to time or power. The area has an average diameter of approximately 2.5 mm varying from 2.2 to 3.2 mm. The depth of damage, on the other hand, is primarily dependent on time of irradiation and less on power density: with ¼ second irradiation time at 20 watts depth was 0.23 mm; at 6 watts for 1 second it was 0.94 mm and at 2.5 watts for 8 seconds was 1.9 mm. Further prolongation of the irradiation period led to only small increases of depth.

The focused laser lesion (spot: 0.6 mm) extends as a fissure to a considerable depth. This reaches a maximum of 4.7 mm at a fissure width of 0.6 mm. The lateral extension of the damaged zone is almost exlusively determined by the length of the pulse (at ¼ second: 0.45 mm; at 1 second: 0.76 mm; at 8 seconds: 0.98 mm), while the depth of the hole seems to correlate with the energy applied.

Defocused application of the Nd:YAG laser results in a hemispherical lesion extending into the brain tissue. With a beam diameter of 2.4 mm, the greatest lesion depth is 3.78 mm with a diameter of 6.8 mm at the surface.

On focusing the beam (spot: 1.2 mm), a very wide faintly wedge shaped lesion is produced. The greatest lesion depth is 2.6 mm with a surface diameter of 2.8 mm.

By comparing the histology of the lesions to the spatial profile of the laser beam, it seems evident that the effective spot size is almost invariably larger than the optical size because of thermal conductivity away from the heated area. Indeed, the scattering effect in tissue is known to be greater for Nd : YAG than for CO_2 laser. Despite these considerations Wharen et al. in 1984[11] have demonstrated that using Nd : YAG laser the low power lesions closely approximated the size of the laser beam even with prolonged duration: 5 watts applied for 8 seconds produced a lesion 1.5 mm in diameter with a beam diameter of 1.2 mm. For this author a higher incident power has a significant scattering effect which can be observed histologically.

1.2. Acute Laser Effects in the Outer Periphery of the Lesion

The experimental studies of Wharen et al. in 1984[11] and Boggan et al. in 1982[2] have demonstrated that a defect of the blood brain barrier exists in the area surrounding a laser lesion.

Using 1% Evans blue solution injected intravenously in the animals following the laser irradiation one-half hour before they were killed, these authors observed that Evans blue staining of the cerebral cortex occurred only in a narrow zone surrounding the area of the laser lesion. No staining was observed in the opposite control hemisphere. The most pronounced blood-brain barrier defect extending 2 mm from the center of the CO_2 lesion was found in the specimens examined at ½ hour[2]. The lesion showed a rapid decline in the intensity of the Evans blue staining during the 24 hours after injury. At all times the blood-brain barrier defect surrounding the subcortical portion of the laser incision was less pronounced and less sharply defined than the staining at the cortical surface. Using Nd : YAG laser there was a distinct zone of staining with a width of 1.0 mm surrounding the 40 watts lesions[11].

These blood-brain barrier defect findings are consistent with those of Toya et al. [10] who used fluorescein angiography to evaluate the epicerebral microcirculation in a region of CO_2 laser-induced brain damage in dogs. Around the focal area of the laser radiation a layer of fluorescein dye nonfilling, in the shape of a long narrow strip ranging in width from 1.0 to 1.5 mm was observed through the arterial and capillary to venous phase. This area coincided with the histological area of coagulation necrosis. Further outside this nonfilling area, from the capillary to the venous phase, extravasation of the fluorescein dye was observed, adjacent to the wall of vessels 200 to 300 microns in diameter. This area (1.0 to 1.5 mm wide) coincides with the histological finding of edema, dilatation or rupture of the

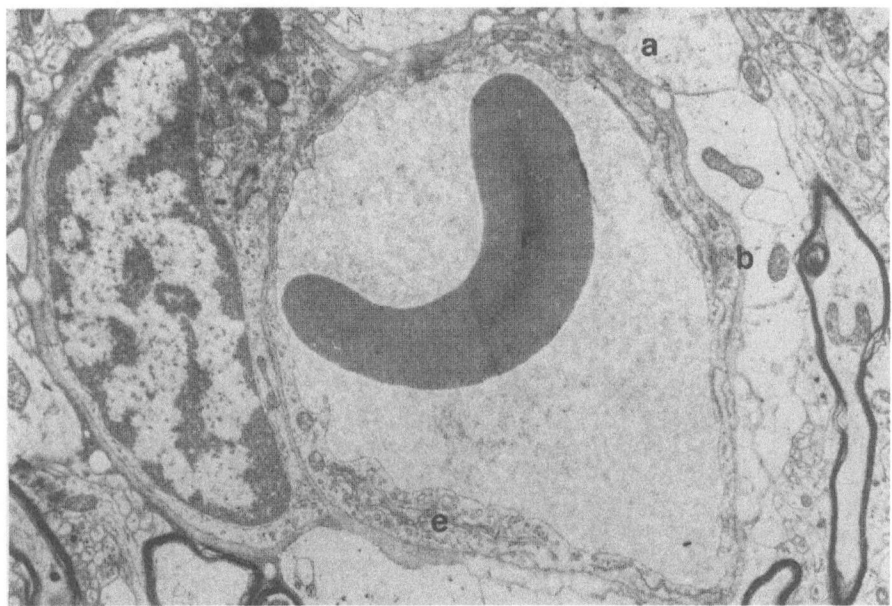

Fig. 1. Transmission electron micrograph of a normal cerebral capillary. (*b* basement membrane; *e* endothelial cell; *a* astrocyte pedicle; *r* red blood cell)

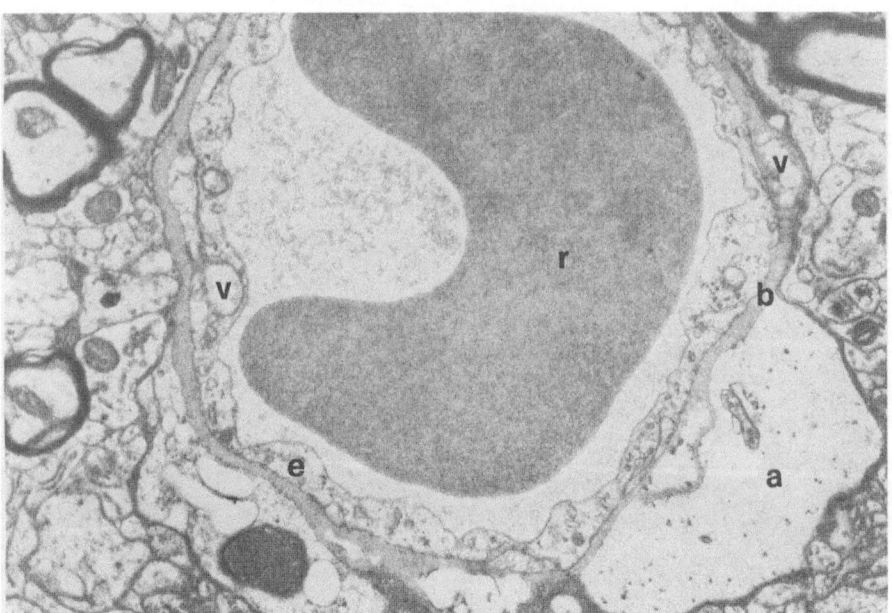

Fig. 2. Transmission electron micrograph of a cerebral capillary after CO$_2$ laser irradiation at 20 watts for 3 seconds. (*b* basement membrane; *e* endothelial cell; *a* astrocyte pedicle; *r* red blood cell; *v* vesicle)

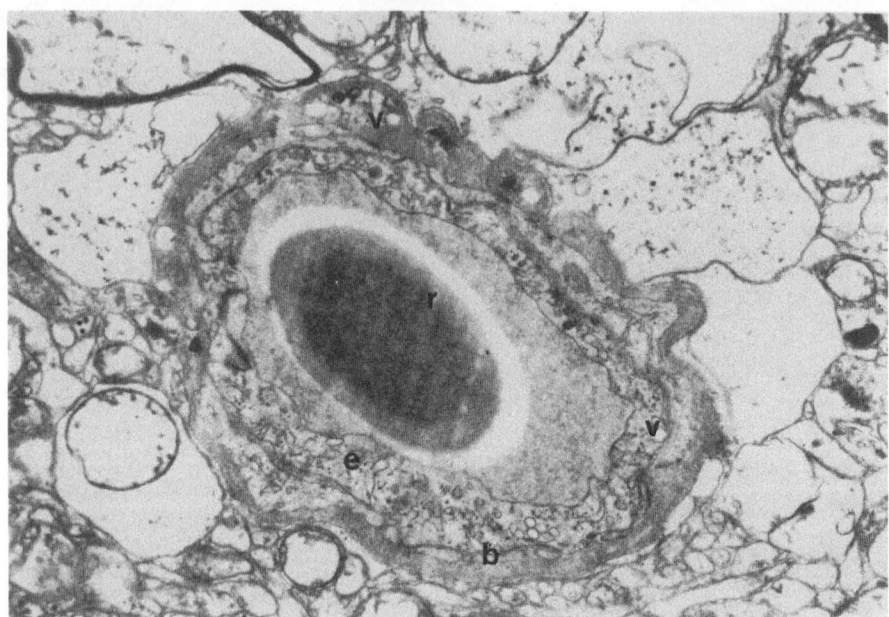

Fig. 3. Transmission electron micrograph of a cerebral capillary after CO_2 laser irradiation at 20 watts for 10 seconds. (*b* basement membrane; *e* endothelial cell; *r* red blood cell; *v* vesicle)

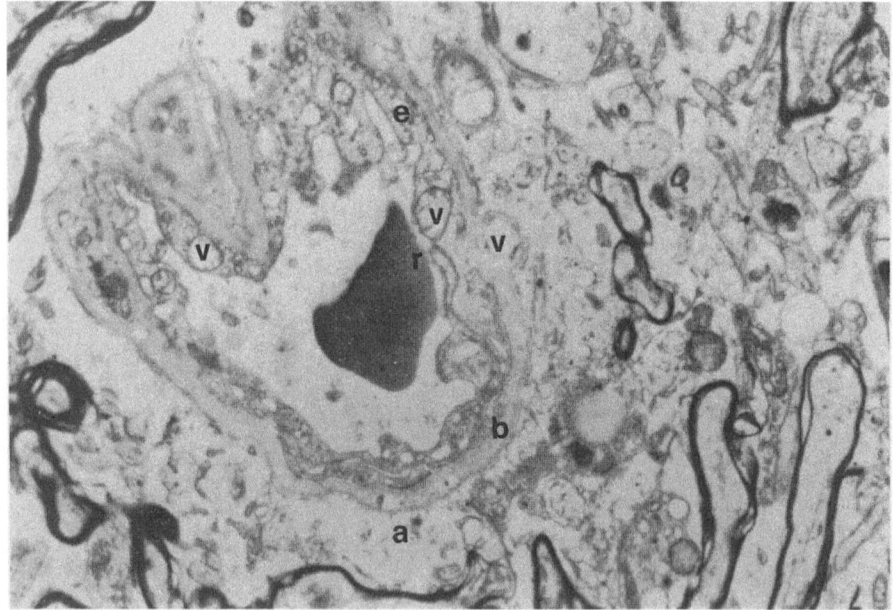

Fig. 4. Transmission electron micrograph of a cerebral capillary after Nd:YAG laser irradiation at 40 watts for 3 seconds. (*b* basement membrane; *e* endothelial cell; *a* astrocyte pedicle; *r* red blood cell; *v* vesicle)

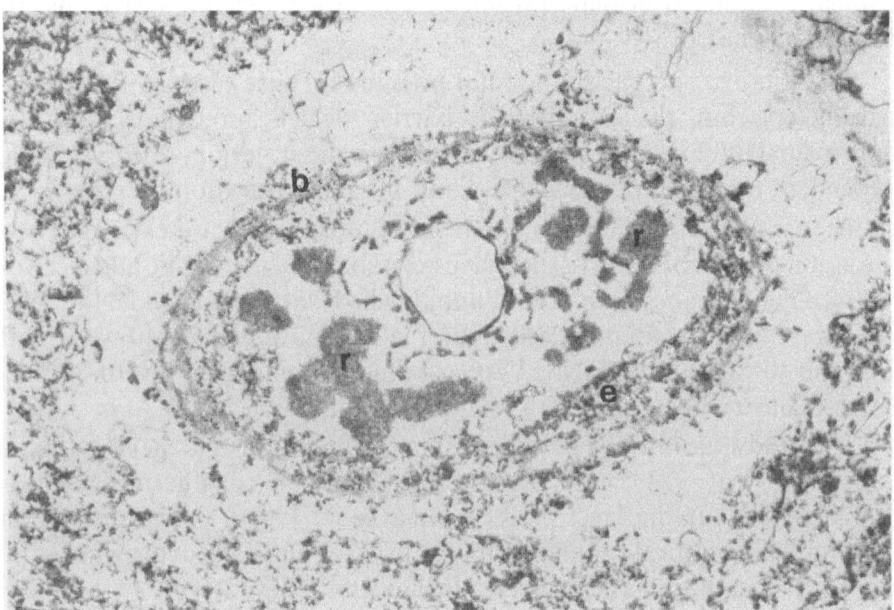

Fig. 5. Transmission electron micrograph of a cerebral capillary after Nd:YAG laser irradiation at 40 watts for 10 seconds. (*b* basement membrane; *e* endothelial cell; *r* red blood cell)

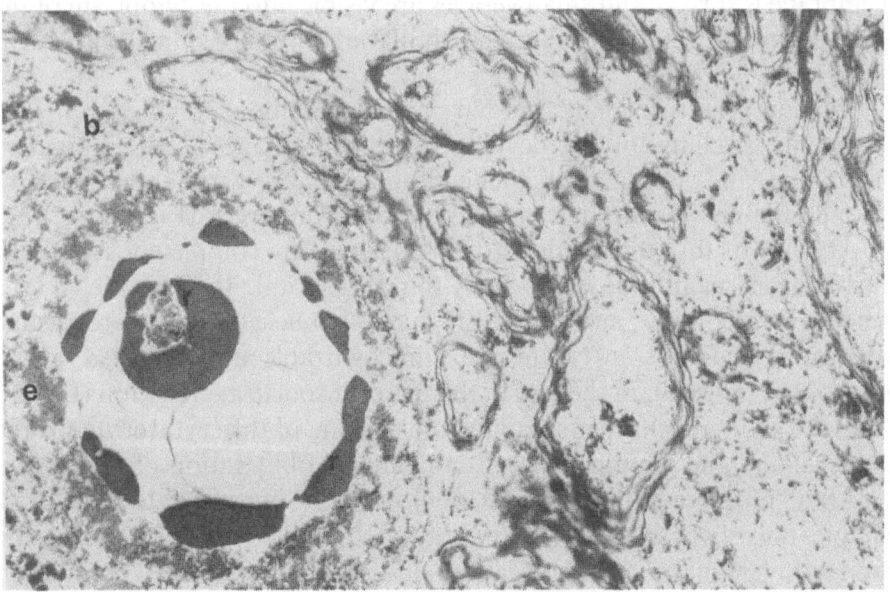

Fig. 6. Transmission electron micrograph of a cerebral capillary after Nd:YAG laser irradiation at 40 watts for 10 seconds (*b* basement membrane; *e* endothelial cell; *r* red blood cell)

capillaries and arteriolar thrombus formation which surrounds the coagulative necrosis.

Quantitative comparison are not possible because of the differences in parameters, but the blood-brain barrier defect appears to exist for approximately 1 to 2 mm surrounding the laser lesion, the size being dependent upon the power density and the pulse duration.

The acute vascular and tissue changes occurring in the outer periphery of the lesion in normal brain tissues have been studied under optic and electron microscope (Fasano *et al*. 1984, unpublished data). CO_2 and Nd:YAG laser were used; irradiation was delivered at a power of 20–40 watts with CO_2 and 40–80 watts with Nd:YAG for times ranging from 3 to 10 seconds; beam diameter was 2 mm with CO_2 and 2.5 mm with Nd:YAG.

The study has been focused on microcirculation and nervous tissue constituents at 1–1.5 mm outside the area of coagulative necrosis, approximately at the level of the edema zone. Fig. 1 shows the normal structure of a cerebral capillary with the perivascular astrocyte pedicles, the basement membrane and the endothelial cells.

CO_2 laser beam produces very limited vessel lesions. At a power of 20–40 watts for 3 seconds slight swelling of astrocyte pedicles and small vesicles into the basement membrane are detectable (Fig. 2).

At a power of 20 watts for 10 seconds the astrocyte pedicles show membrane fragmentation and rupture of the tight junctions; the basement membrane is shrunk and small vesicles are visible into the cytoplasm of the endothelial cells. The patency of the capillaries is preserved in all specimens (Fig. 3).

Damage is more evident after Nd:YAG irradiation. At 40–80 watts for 3 seconds swelling of astrocyte pedicles, shrinkage of the basement membrane and swelling of the endothelial cells with appearance of cytoplasmic vesicles are detectable; patency is preserved (Fig. 4).

At 40 watts for 10 seconds astrocyte pedicles are completely destroyed, the basement membrane is extremely thin and shrunk; the endothelial cells become exceedingly swelled with marked nuclear and cytoplasmic alterations and most of them are unrecognizable and replaced by an amorphous material; in the lumen there is erithrocyte aggregation (Fig. 5).

Fig. 6 shows in another specimen the sticking of the erythrocytes to the endothelium, and in Fig. 7 there is a complete obliteration of the lumen.

After short irradiation time the nervous tissue constituents show in all samples only slight damage. At 20 watts for 10 seconds CO_2 laser irradiation produces cytoplasmic vacuolization and dilatation of the perinuclear cystern; cells are well recognizable (Fig. 8). After Nd:YAG irradiation at power of 40 watts for 10 seconds the cells are no longer recognizable; cellular fragments, granules of pigment, degenerated myelinic sheaths and axons are detectable (Fig. 9).

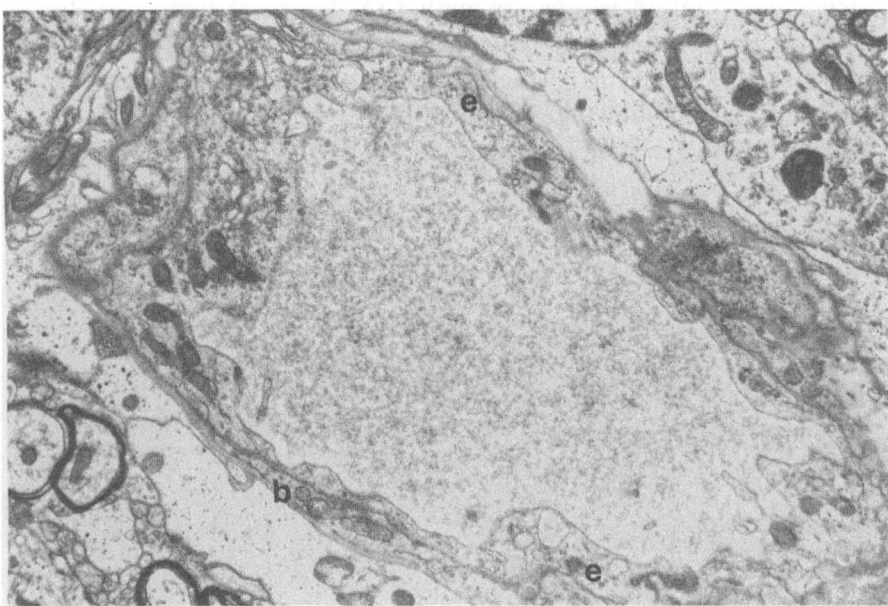

Fig. 7. Transmission electron micrograph of a cerebral capillary after Nd:YAG laser irradiation at 40 watts for 10 seconds. (*b* basement membrane; *e* endothelial cell)

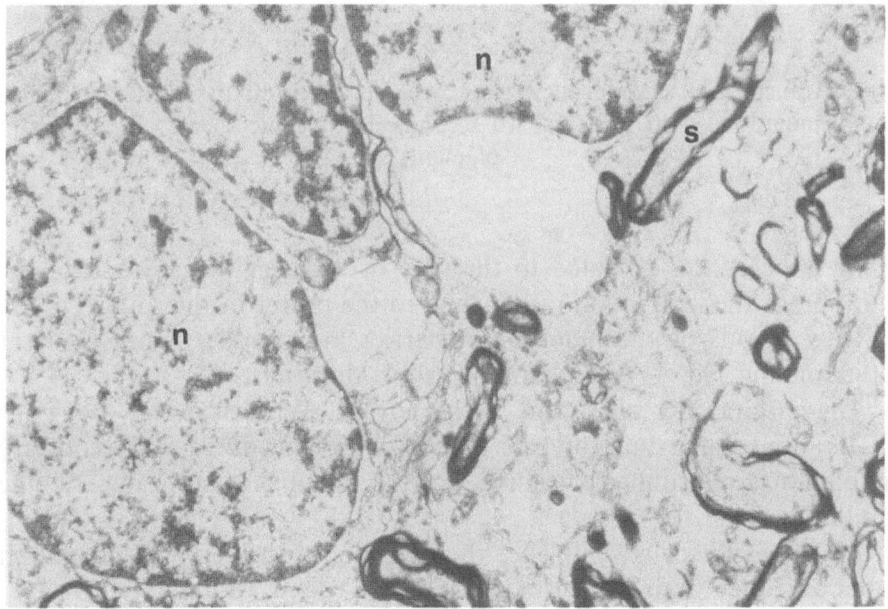

Fig. 8. Transmission electron micrograph of cerebral nervous tissue after CO_2 laser irradiation at 20 watts for 10 seconds. (*n* nucleus; *s* myelinic sheats)

V. A. Fasano:

High peak pulsed irradiation with CO_2 laser produces very limited lesions on both vessels and tissue. Capillaries show a slight swelling of astrocyte pedicles and small vesicles into the basement membrane (Fig. 10). Tissue is preserved showing only cytoplasmic vacuolization.

According to Beck's results the damage of the outer periphery of the

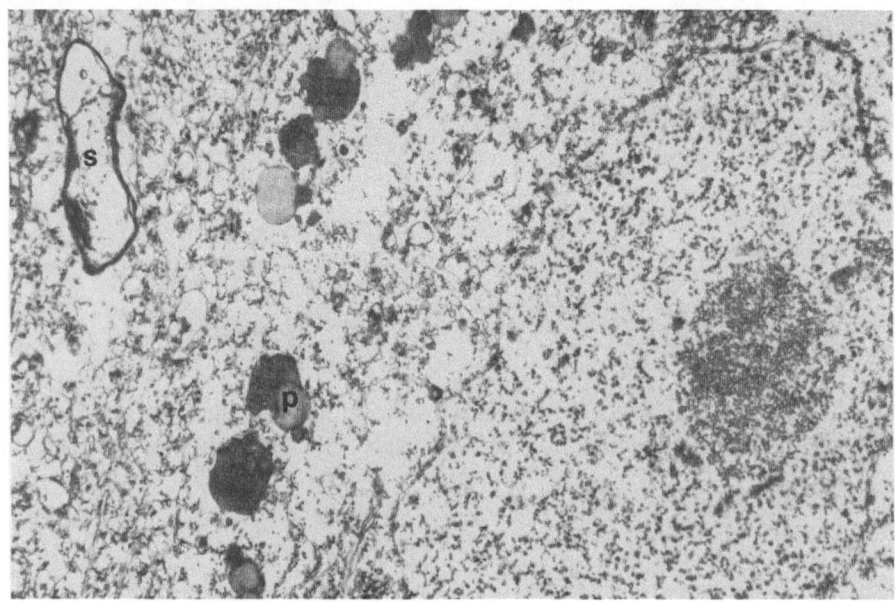

Fig. 9. Transmission electron micrograph of cerebral nervous tissue after Nd : YAG laser irradiation at 40 watts for 10 seconds. (*s* myelinic sheats; *p* granules of pigment)

lesion appears to be related to the type of wavelength used and to the duration of the irradiation rather than to the power of the source.

Only lesions of the blood-brain barrier are produced by CO_2 laser radiation and Nd : YAG radiation of short duration.

These data are consistent with Toya's, Wharen's and Boggan's observations. Long duration Nd : YAG radiation produces on the contrary endoluminal phenomena leading to the complete occlusion of the capillaries.

All these effects can influence the dynamic of the cerebral circulation with consequent impairment of the ICP and edema formation.

The intracranial dynamics after experimental CO_2 laser brain lesions in a rabbit model were studied by James et al. [8]. In this study the behaviour of intracranial pressure (ICP), brain water content, brain edema movement and their response to dexamethasone and furosemide have been analyzed. After a laser impact with a CO_2 unit over the intact dura in a defocused mode with 40 watts for 0.5 seconds for a total of 4 seconds, ICP was increased at 2 hours and remained so at 24 hours. At 2 hours moreover increase in the water content of the surrounding gray matter was seen; it persisted after 6 and 24 hours. At 6 hours a significant increase of water

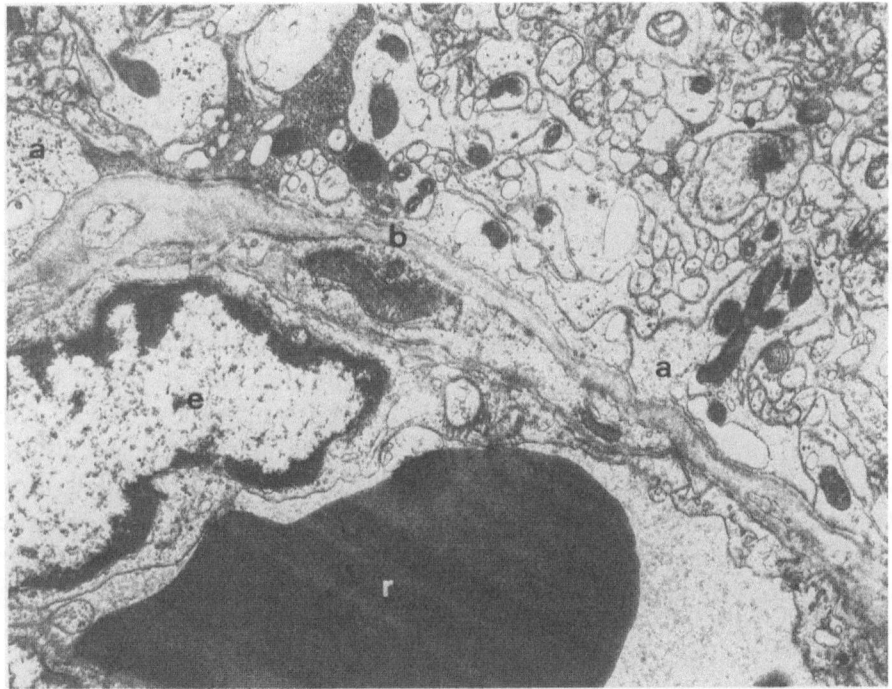

Fig. 10. Transmission electron micrograph of cerebral nervous tissue after high-peak-pulsed CO_2 laser irradiation. (*b* basement membrane: *e* endothelial cell; *a* astrocyte pedicle: *r* red blood cell)

content was seen in the white matter of the ipsilateral hemisphere and at 24 hours water content increased in both gray and white matter of the controlateral hemisphere. This would be explained by the progression of the edema front into the white matter. In the therapy groups a significant decrease of ICP and water content was noted after 24 hours following dexamethasone. No difference was noted in the furosemide subgroup.

Steroids are now felt to improve function after a brain insult primarily by improving metabolism more than by affecting brain edema, while diuretics act directly on the hemodynamics[6]. The lack of action of the furosemide on the brain edema may be due according the authors to the extensive breakdown of the blood-brain barrier which prevents diuretics from mobilizing brain water; infact this is contrary to what is noted in the rabbit edema model with an intact blood-barrier where furosemide reduces brain water significantly[8].

1.3. Morphologic Characteristics of the Chronic Laser Lesion

Chronic lesions are always slightly larger than acute lesions this being even more so at higher incident powers[11].

After 10 days a separation into different zones continues to be distinguishable at the lesion area[1].

The coagulated material remains largerly inert and is surrounded by a border of glial cells and macrophages as well as by abundant vessel proliferation. In the transitional area between the reaction zone and the coagulated material fat granule cells accumulate in varying quantities. The cellular border corresponds to the original edema zone. With the CO_2 laser the reaction zone is distinctly less pronounced and the quantity of coagulated material that cannot be removed initially is likewise smaller. By 1 week there is proliferation of the adjacent meningeal cells (presumably fibroblasts); thin walled channels just deep to the meninges are noted at the margins of the lesion[2]. By 2 weeks, there is significant tissue removal. The meningeal proliferation extends further from the margins of the lesion. Some wallerian degeneration is seen in the white matter deep to the lesion. By 1 month a center of coagulation necrosis is still evident. Much of the adjacent tissue, including the originally necrotic and edematous area, has been replaced by very thin-walled vascular channels that fill much of the collapsed wedge-shaped lesions. There is mild fibrillary gliosis.

1.4. Histochemical Data

To evaluate the physiochemical interaction of laser and neural tissue Burke et al. [3] have employed a technique for catecholamine histofluorescence. The Nd:YAG and CO_2 lesions of identical power densities and radiant exposure were compared in acute and chronic (1 month) preparations.

While the effect of Nd:YAG and CO_2 on rat cerebral tissue are essentially the same, except for the difference in shape and size of the lesions, there are subtle differences between the lasers with respect to the acute response of the catecholamine terminal. In the Nd:YAG lesions, the central coagulation is surrounded by a homogeneous granular zone, devoid of catecholamine terminals, though still appearing viable by hematossilina and eosina stain. Catecholamine fibers abruptly end at the lateral margins of this granular zone, extending the physiologic size of the lesion. By contrast in the CO_2 lesions catecholamine terminals directly abut the central coagulum, and some terminals actually extend within the lesion itself.

After 3 days, dramatic changes in the catecholamine fiber patterns occur in Nd:YAG lesion. The catecholamine terminals now extend directly to the margins of the lesion, where there is no evidence of a granular zone. The chronic preparations continue to show catecholamine fibers up to, and at times extending into the lesion. Thus, the lesion produced by Nd:YAG laser and visualized by light microscope is misleading in terms of size.

2. Nerves

Holzer and Ascher[7] compared cut surfaces severed with focused CO_2 laser and with conventional instruments in 4 sciatic nerves of rabbits. Histological examination revealed that the nerve severed with laser had a smooth cut surface, without damage to endo and perineurium. Conventional cutting with microscissors produces a definite splitting of nerve fibers and damage to endo- and perineurium.

Similar results are reported by Clark et al.[4] in a study on sciatic nerves of rats. Examination of the proximal stumps revealed undamaged myelin and a normal appearance at both 2 and 4 mm proximal to the site of sectioning in nerves severed with CO_2 laser. Myelin changes, consisting mainly in thinning without axonal changes and in a moderate degree of Schwann cell proliferation, occur in nerves sectioned with cutting cautery. Both axonal and myelin degeneration were seen in scalpel sectioning of the nerves. Contrary to the nerves severed with scalpel no sprouting was seen in those nerves sectioned with thermal energy.

Long-term studies on the healing process in nerves cut with conventional instruments and laser were performed by Holzer in sciatic nerves of rabbits severed with both techniques and then sutured[7]. Histological examination after 4 months revealed normal growth of the proximal nerve stump in those nerves severed by scissors and in some cases local neuromas were observed. Analogous growth could not be observed in nerves severed by laser while proximal nerve endings were in a state of degeneration, showing therefore a failure to regenerate.

There are conflicting reports of experimental work on animals involving regeneration of nerves after cutting with laser. There are species differences and regeneration in some lower animals may occur[5].

The effectiveness of laser sectioning in comparison with knife sectioning in the prevention of peripheral nerve regeneration is therefore uncertain.

References

1. Beck, O. J., Wilske, J., Sconberger, J. L., Gorisch, W., 1979: Tissue changes following application of lasers to the rabbit brain. Results with CO_2 and neodymium-YAG laser. Neurosurg. Rev. *1*, 31–36.

2. Boggan, J. E., Edwards, M. S. B., Davis, R. L., Bolger, C. A., Martin, N., 1982: Comparison of the brain tissue response in rats injury by Argon and Carbon dioxide lasers. Neurosurg. *11*, 609–616.
3. Burke, L. P., Rovin, R. A., Cerullo, L. J., Brown, J. T., Petronio, J., 1983: Nd : YAG laser in neurosurgery. In: Neodymium-YAG Laser in Medicine and Surgery (Joffe, S. N., ed.), pp. 141–148. New York-Amsterdam-Oxford: Elsevier.
4. Clark, W. G., Robertson, J. H., Whetsell, W. O., Jr., Rui, J. E., 1983: Comparative observations on effects of carbon dioxide laser induced peripheral nerve lesions in the rats. Surg. Neurol. *19*, 144–149.
5. Day, A., 1982: Effects of CO_2 laser on peripheral nerve regeneration. In: Proceedings of the II Congress on the Laser Neurosurgery, p. 173. Chicago.
6. Harbaugh, R. D., James, H. E., Marshall, L. F., Shapiro, H. M., Laurin, R., 1979: Acute therapeutic modalities for experimental vasogenic edema. Neurosurg. *5*, 656–665.
7. Holzer, P., Ascher, P. W., 1979: Laser surgery of peripheral nerves. In: Laser Surgery III, part one (Kaplan, I., ed.), pp. 149–153. Tel-Aviv: OT-PAZ.
8. James, H. E., Bruce, D. A., Welsh, F., 1978: Citotoxic edema produced by 6-aminonicotinamide and its response to therapy. Neurosurg. *3*, 196–200.
9. James, H. E., Tiznado, E. G., Moore, S., 1984: Experimental high radiation energy Carbon dioxide lesions on the brain: effect on intracranial pressure, EEG, blood-brain barrier and brain water content. Paper presented at the first Congress of LANSI (Laser Association Neurosurgical International). Salzburg, September 27–30, 1984.
10. Toya, S., Kawase, T., Iisaka, Y., Iwata, T., Aki, T., Nakamura, T., 1980: Acute effect of the carbon dioxide laser on the epicerebral microcirculation. Experimental study by fluorescein angiography. J. Neurosurg. *53*, 193–197.
11. Wharen, R. E., Jr., Anderson, R. E., Scheithauer, B., Sundt, T. M., Jr., 1984: The Nd : YAG laser in neurosurgery. Part 1: Laboratory investigations. Dose-related biological response of neural tissue. J. Neurosurg. *60*, 531–539.

Laser Effect on Normal Vessels (CO_2-Nd:YAG-Argon). Histological Data

VICTOR A. FASANO

Institute of Neurosurgery, University of Turin (Italy)

Contents

1. Small Vessels 85
   1.1. CO_2 Laser 85
   1.2. Argon Laser 85
   1.3. Nd:YAG Laser 86
2. Large Vessels 88
   2.1. Acute Changes 89
   2.2. Chronic Changes 91
References 92

1. Small Vessels

1.1. CO_2 Laser

Vessel closure is due to instantaneous vessel shrinkage by thermal collagen contraction and fusion as supported by gross observation and histological examination, blood elements are not damaged and only few cells of the adventitia at the site of impact are shaved off[8].

Schonberger and Beck[8] studied the ability of the CO_2 laser to coagulate blood vessels of different sizes selectively. Optimal coagulation effect on arteries up to 0.8 mm and veins up to 1.2 mm was achieved at a radiation of 25 watts/cm^2; increasing power density there was enhanced risk of vessel perforation.

1.2. Argon Laser

Coagulation experiments with argon laser focused on small blood vessels showed that thrombotic closure of the vessel lumen can be achieved[2, 7]. The basic effects are adherence of coagulated erythrocyte aggregations to the vessel wall and subsequent thrombi formation.

Boergen et al. [2] have studied the effects of the argon laser irradiation on normal small vessels at undisturbed blood flow and reduced flow rates. Vessels up to 0.1–0.25 mm irradiated with a single exposure at low energy (less than 5 mJ) showed at histological examination adhesion to endothelium of clumped and severely damaged erythrocytes, associated to a moderately intense platelet aggregation; endothelium had been only slightly damaged. Occlusion of vessel lumen was not produced in any case. With undisturbed flow, higher energies (more than 10 mJ) must be applied to produce endovascular phenomena. In these cases, short term thrombosis by pronounced platelet aggregation, associated with a lesion of the endothelium and disruption of the internal elastic lamina, can be achieved. Fibrin formation could not be detected.

Longer lasting occlusions were achieved by multiple applications (the first exposure of about 10 mJ, produces a transient occlusion while the second irradiation at lower energy of about 5 mJ, increases the extension of the endoluminal clot). Fibrin formation was observed at electron microscope.

Thermally damaged erythrocytes seem to have the decisive role in the rapid endovascular thrombogenesis while endothelium-free internal elastic lamina and exposed collagen fibers are of less importance. Also blood flow velocity seems to be important. Infact vessel closure was observed only in experiments at undisturbed flow and this is in accordance with the direct relationship existing between rate of thrombocyte aggregation and blood flow velocity[1]. Fibrin formation leads to an additional stabilization of the endovascular thrombus.

On this basis selective vessel obstruction with minimal damage to surrounding tissues may be achieved through multiple exposure with focused argon laser beam at low energy.

Leheta and Gorisch demonstrated that only arteries up to 0.5 mm can be occluded; veins up to 1 mm are easily coagulated[6].

1.3. Nd: YAG Laser

The Nd: YAG laser can produce instantaneous occlusion of arteries up to 1 mm and veins up to 5 mm[6]; it has been reported in literature that closure takes place by continuous narrowing of the vessel walls till complete obliteration and that shrinkage augments other vessel sealing effects such as intravascular thrombosis[4].

Vessel shrinkage is dependent on thermal tightening of circumferencially arranged collagen fibers bundles. This explanation is confirmed by Ewald's and Gorisch's studies.

Ewald[3] demonstrated that purified collagen fibers of the rat tail tendon show the ability to shrink to about a tenth of their original length when held at a temperature of 65 °C over a period of 20 seconds.

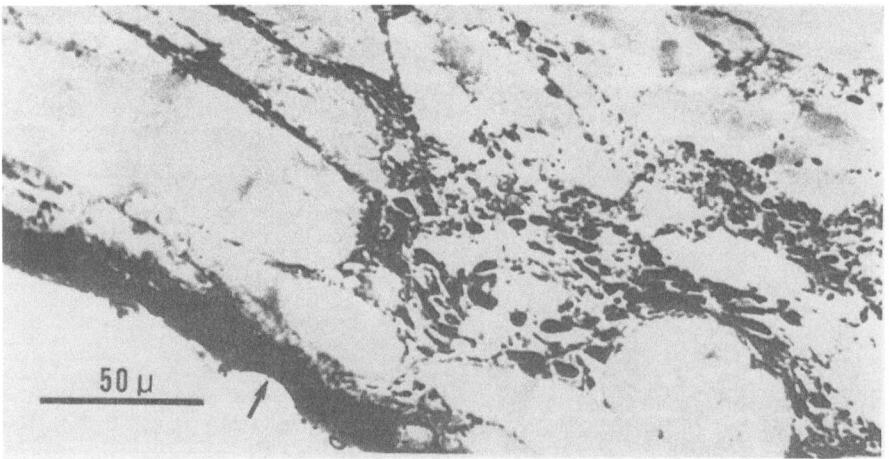

Fig. 1. Rabbit carotid irradiated with Nd:YAG laser. Arrow indicates a superficial dense adventitial layer. Numerous altered cells are detectable

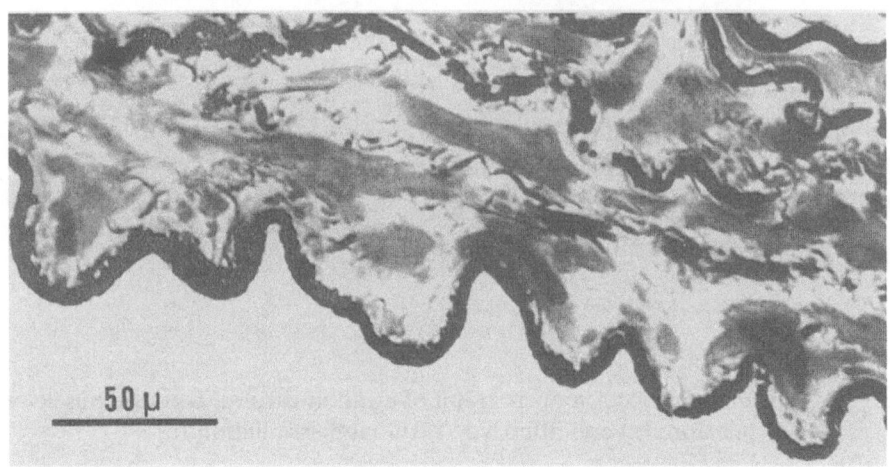

Fig. 2. Rabbit carotid irradiated with CO$_2$ laser: a tract of the intima without endothelial cells

Gorisch[5] evaluated in mesenteric vessels the change in diameter occurring after irrigation of the vessel with saline solution heated to preselected temperature (between 40 and 90°C). During irrigation both veins and arteries shrank at high temperature. Vein diameter decreased to approximately 20% of the original value in cases where temperatures above 70°C were applied. Most of the collapsed veins slightly dilated during the following 8 minutes. In contrast, heating over 75°C was required for arteries to constrict. The amount of shrinkage did not exceed that of veins. The narrowed arterial lumen relaxed considerably after heating in most cases.

V. A. Fasano:

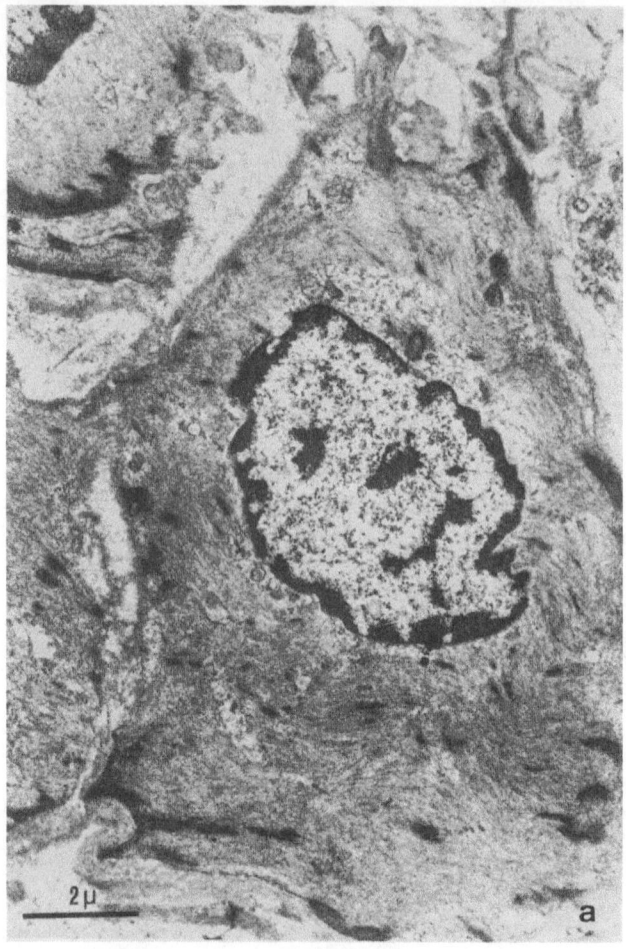

Fig. 3. Transmission electron micrograph of a rabbit carotid. Smooth muscle cell
before (a) and after Nd : YAG laser irradiation (b)

2. Large Vessels

The effects of laser irradiation on vessels up to 3 mm (rabbit carotid
arteries) have been studied after CO_2 argon and Nd : YAG under optic and
electron microscope (Fasano *et al.* 1983 unpublished data). Power, spot and
exposure time were chosen in preliminary experience to avoid the
perforation or carbonization of the vessels. The following parameters were
used: CO_2 laser: 40 watts for 2–3 seconds, spot size five times the vessel
diameter; argon laser: 5 watts for 10 seconds, spot size three times the vessel
diameter; Nd : YAG laser: 60 watts for 2 seconds, spot size three times the
vessel diameter.

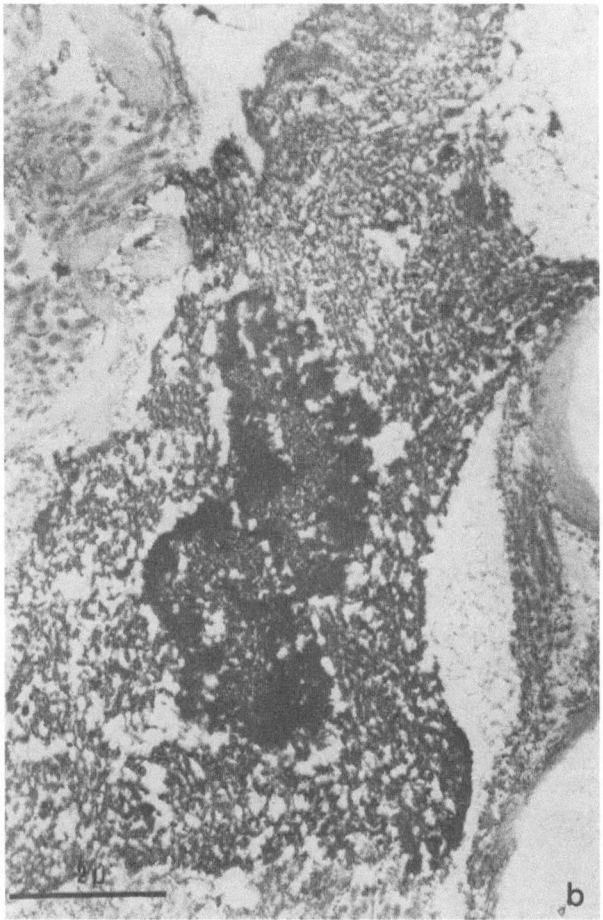

Fig. 3 b

2.1. Acute Changes

Irradiation produced instantaneous vessel shrinkage of about 20% of the original diameter.

The optical study of areas irradiated with the three lasers have similar adventitial alterations: the architecture of the external layer of the adventitia is lost, appearing vacuolated (Fig. 1). The vasa vasorum are rarely detectable and if so, appear full of dense material probably of hematic origin; frequently destroyed cells are visible. The tunica media has no evident alterations. In CO_2 and argon lesions only a slight detachment of the endothelial cells in the target area occurs whereas in Nd:YAG lesions the endothelial cells of both the target and the opposite area are completely lost (Fig. 2); numerous little thrombi adhering to the elastic lamina are also seen.

The ultrastructural study shows evident alterations of the whole vessel

V. A. Fasano:

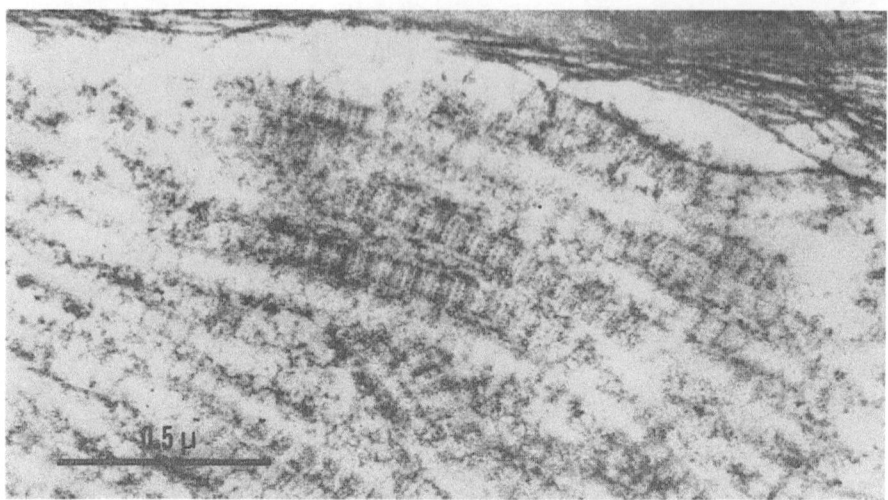

Fig. 4. Transmission electron micrograph of a rabbit carotid. Normal collagen
fibers

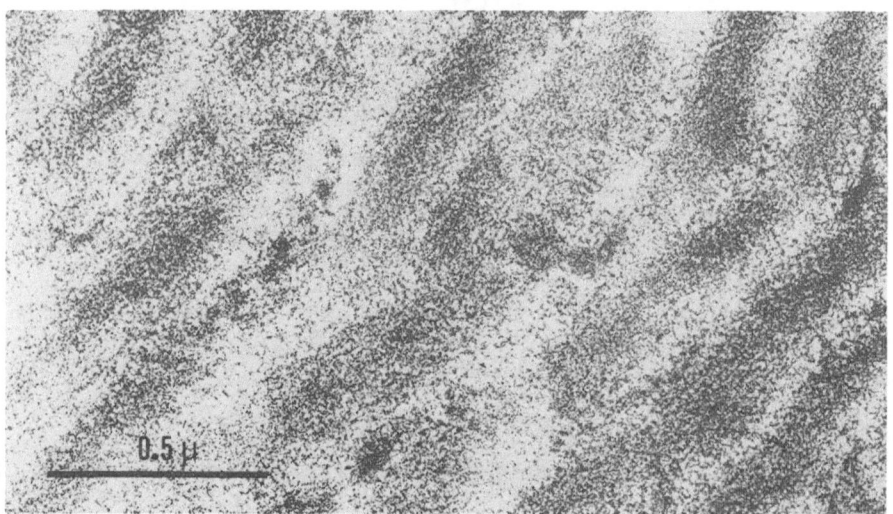

Fig. 5. Transmission electron micrograph of a rabbit carotid. Collagen fibers after
Nd : YAG laser irradiation

wall. In the external layer of the adventitia the cells are unrecognizable,
while in the internal ones and in the tunica media there is a disarrangement
of the cellular structures which are nevertheless still recognizable. The
cytoplasm appears dense and floccular, the nucleus has an irregular outline
and clumped chromatine, and the cytoplasmic organules are markedly
altered (Fig. 3). The collagen fibers are swollen with a diameter 3 or 4 times

normal and frequently fused. In the longitudinal sections, they show a complete disarrangement and their characteristic transversal periodicity is lost (Figs. 4 and 5). Minimal damage of the endothelial cells occurs after CO$_2$ and argon irradiation. Platelet aggregation is not detectable. Marked lesions are produced by Nd:YAG laser. In the target area endothelial cells are almost completely lost and when present damaged. Small thrombi close

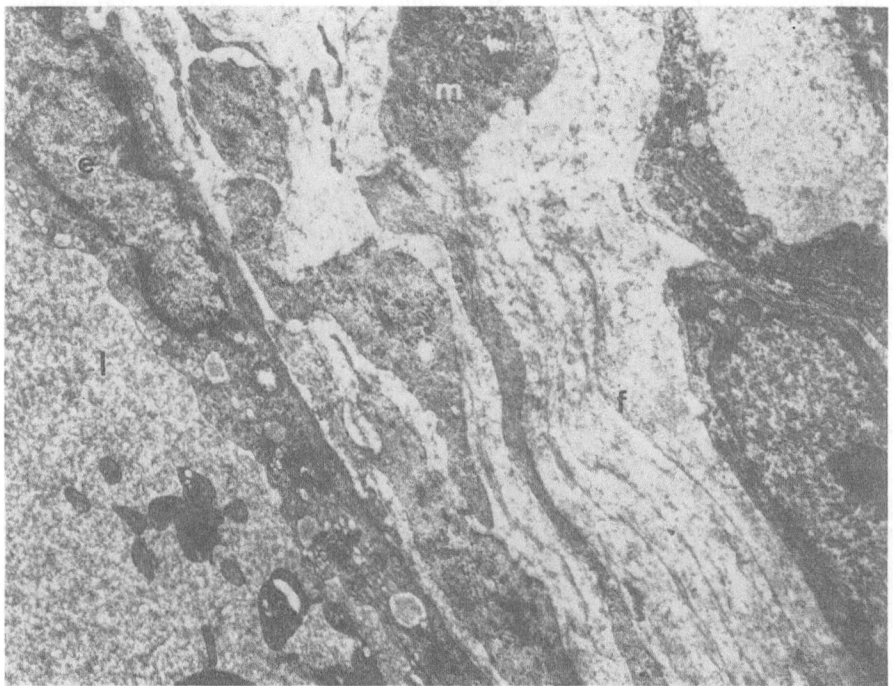

Fig. 6. Transmission electron micrograph of a rabbit carotid. Observations after 60 days. (*e* endothelium; *l* lumen; *m* muscolar cells; *f* collagen fibers)

to the damaged areas are frequently detectable. In all irradiated samples elastic fibers appear normal.

2.2. Chronic Changes

Gross observations at 10 days, 1 month and 2 months after irradiation show the persistence of the vessel narrowing in all arteries irradiated with CO$_2$ and argon lasers; vessel patency is preserved. After 10 days all arteries irradiated with Nd:YAG laser show complete endoluminal thrombosis.

60 days after irradiation with CO$_2$ and argon laser, irradiated areas were taken away for histological analysis. Macroscopic damage was not evident. Optic microscope showed an increse in width of the vessel walls mostly

concerning collagen components. Electron microscope did not show any endothelial lesion and there were no signs of thrombosis. Adventitia and media were preserved (Fig. 6).

References

1. Baumgartner, H. R., 1973: The role of blood flow in platelet adhesion, fibrin deposition, and formation of mural thrombi. Microvasc. Res. *5*, 167–179.
2. Boergen, K. P., Birngruber, R., Hillenkamp, F., 1981: Laser-induced endovascular thrombosis as a possibility of selective vessel closure. Ophthalmic Res. *13*, 139–156.
3. Ewald, A., 1918: Beiträge zur Kenntnis des Collagens I: Über die Quellung und Verkürzung der leimgebenden Fibrillen des Bindegewebes in heißem Wasser. Hoppe-Seyler's Z. Physiol. Chem. *104*, 115–134.
4. Gorisch, W., Boergen, K. P., McCord, R. C., Weinberg, W., Hillenkamp, F., 1978: Temperature measurements of isolated mesenteric blood vessels of the rabbit during laser irradiation. In: Laser Surgery III (Kaplan, I., ed.), pp. 202–207. Jerusalem: Jerusalem Academic Press.
5. Gorisch, W., Boergen, K. P., 1979: Thermal shrinkage of collagen fibres during vessel occlusion in laser surgery. In: Laser Surgery II, part two (Kaplan, I., ed.), pp. 123–127. Tel-Aviv: OT-PAZ.
6. Leheta, F., Gorisch, W., 1976: Coagulation of blood vessels by means of Argon ion and Nd: YAG laser radiation. In: Laser Surgery I (Kaplan, I., ed.), pp. 178–184. Jerusalem: Jerusalem Academic Press.
7. Lenz, H., Eichler, J., 1975: Wirkung des Argon-Lasers auf die Gefäße, Mikro- und Makrozirkulation der Schleimhaut der Hamsterbackentasche. Laryng. Rhinol. *54*, 612–619.
8. Schonberger, J. L., Beck, O. J., Gorisch, W., Bise, K., 1979: Selective blood vessel coagulation with carbon dioxide laser at various irradiance. In: Laser Surgery III, part one (Kaplan, I., ed.), pp. 9–11. Tel-Aviv: OT-PAZ.

Laser. A Progress of the Traditional Surgical Procedure

VICTOR A. FASANO

Institute of Neurosurgery, University of Turin (Italy)

Contents

1. Histological Studies.. 93
2. Functional Studies 94
References 95

The use of lasers on nervous structures and activity have been compared with the use of traditional surgical instruments in many works.

1. Histological Studies

The morphologic characteristics of the lesion and the extension of the coagulative necrosis have been compared after laser irradiation and the use of electrosurgery by Keiditsch et al. [3]. Lesions were equally extended when the two methods were compared in homogeneous tissues (liver): a sharp demarcation of the surrounding structures was observed.

In heterogeneous tissues (urinary bladder wall) electrocoagulation produced necrosis with irregular margins whose extension increased at higher powers. Laser irradiation produced a demarcated lesion the extension of which remained invaried at different powers. The irregular spread of necrosis in heterogeneous tissues is due to the tendency of the high frequency currents to follow the paths of least resistance, such as across the tissue surface and along the larger vessels. However, electromagnetic energy is distributed equally and independently to tissue structure thus producing sharp lesions with predictable and controllable penetration depth and extension.

The changes produced by CO_2 laser irradiation and electrocoagulation have been studied in brain under optic and electron microscope by Takizawa [7].

The lesion produced by CO_2 laser at 15–25 watts with spot of 0.5 mm and pulsed wave of 1 second on the surface of the brain or spinal cord consisted of a charred layer 10–20 microns thick, a honeycomb structure layer about 20–30 microns wide, a layer of edema 250–300 microns thick.

The lesion produced by monopolar electrocoagulation was considerably larger. The diameter on the cortical surface measured 4.5 mm. The width of the necrosis and the edema zone was twice as large as that produced by laser. In comparison with monopolar coagulation the lesion produced by bipolar coagulation was much smaller than expected. The diameter was confined to the distance between the two ledges of the bipolar electrodes. Contrary to laser the depth of the necrosis increased proportionately to the output power and the duration of the current while, as for the laser, the edema thickness remained the same.

The temperature measurement 1 mm from the focus of the CO_2 laser showed that the maximum increase was about 10 °C. Temperature reached peak value in 2 seconds but it tooked about 30 seconds to drop down to the previous level. In bipolar coagulation the temperature rise was 2.5 °C at 3 mm from the electrode and the change lasted for 23 seconds. In monopolar coagulation the rise was about 18 °C at 3 mm from the electrode and the change lasted for 23 seconds.

Cozzens[2] compared conventional techniques of cutting and coagulating neural tissue with CO_2 laser. The Evans blue model was used to document and quantify the extent of blood-brain barrier disruption by thermal trauma. It was found that there was statistically significantly less staining of the brain in laser lesions than bipolar lesions.

The cerebral edema occurring after laser vaporization was quantitatively evaluated by Saunders et al. [6]. Bifrontal craniectomies were performed in cats and a laser lesion was formed on one side by vaporizing approximately 125 mm² of the hemisphere with 35 watts, continuously, at a beam diameter of 0.77 mm. A scalpel lesion was placed in the controlateral hemisphere by inserting a no. 11 blade perpendicular to the surface, then coagulating the pial margins with bipolar electrocautery. Animals were sacrified at 24–48 hours. The white and gray matter at the margin of the lesion as well as from the occipital cortex (for control) was studied to determine the percentage of water per gram of tissue using the density gradient technique. The edema associated with laser-induced lesions was consistently lower than that with steel-induced lesions at all sampling times in both gray and white matter.

Cozzens and Cerullo[1] report similar results in a comparative study between CO_2 laser and bipolar cerebrotomy showing that edema of the surrounding tissues is significantly reduced when using laser.

2. Functional Studies

Saunders et al. [6] wished to determine whether the CO_2 laser was capable of vaporizing specific neural structures precisely without functionally impairing or morphologically altering adjacent tissue; authors used somatosensory evoked potentials as functional test, the elaboration of this response requiring functional integrity of a certain neural population within the spinal dorsal column. By vaporizing tissue in the cat cervical spinal cord in the dorsolateral funiculus contiguous with the dorsal column the authors could assess the quantitative effect of known radiant exposure upon the ipsilateral sensory evoked potentials. Single or multiple lesions of radiant exposure from 287 to 43,750 joules/cm^2 could be placed contiguous to the dorsal column without permanent impairment of that response. Olson et al. [5] studied if specific changes might occur into activity of nerve roots and specific cranial nerves as result of close proximity laser irradiation using evoked potential monitoring. When utilizing laser vaporization in course of laminectomy in and around specific nerve roots, the evoked latency increased during irradiation but returned to pre-laser state within a period of 2 to 10 minutes. Similar results were noticed when operating around optic nerves (monitoring of visual evoked response) or in the course of spinal and cranial surgery (monitoring of somatosensory evoked response). When using adequate protective mechanisms such as cloth, paddies etc. no appreciable neuroeffect was noted as recorded by evoked potential.

Lanner et al. [4] undertook investigations on whether the patho-morphological changes brought about by the CO_2 laser and by the diathermy needle are reflected in the functional bioelectric activity of the brain. In 13 patients with cerebral tumors cortical activity was recorded before, during and after incision with the CO_2 laser and diathermy needle. Following incision with diathermy needle several patients showed a flattening of the amplitude of cortical activity as well as the appearance of slow frequencies of theta and delta wave type as an indication of the spread of collateral edema. These changes could be detected using laser in 3 cases only confirming that edema can be kept under control with the use of laser beam.

The effects on the different laser wavelengths on electrocorticographic pattern have been studied during tumor resection (Urciuoli et al. 1981)[8]. Voltage reduction of electrical brain activity appeared more frequently when using CO_2 laser in combination with Nd : YAG laser than with CO_2 laser alone. The cases treated with an argon laser did not show any modifications in the peritumoral cortical pattern.

In the surgical experience, ECG monitoring during surgical procedures near the brainstem did not reveal modifications of the cardiac activity in any case when using laser.

References

1. Cozzens, J., Cerullo, L. J., 1981: Comparison of CO_2 laser and bipolar cerebrotomy: measurement of brain edema. In: Laser Tokyo 81 (Atsumi, K., Nimsakul. N., eds.), (4) 25. Tokyo: Inter Group Corp.

2. Cozzens, J., 1981: Evans blue brain edema model for comparison of CO_2 and bipolar lesions. In: Proceedings of the First American Congress on Laser Neurosurgery, pp. 49–50. Chicago.
3. Keiditsch, E., Maiwald, H., Hofstetter, A., Rothenberger, K., Pensel, J., Frank, F., 1979: Comparison of the effects of the Nd-YAG laser and electrocoagulation in experimental animal research. In: Laser Surgery III, part two (Kaplan, I., ed.), pp. 181–194. Tel-Aviv: OT-PAZ.
4. Lanner, G., Heppner, F., Ascher, P. W., 1979: Cortical activity—is there some biochemical interference with the CO_2 laser? In: Laser Surgery III, part one (Kaplan, I., ed.), pp. 156–157. Tel-Aviv: OT-PAZ.
5. Olson, D. R., Warpinski, M., Hammargren, L. L., Lewin, R., 1982: Intraoperative evoked potential monitoring during laser surgery. In: Proceedings of the II Congress on Laser Neurosurgery, pp. 195–196. Chicago.
6. Saunders, M. L., Young, H. F., Becker, D. P., Greenberg, R. P., Newlon, P. G., Corales, R. L., Ham, W. T., Povlishock, J. T., 1980: The use of the laser in neurological surgery. Surg. Neurol. *14*, 1–11.
7. Takizawa, T., 1977: Comparison between the laser surgical unit and the electrosurgical unit. Neurol. Med. Chir. *17*, 95–105.
8. Urciuoli, R., Bergamasco, B., Benna, P., Lo Russo, G., 1981: ECoG Changes during cerebral tumor laser surgery. In: Laser Tokyo 81 (Atsumi, K., Nimsakul, N., eds.), (4), pp. 16–19. Tokyo: Inter Group Corp.

Principles of Laser Surgery

VICTOR A. FASANO

Institute of Neurosurgery, University of Turin (Italy)

Contents

1. General Considerations.. 97
2. Cutting 98
3. Vaporization and Tissue Removal... 98
4. Hemostasis 99
5. Tissue Welding... 100
6. Laser Microscope Coupling.. 101
References... 101

1. General Considerations

Lasers have provided the means to operate on tissue without mechanical contact thus reducing the manipulation of the surrounding healthy structures and the need for tissue retraction. The operative field is under constant vision without obstruction by solid instruments which are used much less in laser surgery. Hemostasis is improved and laser permits surgery in coagulopathies.

The main advantage of the laser consists however in the possibility to produce very limited lesions whose extension and depth are predictable with a fair degree of accuracy. This is in contrast to the use of mechanical and electrical instruments and arises from the tissue absorption characteristics for the different wavelengths. It has been reported that the volume of the lesion can be increased by thermal spreading which is related to the amount of energy delivered and more precisely to the time of irradiation; tissue damage instead can be markedly reduced by using very short exposure time[2, 3, 11].

Atsumi et al.[1] have studied the advantages of high peak pulsed irradiation and report that with super pulsed mode similar lesions can be attained at energies ranging from a half to a third of those delivered with continuous wave irradiation; side effects are minimal and carbonization is not produced because the thermal effect on the surrounding area is slight.

On these bases therefore high power density and long irradiation time can be used to produce larger lesions; this maneuvre is suitable for tumor resection when operating at distance from the healthy tissues. High power output and short irradiation time limit however the damage on the surrounding structures and must be used to obtain a sharp cutting or a more selective dissection. Short intermittent pulses at low power, focused upon blood vessels, must be used to produce a safe coagulation within brain tissue.

2. Cutting

CO_2 laser is the ideal cutting tool because it produces less damage to surrounding tissues than cautery and scalpel. To achieve a sharp cutting power density should be 1,000 watts/cm² or higher and the beam should be focused to the smallest spot possible. In this way tissue water is instantaneously converted to steam with explosive distruption expansion along the incision line. Depth can be controlled by varying time or power and at a given power density the slower the beam is moved the deeper the incision will be. For example CO_2 laser at 25 watts and spot of 0.6 mm produces an incision depth of 3.5 mm with a fissure width of a few tenths of mm when moved at a speed of 1.5 mm/s.

Because of the high scattering argon and Nd:YAG lasers are not suitable for cutting as CO_2, producing very wide faintly wedgeshaped incisions.

3. Vaporization and Tissue Removal

At power density inadeguate to produce boiling of the fluids, tissue temperature rises rather slowly and fluids vaporize gradually, drying and shrinking the tissue.

Vaporization is typical of the laser. It can be achieved with any of the three wavelengths used but, because of the lower absorption in water it is a tremendous waste of energy to vaporize a mass with argon and Nd:YAG as compared with the CO_2 laser. After evaporation of the tissue fluids CO_2 laser dehydrates the nonwater tissue constituents with smoke and gas generation leading to tissue ablation. In contrast with the cautery loop removal is achieved by means of successive exfoliation from the outside in wards thus enabling to keep accurate control of the successive planes and adjacent structures. Because of the limited penetration (few thents of mm) removal is very slow. At 25 watts it takes 2 minutes to vaporize 1 g of soft tissue; firm tumors require higher power (up to 80 watts) to be ablated. The beam must be swept across the area in orthogonal planes and the lines are kept mutually perpendicular. This is important in ablating tumors as small islands of unvaporized tissue in the middle may contain viable cells. Capillaries and lymphatic are sealed as tumor is evaporated and this may reduce the spilling of neoplastic cells into the circulation; the local spilling however is not eliminated. For example during ablation of medullo-blastomas some cells may fall into CSF pathways and seat elsewhere.

Contrary to CO_2 laser, most energy of the Nd : YAG is directly absorbed by nonwater tissue constituents, producing a complete coagulative necrosis and a fair hemostasis. A short pulse of 2–3 seconds at 40–50 watts achieves a necrosis depth of 3–4 mm[6]. By increasing the time of irradiation or the power density, temperature rises up to 100 °C and carbonization occurs with consequent enhanced surface absorption which prevents a further deepening of the lesion; lateral extension of the damage, however, enlarges because of the high thermal spreading. Greater lesions depths are therefore achieved by using separate pulses of 2–3 seconds with cooling periods of 20–30 seconds[6].

4. Hemostasis

Vessel closure takes place by shrinkage of the walls and sticking of endoluminal surface depending on vessel diameter, thickness of the wall and hemodynamic characteristics of flow. Only small arteries can be occluded since most of the energy is lost in overcoming the heat dissipation in blood flow and the intraluminal pressure distending the wall.

CO_2 laser seals off small blood vessels as it cuts, hemostasis, however, is ineffective in larger vessels and the focused beam can perforate the wall with consequent flooding of the operating field. Mechanical constriction by tissue edema and wall shrinkage are involved in vessel closure.

Argon laser, because of the high absorption in hemoglobin, can produce at low power density a selective coagulation mostly by endoluminal thrombosis.

Irradiation with Nd : YAG laser involves the whole wall producing shrinkage of the vessels and endoluminal processes. Coagulation is immediate in arteries up to 1–1.5 mm while, in arteries larger than 2 mm, a delayed occlusion occurs within a few days. Veins are easily coagulated with the different laser sources because of the thin wall and the low volume of flow inside. Blood vessels submerged in fluids can be coagulated by Nd : YAG and argon laser because of their poor absorption in water, thus enabling the hemostasis of intraventricular tumors.

Contrary to electrocoagulation laser does not produce any squeezing of the vessels and avoids mechanical damage of the walls; there are no effects of neurostimulation by leakage of electric currents. Bipolar coagulation is, however, still necessary because it enables obliteration of bleeding vessels and arteries larger than 3 mm, which cannot be otherwise coagulated. Presently, various disadvantages are avoided by the recent innovation in electrocoagulation[8, 10]. Bipolar coagulators provided either damped trains of sine or square waves, or simply repetitive pulses. The synchronizing of these pulses or waves increased undesiderable cutting or perforating of vessels being coagulated, as a result of molecular resonance. These effects are avoided by the Malis Bipolar Coagulator CMC I; spark-gap generators are used to produce coagulating aperiodic waveform which results in the elimination of molecular resonance. However, the initial spike of each damped train is always much higher in voltage than the rest of the train and this high voltage initial spike is responsible for the indesiderable sparking at the forceps tips, and monitoring equipment interference. In the Malis Bipolar Coagulator and Bipolar Cutter System CMC II the leading spike is proportional to the remainder of the damped asynchronous train resulting in marked reduction or sparking of the forceps and interference with other equipments. In addition the waveform parameters are specifically programmed for the smoothest coagulation, the least neuromuscolar stimulation and the least charring and sticking[8].

Similar advantages are offered by Computerized Bipolar Coagulators[10]. Laboratory tests proved that strong seals were achieved when the coagulation was interrupted soon after minimum impedance. Good seals were also achieved with later interruption of the heating but the well-known phenomena of sticking of the forceps to tissues and charging of the tips with charred tissue became more prominent. Based on these results, microcomputerized equipment was built which cutt off the coagulation soon after minimum impedance, i.e., when good strength without sticking was achieved.

The main advantage of the laser is however in the predictability of the lesion which permits a graduation of penetration and minimizes the damage of the surrounding tissues according to the energy delivered and the wavelength used. Both effects are of great importance in the treatment of the cerebral vascular malformations and when a selective hemostasis in high functional areas is required.

5. Tissue Welding

Heating of tissue produces physiochemical changes in the collagen fibers of the connective tissue at energy lower than for coagulative necrosis. This effect produces a gluing of tissue constituents and practical applications are in microvascular surgery for anastomizing blood vessels. By changing the morphological configuration of such elastic elements welding involves the elastic response of the vessel walls to strain. The problem will be discussed in the chapter on the treatment of the arterial aneurysms.

6. Laser Microscope Coupling

For microsurgical purposes the laser beam can be directed to a microscope attachment by a beam-manipulating arm (CO_2 laser) or fiberoptic system (argon and Nd : YAG lasers). Flexible delivery systems for CO_2 laser are in progress.

In our experience the main indications for the use of the laser associated to the operating microscope are:

a) The dissection of remaining mass from adjacent tissues in critical or high functional areas. The beam is inserted into the microscope and directed by joystick. Selectivity can be increased with the use of a microscan microprocessor controlling the application of the laser energy on tissue; the maneuvre is automatically performed by microprocessor memory consenting maximal delivers precision and uniformity of irradiation within selected boundries; automatic lasing can be terminated at any point by simply removing foot from footswitch consenting in this way a controlled layer by layer dissection by progressive exfoliation.

b) The coagulation of arterio-venous malformations and arterial aneurysms. In these cases defocused irradiation is required and therefore the laser is used freehand under direct control of the microscope.

c) The removal of some larger lesions in high functional areas when a greater accuracy is required; laser is used freehand under direct control of the microscope.

References

1. Atsumi, K., Nakajima, M., Ihara, A., Tsukagoshi, S., Inone, H., Toida, M., Sugiyama, S., Suenaga, N., 1981: Practical application of high peak powered CO_2 surgical laser unit. Laser Tokyo 81 (Atsumi, K., Nimsakul, N., eds.), (19), pp. 12–15. Tokyo: Inter Group Corp.
2. Beck, O. J., Wilske, J., Schonberger, J. L., Gorisch, W., 1979: Tissue changes following application of lasers to the rabbit brain. Results with CO_2 and Nd : YAG lasers. Neurosurg. Rev. *1*, 31–36.
3. Burke, L. P., Rovin, R. A., Cerullo, L. J., Brown, J. T., Petronio, J., 1983: Nd : YAG laser in neurosurgery. In: Neodymium-YAG Laser in Medicine and Surgery (Joffe, S. N., ed.), pp. 141–148. New York-Amsterdam-Oxford: Elsevier.
4. Fasano, V. A., 1983: Experiences on the use of various laser sources (CO_2-argon-Nd : YAG) in neurosurgery. In: New Frontiers in Laser Medicine and Surgery (Atsumi, K., ed.), pp. 188–195. Amsterdam-Oxford-Princeton: Excerpta Medica.
5. Gong-Bai, C., 1981: Laser vaporization on intracranial tumors. Lasers Surg. Med. *1*, 235–240.
6. Hofstetter, A., Frank, F., 1979: Der Neodym-YAG-Laser in der Urologie. Editiones Roche.

7. Leheta, F., Gorisch, W., 1976: Coagulation of blood vessels by means of argon ion and Nd : YAG laser radiation. In: Laser Surgery I (Kaplan, I., ed.), pp. 178–184. Jerusalem: Jerusalem Academic Press.

8. Malis, L. I., 1967: Bipolar coagulation in microsurgery. In: Microvascular Surgery (Donaghy, R. M. P., Yaşargil, M. G., eds.), p. 126. Stuttgart: G. Thieme.

9. Schonberger, J. L., Beck, O. J., Gorisch, W., Bise, K., 1979: Selective blood vessel coagulation with carbon dioxide laser at various irradiance. In: Laser Surgery III, part one (Kaplan, I., ed.), pp. 9–11. Tel-Aviv: OT-PAZ.

10. Vallfors, B., Bergdahl, B., 1984: Automatically controlled bipolar electro-coagulation-"COA-COMP". Neurosurg. Rev. 7, 187–190.

11. Verschueren, R., 1976: The CO_2 laser in tumor surgery. Medical Series NR 232. Assen-Amsterdam: Van Gorcum.

Laser Safety

Victor A. Fasano

Institute of Neurosurgery, University of Turin (Italy)

Contents

1. Laser Controlled Area 103
2. Appropriate Use and Training Procedures... 103
3. Identification of Danger and Safety Precautions.................................... 104
   3.1. Mechanical Hazards 104
   3.2. Electrical Hazards.. 104
   3.3. Damage to the Eyes 104
   3.4. Damage to the Skin.. 105
   3.5. Inhalation of Toxic Vapours with CO_2 Laser............................. 105
   3.6. Microbiological Contamination of the Target Area 105
   3.7. Investigations of Carcinogenic Effects of the Laser...................... 106
   3.8. Fire Hazards... 106
References 106

1. Laser Controlled Area

The area in which the laser is used should be defined as a laser controlled area and access to this area should be limited to personnel whose presence at the operation is essential. Ideally the dors of the laser controlled area should be latched shut by a remote interlock which comes into operation when laser is switched on; appropriate warning notices bearing the words, *Danger—visible and invisible laser radiation—avoid eye or skin exposure to direct or scatter radiation-class IV laser product,* must be displayed at all points of access to the area.

2. Appropriate Use and Training Procedures

Lasers offer unique advantages to patient and surgeon but it is essential to ensure that lasers are only used where they offer scientifically proven advantages over established surgical techniques. To achieve this National

Medical Laser Groups must be set up to supervise and to control the use of lasers. Membership of National Medical Laser Groups must be an essential for all who wish to use these valuable machines in order to ensure that "safe" lasers are used on appropriate clinical conditions by fully-trained laser surgeons following an approved laser safety code for all lasers in all their various clinical roles.

3. Identification of Danger and Safety Precautions

Lasers used in surgery and in some other biomedical applications can pose potential hazards to both the patient and the laser operating personel. They can be divided into different types: mechanical, electrical, damage to the eyes and skin, inhalation of toxic vapours with CO_2 laser, microbiological contamination of the target area and the possibility of fire.

3.1. Mechanical Hazards

The laser apparatus must be handled with appropriate care because they are heavy and may damage feet and fingers of the operating personnel.

3.2. Electrical Hazards

The laser tube itself operates on extremely high voltages and fairly high currents, and the connections to the laser chambers must be protected in order to avoid accidental touching.

3.3. Damage to the Eyes

The eye is a frequent target organ for damage by lasers. Visible and near-infrared lasers are focused on the retina causing a local heating and sometimes pigmented epithelium, rods and cones may be burnt. Ultraviolet and far-infrared lasers are a particular hazard to the cornea and anterior chamber. The laser radiation at these structures will cause corneal burn and cataract formation. Generally these hazards are due to beam reflection by shiny metallic surfaces. In particular reflection from a concave surface is to be avoided because a high-power density results. In order to reduce this phenomenon, it is possible to use blackened instruments, but they absorb the beam and become hot.

Eye protection from the lasers is, therefore, of vital importance. The patient's eyes must be protected and operating room personnel must wear glasses. It is important to know for each glass the wavelengths against which protection is afforded and the maximum radiant exposure possible. If the CO_2 laser is used with the operating microscope, surgeon's eyes are protected only while looking into the microscope. When argon and Nd:YAG lasers are used a protective shutter is necessary.

The He-Ne laser guide beam, though of very low power, should not be pointed at eye level as it may cause damage. This beam is harmless to skin and other structures.

The eye injury may be cumulative effect of chronic exposure to low levels of laser radiation.

3.4. Damage to the Skin

Damage to the skin depends on the laser wavelength. The most common lesions include: photosensitivity reactions, skin burn, erythema, increased pigmentation and accelerated ageing. It is extremely rare that a direct beam may injure the skin of the operator or operating theatre staff. However it is possible that a laser beam is reflected from an instrument or a retractor, but in these cases the power of the laser falls off beyond the focal point, so the skin lesions are minimal. For these reasons normal clothing is sufficient to provide an adequate protection.

Protection must be provided on all areas around the operative site in order to avoid damage to the patient. When CO_2 laser is used this result is achieved by moistened gauze.

3.5. Inhalation of Toxic Vapours with CO_2 Laser

Recently it has been suggested that the vapour and smoke released when CO_2 laser is used may be toxic or even carcinogenic. Analysis of smoke from lasing tumors in some studies has shown that some cells escape destruction, but culture studies have shwon that they are not viable[3, 5].

Another problem of smoke is the obscuration of the surgeon's view, particularly in microsurgery and the contamination of mirror and lenses.

It is therefore necessary to remove this vapour by a strong suction, very close to the operative site.

3.6. Microbiological Contamination of the Target Area

One of the advantages claimed for use of the laser beam as a surgical tool is its sterilization capability[1]. The high laser energy kills the microbial population at the site of irradiation[4], thus lowering the risk of microbial contamination and ensuing infections. However experiments dealing with the effects of laser on bacterial population were conducted by Eli et al.[2] demonstrating that laser contaminates the working surface in the area immediately around the irradiating probe. The source of the contamination was found to be the stream of gas which is emitted during irradiation near the laser lens to cool it. To examine this problem steril agar plates containing bacteriological growth medium were placed beneath the laser probe at 6 cm from focus and exposed to 60 or 120 seconds of gas emission with laser energy setting on 0 watt. As control identical sterile agar plates were opened to the atmosphere in the same room for equal time. Differently from controls the authors always found substantial contamination of irradiated plates by viable bacteria and fungi. In order to overcome this problem the following steps were taken:

a) A sterile filter was inserted on the end of the plastic tube at the entrance to the probe handle.

b) The plastic tip of the probe handle was sterilized by autoclave.

e) The laser lens was sterilized with a 70% ethanol solution.

Following these simple procedures, the level of contamination dropped to negligible values.

On the basis of these data Eli *et al.* recommend that similar simple procedures be implemented in order to eliminate the possibility of contamination during surgery.

3.7. Investigations of Carcinogenic Effects of the Laser

Investigation into the biological interaction of laser energy and tissue and specifically long-term laser safety in relation to possible carcinogenesis is still underway. Heteroploid mouse fibroblast cell line of the BALB/3 T 3 strain has been used by Apfelberg *et al.*[2] to quantify the carcinogenic effect of argon laser, CO_2 laser and as control X-ray. In this study lasers did not produce a significant malignant transformation.

3.8. Fire Hazards

It is important that no inflammable material lies in the laser target area. Drapes and protective gauze around the operative field must be well moistened to avoid the risk of fire.

References

1. Adrian, J. C., Gross, A., 1979: A new method of sterilization. The carbon dioxide laser. J. Oral. Pathol. *8*, 60–61.
2. Apfelberg, D. B., Mittelman, H., Chadi, B., Maser, M. R., Lash, H., 1984: Investigation of carconogenic effects of in vitro argon and CO_2 laser exposure of fibroblasts. Lasers Surg. Med. *4*, 173–179.
3. Eli, I., Judes, H., Rosenberg, M., 1983: Microbial contamination by a medical carbon dioxide laser. Lasers Surg. Med. *3*, 39–44.
4. Osterhius, J. W., Verschuern, R. C. J., Eidergen, R., 1982: The viability of cells in waste products of CO_2 laser vaporization of Cloudman mouse melanoma. Cancer *49*, 61.
5. Stellar, S., Polany, T. G., Bredemeier, A. C., 1974: Lasers in surgery. In: Laser Application in Medicine and Biology (Wolbarsht, M. L., ed.), *2*, 265–268. New York: Plenum Press.
6. Voorhies, R. M., Lavyne, M. H., Strait, T. A., Shapiro, W. R., 1984: Does the CO_2 laser spread viable brain-tumor cells outside the surgical field? J. Neurosurg. *60*, 819–820.

Laser Neurosurgical Techniques

VICTOR A. FASANO

Institute of Neurosurgery, University of Turin (Italy)

Contents

Laser Surgery of the Nervous Tissue Tumors.. 108
1. General Considerations.. 108
2. Operative Technique in Extraaxial Tumors.. 116
    2.1. Meningiomas 116
        2.1.1. Convexity Meningiomas.. 116
        2.1.2. Parasagittal Meningiomas... 117
        2.1.3. Basal Meningiomas... 117
    2.2. Pituitary Adenomas, Craniopharyngiomas and Tumors of the Pineal
        Region 117
    2.3. Acoustic Tumors 118
3. Operative Technique in Intraaxial Tumors.. 118
    3.1. Supratentorial Tumors 118
    3.2. Infratentorial Tumors... 119
4. Operative Technique in Brain Stem Tumors 119
5. Operative Technique in Spinal Cord Tumors... 119
6. Surgical Results... 120
7. Conclusive Considerations 123

Laser Surgery of the Cerebral Vascular Malformations 124
1. Arteriovenous Malformations.. 124
    1.1. General Considerations 124
    1.2. Operative Technique... 125
    1.3. Surgical Results 125
    1.4. Conclusive Considerations... 127
2. Arterial Aneurysms 127

Miscellaneous Indications for Laser Surgery 135
1. Syringohydromyelia: Laser Fenestration 135
2. Chronic Pain of Spinal Origin: Dorsal Root Entry Zone Lesions.......... 136
3. Discectomy.. 136
References.. 137

Laser Surgery of the Nervous Tissue Tumors

1. General Considerations

In comparison with the traditional techniques the main characteristics of the laser in the treatment of the nervous tissue tumors consist in the no-touch surgery, in the limited effect on restricted areas and in the possibility to obtain a shrinkage of the mass by drying of the tissue. These properties consent a sharp dissection which is peculiar of the CO_2 laser; local cooling methods (N_2 gas, Freon gas, gauzes soaked with saline solution, chilled water) can be used to limit the thermal spreading, thus increasing the selectivity of the maneuvre[33, 34].

The width of the laser lesion represents in the resection of large tumors a disadvantage, which is partly balanced by the association of a fair hemostasis to the tissue sloughing. This effect is typical of the Nd:YAG laser.

On this basis the aim of most clinical reports was to demonstrate that laser is able to remove a tumor with acceptable surgical results offering some advantages in comparison with the traditional techniques. In some works lasers and conventional techniques were compared in specific neurosurgical pathologies to evaluate when laser led to a true improvement of the surgical procedure. In all reports lasers have been used on the basis of the knowledge of their effects on normal brain tissues and the problem of the interaction between laser and tumors has not been considered. There are very few studies on this subject.

The absorption coefficients of meningiomas, high grade gliomas and metastatic tumors have been evaluated (de Tommasi et al.[32]). Optical absorption to the argon laser resulted three times greater than the normal brain and was still more considerable in highly vascularized tumors.

Absorption coefficient does not consent the determination of the light penetration in tissue since scattering is another important factor in attenuating electromagnetic energy. The penetration of the laser radiation in neoplastic human brain tissue has been studied for blue light (488 nm), green light (514 nm), red light (635 nm) and near-infrared radiation (1,060 nm) by Svaasand and Ellingsen[29]. In comparison with the normal brain, penetration depth was somewhat higher in meningiomas significantly higher (2–3 times larger) in rapidly growing glioblastomas and equal to the corresponding values in normal tissues, in metastatic tumors.

The extent of thermal penetration of Nd:YAG laser was studied histologically by Yamagami et al.[37] in meningiomas and gliomas. In general, histological findings of brain tumor tissue irradiated with the Nd:YAG laser were those of an acute thermal coagulative injury. Beneath the vaporized crater and the carbonized surface, a vesicular layer caused by rapid dehydration was seen. This layer was, in turn, surrounded by a necrotic layer and than an edematous layer. A decrease in cell population and changes in staining properties were noted in the edematous layer. There was an ill-defined border between the edematous layer and the intact tumor cell layer which included eosinophilic fiber and increased cell population. There was a clear relationship between the irradiated energy and the thermal injury both in depth and in width. The maximal thermal injury was observed 6 mm in depth and 10 mm in width when the tumor tissue was irradiated four times for 2 seconds at 90 watts.

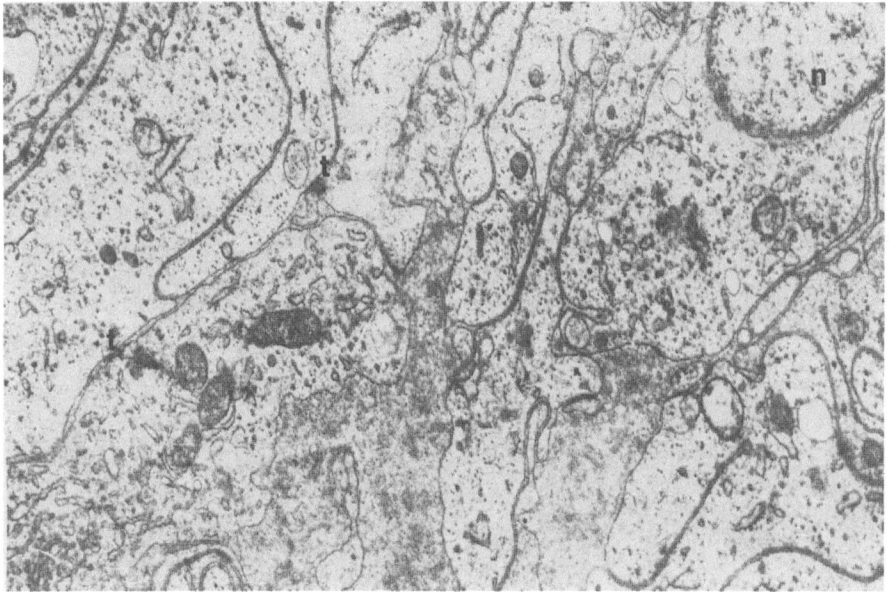

Fig. 1. Transmission electron micrograph of a meningioma. (n nucleus; t tight junctions)

The changes occurring in the outer periphery of the lesion after laser irradiation have been described for normal brain. See: Laser effect on normal nervous tissue (CO_2, Nd : YAG). Histological data. At this level lesions of the constituents of the blood-brain barrier and vessel occlusions can affect the microcirculation and modify the extension of the lesion. This is particularly important in tumor surgery. For these reasons a similar study has been carried out during neurosurgical operations in different tumors: meningiomas and high grade gliomas (Fasano et al. 1984 unpublished data). Irradiation was delivered according to the surgical experience: high power and short irradiation time were used (40 watts for 3 seconds with CO_2, 80 watts for 3 seconds with Nd : YAG). In all cases the beam diameter was 2 mm with CO_2 and 2.5 mm with Nd : YAG. The portion of the irradiated tumor including the surrounding tissue was removed for histological analysis. Fig. 1 shows the normal structure of a meningioma. Nuclei, mitochondria, lysosomas and tight junctions are detectable.

After irradiation with CO_2 and Nd:YAG lasers a complete disorganization of the tumor structure occurs in the outer periphery of the lesion (Fig. 2). Marked morphologic alterations of cytoplasmic organules

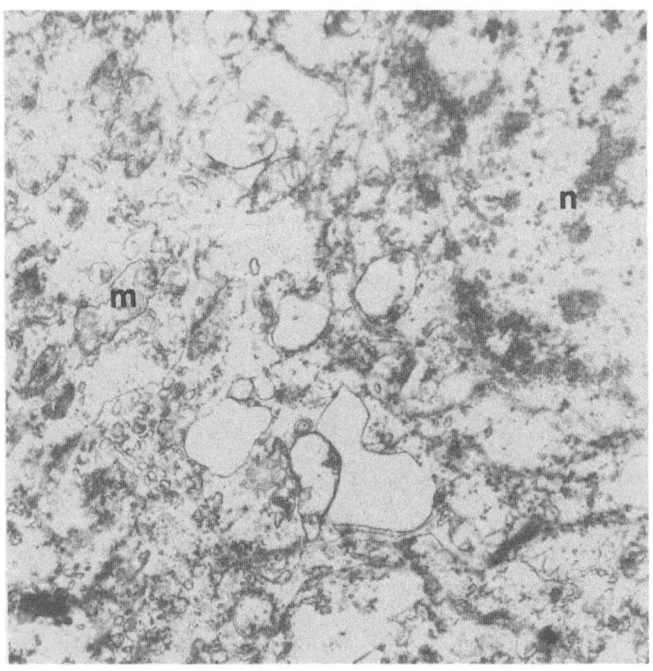

Fig. 2. Transmission electron micrograph of a meningioma after CO_2 laser irradiation at 40 watts for 3 seconds. (*n* nucleus; *m* mitochondria)

(mitochondria, lysosomas) and nuclei are detectable. CO_2 laser does not produce any significative damage of the vascular network.

After Nd:YAG irradiation capillaries show almost complete destruction of the endothelial cells and intraluminal eryhrocyte aggregation; basement membrane, although thin is preserved in all samples (Fig. 3).

Fig. 4 shows the normal structure of a glioma at optic microscope. After CO_2 laser irradiation the conventional histologic examination does not show any tissue damage at the level of the outer periphery of the lesion; electron microscope shows complete disorganization of the tumoral architecture; subcellular structures (nuclei, mitochondria) are damaged but still recognizable (Fig. 5). The vascular network does not show important lesions. High peak pulsed CO_2 laser irradiation does not produce important

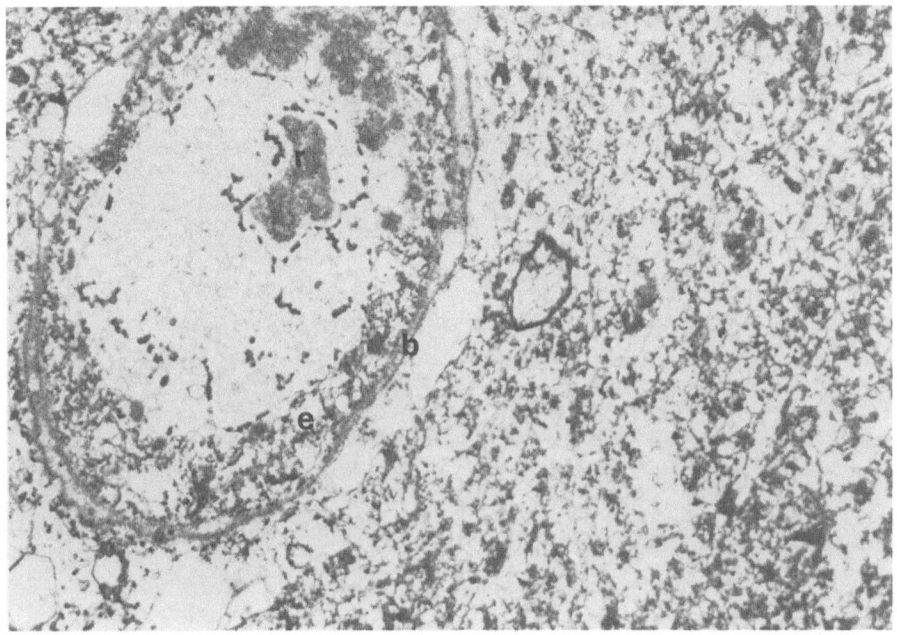

Fig. 3. Transmission electron micrograph of a tumor capillary after Nd : YAG laser irradiation at 80 watts for 3 seconds. (*b* basement membrane; *r* red blood cell; *e* endothelial cell)

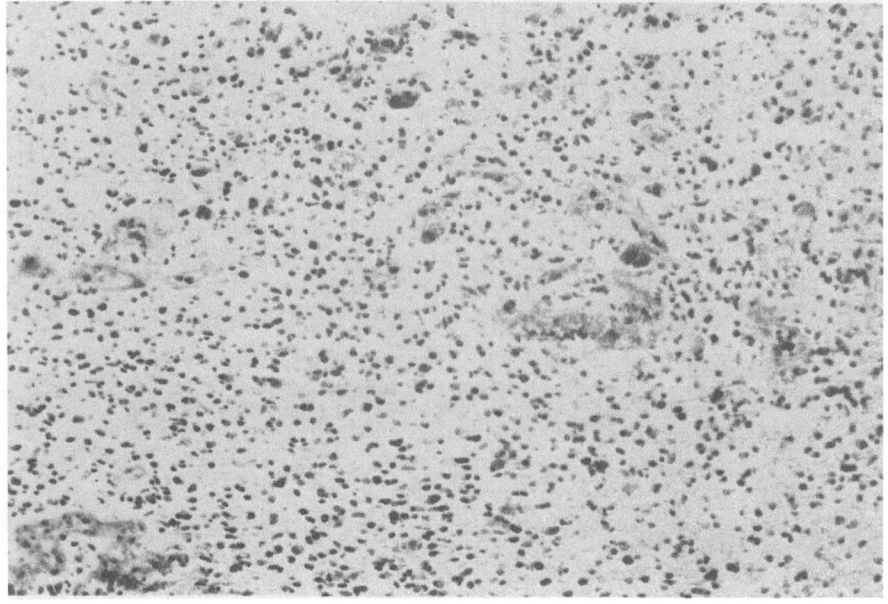

Fig. 4. Histological finding of a cerebral astrocytoma. Hematos Eos

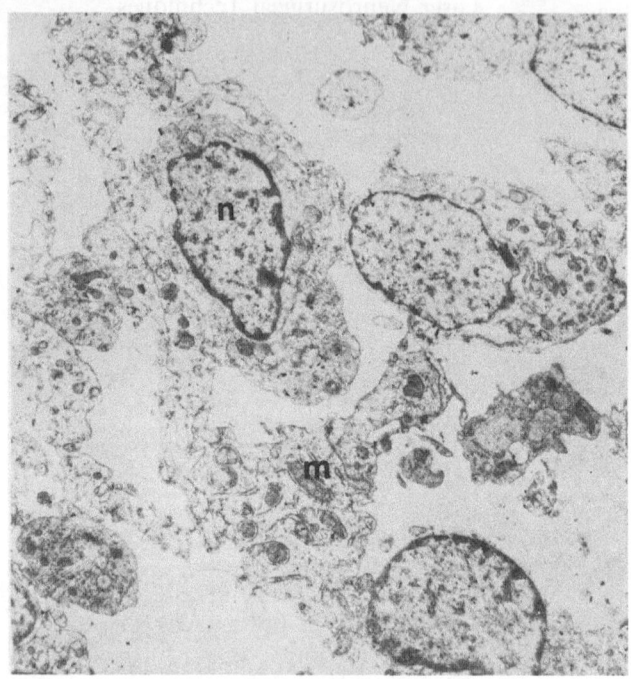

Fig. 5. Cerebral astrocytoma after CO_2 laser irradiation at 40 watts for 3 seconds. Electron micrograph. (*n* nucleus; *m* mitochondria)

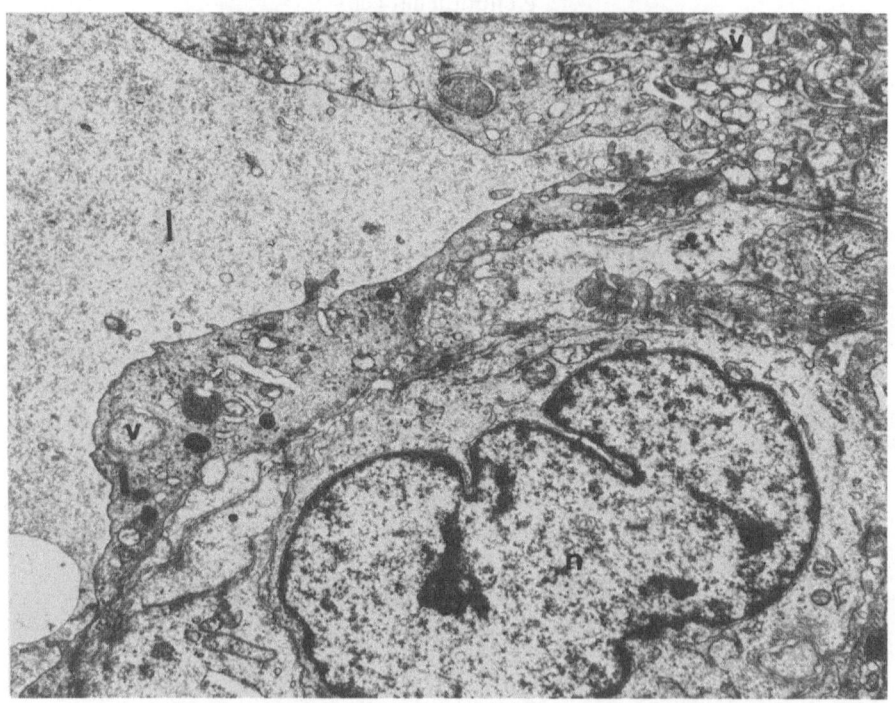

Fig. 5 a. Cerebral astrocytoma after high peak pulsed CO_2 laser irradiation. (*n* nucleus; *l* lumen; *v* vesicles)

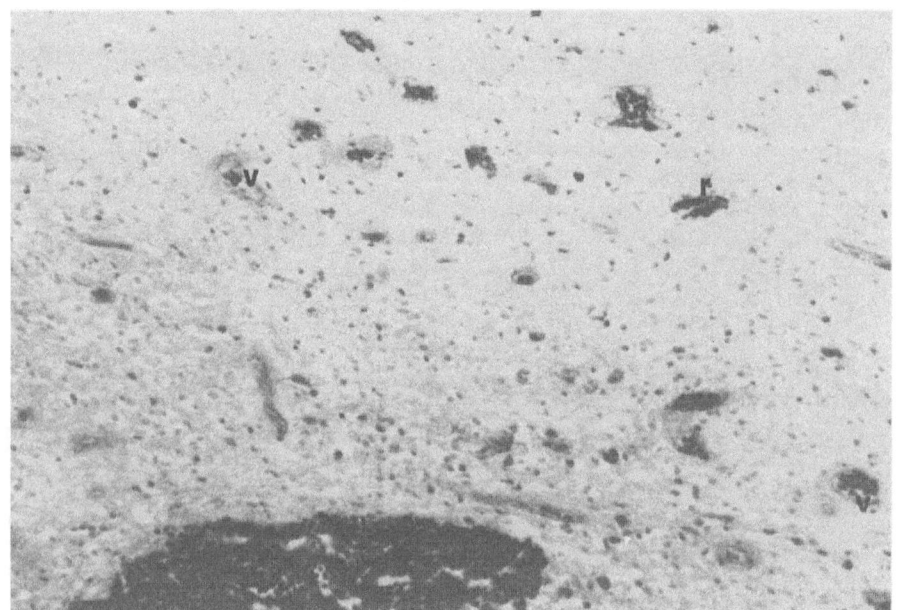

Fig. 6. Cerebral astrocytoma after Nd:YAG laser irradiation at 80 watts for 3 seconds. Histological finding. Hematos Eos (*v* vessel; *r* red blood cells)

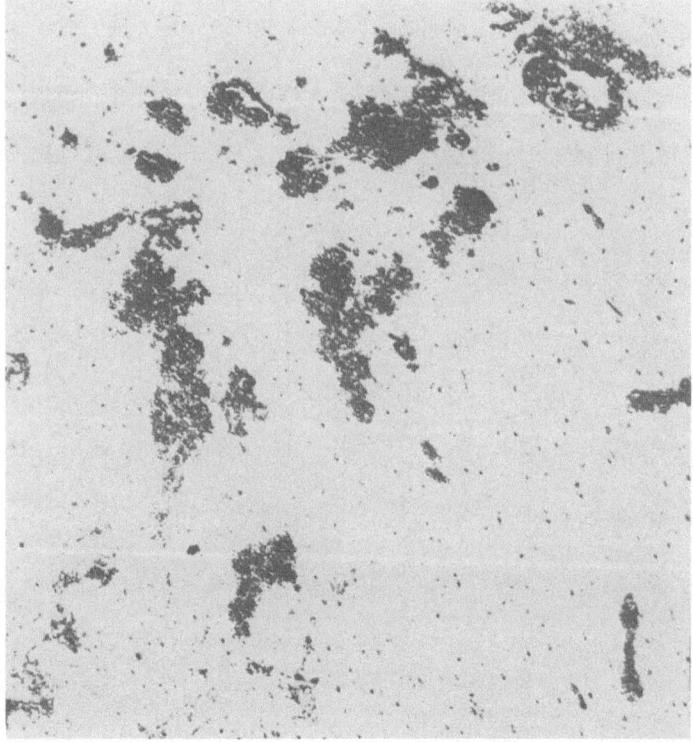

Fig. 7. Cerebral astrocytoma after Nd:YAG laser irradiation at 80 watts for 3 seconds. Hematos Eos. Histological finding at high magnification

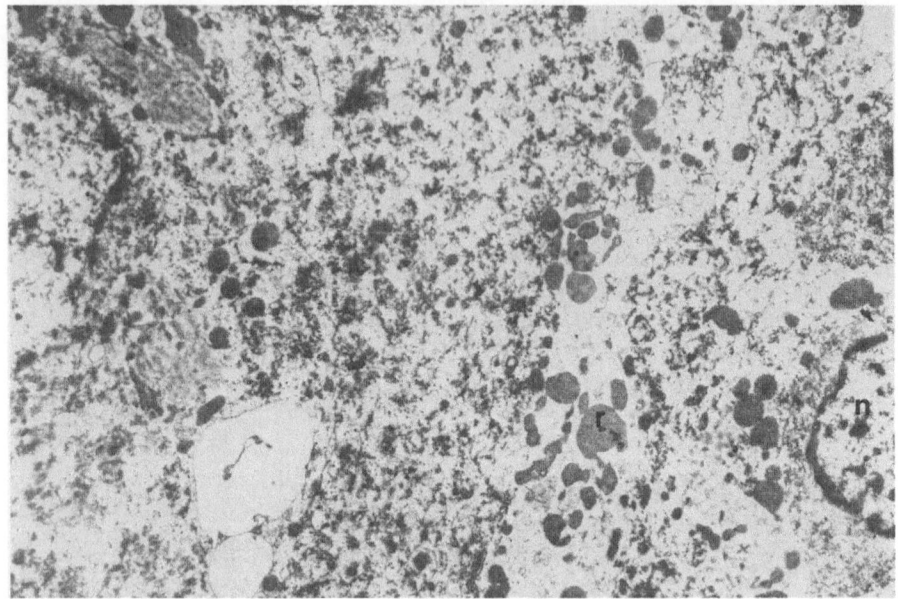

Fig. 8. Cerebral astrocytoma after Nd : YAG laser irradiation at 80 watts for 3 seconds. Electron micrograph. (*n* nucleus; *r* red blood cells)

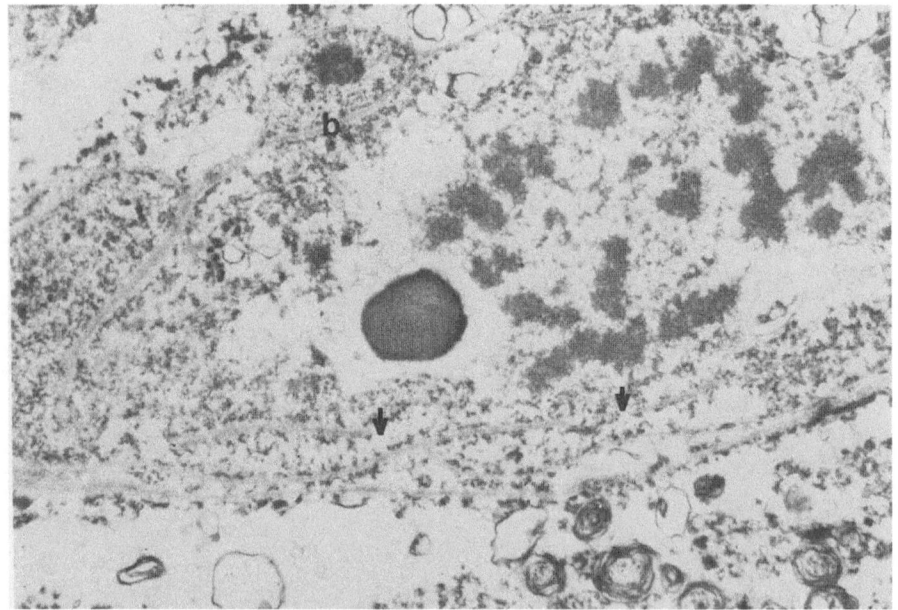

Fig. 9. Transmission electron micrograph of a tumor capillary (astrocytoma) after Nd : YAG laser irradiation at 80 watts for 3 seconds. (*b* basement membrane; arrow: interruption of basement membrane)

vascular or tessutal damages; only intracellular vesicles are evident (Fig. 5a). After Nd:YAG irradiation all samples show at optic microscope thrombized arterioles and perivascular intraparenchimal hemorrhage (Figs. 6 and 7). Electron microscope shows the loss of the normal tumor structure; multiple microhemorrhages are moreover detectable (Fig. 8). Capillaries show almost complete destruction of endothelial cells; the basement

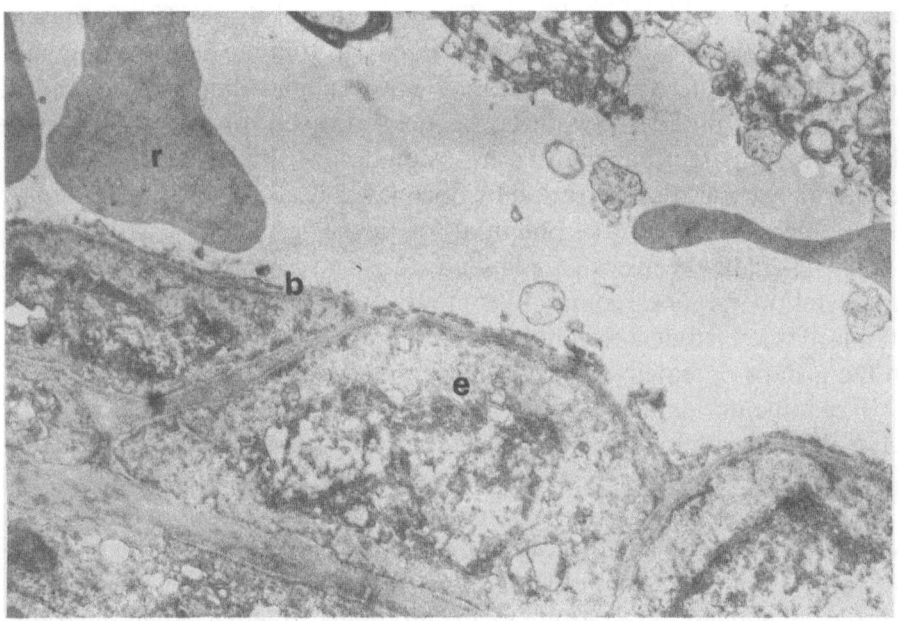

Fig. 10. Transmission electron micrograph of a tumor capillary (astrocytoma) after Nd:YAG laser irradiation at 80 watts for 3 seconds. (*b* basement membrane; *e* endothelial cell; *r* red blood cell)

membrane is interrupted in some points (Fig. 9) and perivascular microhemorrhages are visible (Fig. 10).

More marked lesions are, therefore, produced in neoplastic brain tissue in comparison with normal brain, on both parenchima and vascular network, especially after Nd:YAG laser irradiation. This depends probably to the different structure of the pathological vessels and the different optical characteristics of the tumor. The damage of the microcirculation is evident after Nd:YAG irradiation. Endoluminal obliteration is observed in the outer periphery of the lesion in hard tumors after irradiation at 80 watts for 3 seconds, and at this power, in highly vascularized gliomas perivascular hemorrhages occur. Therefore in case of repeat irradiations with Nd:YAG laser, as used in surgery, there is a risk of postoperative hemorrhage. This has been confirmed in some patients with glioblastomas who developed delayed intracerebral hemorrhages after surgery.

On this basis the predictability of the lesion cannot be absolute in the early stage and even less in the laste stage. From a surgical point of view the greater absorption of the tumor in comparison to the normal brain may increase the selectivity of the laser.

The thermal spreading ensuing from the resection of the tumor may produce delayed biologic effects. Temperatures of 40–43 °C are present around the laser site. Because of the greater sensitivity to heat of malignant cells this moderate hyperthermia may cause cellular damage and a local inflammatory processes with consequent delayed fibrosis[4]. One may therefore suppose that after laser irradiation a similar response could replace the neoplastic infiltration by fibrous tissue, although nests of tumor cells could survive with the potential for further growth.

This effect has been evaluated by Edwards and coworkers in rats bearing intracerebral 9 L gliosarcomas. In comparison with the group operated with standard microsurgical techniques no difference in survival were observed in the groups operated with CO_2 and argon lasers[7].

Experimental data regarding the benefit of surgical removal by laser when dealing with lower grade intracranial glial tumors are not reported in literature.

According to the experimental results there is no evidence in the surgical practice that laser can in any way influence the survival time. In Beck series[2] on 14 patients with high grade gliomas 10 have not survived more than 1 year. In all patients of this group recurrent tumor growth was demonstrated on follow-up CT studies.

2. Operative Technique in Extraaxial Tumors

2.1. Meningiomas

2.1.1. Convexity Meningiomas

These tumors have often a considerable size; the most important problem is to limit the manipulation of the healthy tissues during surgery especially when the mass is broad based in critical areas.

Initially the borders of the tumor are irradiated with CO_2 laser at maximal power defocused, in separate short pulses, to obtain shrinkage and retraction of the external part of the tumor capsule away from the close structures; a fair amount of hemostasis is present because of the sealing of the smaller blood vessels.

Resection of the tumor by laser is very slow and thermal spreading notable, therefore we prefer to open the capsule, empty the tumor by progressive fragmentation and suction with ultrasonic aspirator and then draw the capsule dissecting it from the deeper planes by CO_2 laser focused at low power. By this procedure tumor can be removed readily with minimal manipulation of neural structures.

2.1.2. Parasagittal Meningiomas

These tumors present some problems because of the high vascularization and the frequent involvement of the superior sagittal sinus. Following the incision of the capsule, debulk is attained with minimal bleeding alternating to suction by ultrasonic aspiration, the irradiation of the tumor planes by defocused Nd : YAG laser at low power in separate short pulses to obtain devascularization of the mass. The dissection of the implant from the sinus is made with focused CO_2 laser at low power.

According to Beck's technique[2], in cases of infiltration of the sinus wall by tumor growth, the wall is irradiated with defocused Nd : YAG laser at 30–40 watts in separate short pulses. Because of the thick wall there is no risk of thrombosis of the sinus. When the sinus is obliterated, the part of the tumor bulging into it is irradiated with defocused Nd : YAG laser at 50–60 watts in separate short pulses to produce a complete necrosis of the mass and a segmental coagulation of the sinus. In these cases Beck's technique[2] consists in cutting open the sinus and removing the tumor from the inside with the use of the laser beam; the wall of the sinus is then closed again by continuous suture technique.

2.1.3. Basal Meningiomas

The use of the laser is particularly useful in meningiomas arising from the olfactory groove or the planum sphenoidale as well as in medial and lateral sphenoid ridge meningiomas and in tentorial meningiomas.

After incision of the capsule, the tumor is debulked with ultrasonic aspirator; defocused Nd : YAG laser at 40–50 watts in separate pulses is used in some cases to devascularize the mass or in harder tissues to facilitate the suction by sloughing of the tumor. Subsequently the tumor is separated from its base by using focused CO_2 laser at 30–40 watts. Thus it is possible to cleave the tumor from the optic nerves, the chiasma, the carotid arteries and their tributaries, the adjacent brain parenchima and the cavernous sinus. The placement of well-soaked cottonoid strips on these structures protects them completely from the laser beam. Finally all parts of the dura with dural infiltration are irradiated with Nd : YAG laser defocused at 40–50 watts in separate pulses.

2.2. Pituitary Adenomas, Craniopharyngiomas and Tumors of the Pineal Region

All these tumors are soft and poorly vascularized and therefore rapidly removed with ultrasonic aspirator which is particularly helpful in pinealomas operated through supracerebellar infratentorial approach.

Focused CO_2 laser at low power is useful in pituitary adenomas to dissect the remnants of the tumor without damaging chiasma and optic nerves.

In transphenoidal approach of pituitary adenomas Nd:YAG laser (defocused at 50–60 watts) is used to open the bony floors of sphenoid sinus and *Sella turcica*. The dura is then opened and tumor removed by rapid coagulation of the mass without blood loss. The advantages consist in easy control of the bleeding from the spongy bony matrix and in the absence of traction on nearby structures in the opening of the bone.

2.3. Acoustic Tumors

In the first step of the surgical procedure the capsule of the tumor is opened and then internal decompression is obtained by reduction in size of the mass with ultrasonic aspirator. The cavitation of the tumor thus obtained facilitates the separation of the capsule from the adjacent structures of the cerebello-pontine angle which is attained with the conventional microsurgical techniques. Laser has not been particularly useful in our hands in these procedures.

A technique for removal of extraaxial neoplasms using CO_2 laser only has been proposed by other authors[6]. Following tumor exposure the capsule is opened and a gradual excavation which proceeds from the centrum of the neoplasm to the periphery is attained by progressive vaporization. Capsule is also vaporized at a readily accessible area and this results in capsule shrinkage which further diminishes the surface area of the tumor. As a consequence of both effects the neoplasm pulls itself from surrounding structures at the arachnoid/arachnoid interface. Eventually tumor remnants can be vaporized in toto.

The specific surgical procedures for the different types of tumor are described in another chapter.

3. Operative Technique in Intraaxial Tumors

3.1. Supratentorial Tumors

The cortical incision is made with focused CO_2 laser at low power over the external surface of the tumor. Then the neoplasm is progressively removed with ultrasonic aspiration. In highly vascularized tumors a layer by layer irradiation with defocused Nd:YAG at low power in separate pulses is associated to the suction in order to achieve a devascularization of the neoplasm.

Defocused CO_2 laser at low power in short pulses can be used to remove tumor remnants in highly functional areas. The technique consents a rapid tumor resection with limited blood loss. Choroid plexus papillomas and ependimomas of the lateral ventricles can be easily coagulated by Nd:YAG laser defocused at low power in short pulses after the opening of the ventricle and then removed with ultrasonic aspirator.

3.2. Infratentorial Tumors

Intraaxial infratentorial lesions can either extend into the brain stem or occupy a position bordering the fourth ventricle. They are removed with ultrasonic aspirator after cutting of the cerebellar cortex with focused CO_2 laser at low power.

In cystic astrocytoma of the midline the mural node is often in connection with the brain stem and important vascular structures; it can be dissected with focused CO_2 laser at low power. Cerebellar hemangioblastomas are irradiated with Nd:YAG at 40–50 watts, defocused in separate short pulses in order to produce a layer by layer tumor coagulation; this allows a step by step nonmanipulative excission of the tumor by curette with reduced blood loss.

4. Operative Technique in Brain Stem Tumors

Brain stem tumors are represented by two different types:

a) Those originating from the brain stem which protrude into the 4th ventricle; they can extend out into the cerebello-pontine angle and may down over the dorsal surface of the cervical spinal cord. In these cases an obstruction of the CSF pathways often occur.

b) Those infiltrating the brain stem without extraaxial extension.

In the past surgery has been limited to the excision of the portion of the tumor protruding out from the axis or to the evacuation of an intrinsic tumoral cyst. New technologies have made possible a direct approach in intrinsic solid tumors. Surgical technique consists in traditional approach to posterior fossa. The floor of the 4th ventricle is reached through incision of vermis cerebellaris thus consenting to identify the mass with the aid of the tessutal A-mode echoencephalography. Tumor is then vaporized layer by layer under sonographic control which enables to differentiate neoplasia from surrounding normal tissues. Tumors protruding out from the axis into the cerebello-pontine angle were reached through a lateral approach. The extrinsic part is removed with CUSA; the intrinsic one is then vaporized.

5. Operative Technique in Spinal Cord Tumors

The focused CO_2 laser is useful for incision of the fascia and muscle and exposure of spinous processes and vertebral lamina. The procedure is rapid and blood loss reduced.

Extradural tumors, mainly sarcomas, are often very vascularized; they are quickly debulked with CUSA; Nd:YAG laser is associated to obtain a satisfactory devascularization of the mass. Aspiration is ineffective in very hard tissues; in these cases focused CO_2 laser, can as a cutting tool, remove large tumor chunks and this action is facilitated by a slight traction.

Intradural meningiomas are soft and poorly vascularized tumors and are therefore easily removed with ultrasonic aspirator; defocused Nd:YAG irradiation at low power in short pulses can be associated to achieve hemostasis of the tissue before suction. The remnants are dissected from the surrounding structures by a low power focused CO_2 laser; the infiltrated dura is then irradiated with Nd:YAG laser defocused at 30–40 watts in separate pulses. Because of the high water content neurinomas are easily removed by a layer by layer vaporization with defocused CO_2 laser.

In intramedullary tumors mielotomy is performed with focused CO_2 laser at low power tumor is then removed by ultrasonic aspirator which is able to distinguish, by tactile feedback, the interface between neoplastic and spinal cord.

6. Surgical Results

The review of literature on the use of the laser in neurosurgery provides important data. Extended clinical studies on the use of the CO_2 laser are presented by Heppner and Ascher, Inaba, Takizawa, Mattos Pimenta, Perria, Strait[15, 16, 21, 23, 27, 30]. These works report the main advantages of the technique which can be summarized as follows:

a) Reduction of blood loss.

b) Reduction of the use of brain retractors.

c) Possibility of accurate dissection of the tumor from adherent structures without lesion.

d) Limitation of neurological impairment in the postoperative course.

e) Faster recovery with less time of hospitalization.

Bartal et al.[1] provide important observations in a preliminary experience on the use of the CO_2 laser in the surgery of basal meningiomas. The main difficulties encountered while working with the laser were:

a) Cancelling of the guidelight by coaxial light source of the operating microscope (this incovenience is at present overcomed in the more recent models having a brighter guidelight).

b) Loss of feeling and appreciation of the texture and consistency of tissues usually experienced with forceps.

c) Length of time because the limited penetration of the beam.

d) Difficulty in the use of the laser with a fixed-coordinate system attached to the microscope. For the authors the freehand use of the handpiece is mandatory to consent an easier maneuvre in directing the beam at different angles to the target site without readjustments and repositioning of the microscope which are required when using joystick-guided unit.

The authors conclude that these tumors can be removed completely with bipolar coagulation and dissection alone but they have the feeling, however, that whenever the laser is not available they are deprived of a most useful tool.

The use of CO_2 laser in the treatment of the acoustic tumors is described by Robertson et al.[25] in a series of 28 cases. Preservation of the facial nerve was possible in 92.9% of cases. No blood transfusion was needed for any tumor.

The results of the treatment of intraaxial neoplasms by stereotactic CO_2 laser system (Kelly)[17] are reported in another chapter. Hara et al.[14] have evaluated the degree of necessity for neurosurgical use of the laser unit (CO_2) in 20 cases, including mostly meningiomas and gliomas, on the basis of the extent of tumor removal, volume of blood transfused during surgery and duration of the surgical operation. The results in 20 cases in which laser was not utilized were used as control. The authors established three grades of evaluation: grade 1 (adjuvant), grade 2 (also necessary), grade 3 (indispensable). A grade 1 or 2 is ascribed for most convexity and parasagittal meningiomas; in cases of meningiomas of the basal skull (especially sphenoid ridge meningiomas) the necessity grade is 3. In subcortical gliomas the necessity grade is also 3.

The results on the use of the Nd : YAG laser are reported by Beck[2] in 103 cases (meningiomas, gliomas, intrinsic brain tumors, metastatic brain tumors, spinal tumors). In the group of meningiomas (51 cases) most patients left the hospital without neurologic deficits and in about half of the cases no blood transfusion were required. CT follow-up studies failed to show any evidence of recurrent tumor growth. The results of the treatment of the gliomas are reported previously (General considerations). Spinal cord tumors include 6 intradural tumors and 2 ependymomas of the cauda equina. In all patients with intradural tumors a good recovery of paraplegic symptoms was noted over the subsequent weeks following surgery. In both patients with intramedullary tumors over a 2-year follow-up period there has been no evidence of recurrent tumor growth.

Similar results are reported by Handa et al.[13] in a series of 72 cases treated with Nd : YAG laser.

A series of 68 neurosurgical procedures performed with argon laser is reported by Edwards et al.[8]. In this study laser is considered very helpful, when comparing surgical results with that obtained with standard microsurgical technique, in 48 cases including mostly spinal procedures, acoustic neurinomas, intracranial meningiomas, cerebellar tumors and pituitary adenomas. Technique in the treatment of various neurosurgical pathologies with argon laser is described in another chapter.

Our series of case is reported in Table 1.

Table 2 shows postoperative morbidity and average volume of the tumor (determined on CT scan).

On CT scan control the extent of removal was complete in all cases of

Table 1. *Tumors Operated with Laser Sources*

Tumor location	Number of cases
Superficial gliomas	71
Subcortical gliomas mostly extended in white matter	50
Deep-seated gliomas mostly extended around the basal structures	10
Tumors of the lateral ventricles	4
Midline tumors (pinealomas)	3
Superficial meningiomas	55
Parasagittal meningiomas	24
Convexity endotheliomas	22
Falx meningiomas	9
Basal meningiomas	30
Adjoining vessels	14
Adjoining vessels and nerves	16
Tentorial meningiomas	4
Orbital meningiomas	2
Cerebellar tumors	16
Medulloblastomas	7
Spongioblastomas	6
Hemangioblastomas	3
Tumors of the IVth ventricle	3
Tumors of the pontocerebellar region	7
Acoustic neurinomas	3
Meningiomas	4
Brain stem tumors	11
Intrinsic tumors	7
With extraaxial extension	4
Intramedullary tumors	3
Intradural spinal cord tumors	14
Neurinomas	8
Meningiomas	6
Extradural spinal cord tumors (sarcomas)	7
Metastatic tumors	14

superficial and subcortical gliomas, midline and lateral ventricle tumors, superficial meningiomas, meningiomas of the tentorium and orbit, tumors of the ponto cerebellar region, metastatic tumors. The percentage of complete removal in tumors located in other areas was the following: 90% in deep-seated gliomas, 83% in meningiomas of the base of the skull, 93% in cerebellar tumors, 66% in tumors of the 4th ventricle.

Cortical incision never exceeded 3–4 cm.

Blood transfusion ranged from 200 to 600 ml.

Table 2. *Surgical Results in 425 Tumors Operated with Laser Sources*

Tumor location	Average tumor volume on CT scan	postoperative morbidity
Superficial gliomas	2.5 × 4 cm	no morbidity
Subcortical gliomas	2.7 × 4.6 cm	no morbidity
Deep-seated gliomas	2.5 × 3.8 cm	10% of cases
Tumors of the lateral ventricle	1.1 × 2.3 cm	25% of cases
Midline tumors	—	no morbidity
Superficial meningiomas	4.3 × 6.2 cm	no morbidity
Basal meningiomas	4.7 × 5.32 cm	10% of cases
Tentorial meningiomas	2.2 × 3.1 cm	no morbidity
Orbital meningiomas	1.5 × 2.1 cm	no morbidity
Cerebellar tumors	2.2 × 2.6 cm	no morbidity
Tumors of the IVth ventricle	1.7 × 2.2 cm	no morbidity
Brain stem tumors	—	no morbidity
Tumors of the pontocerebellar region	2.3 × 3.2 cm	no morbidity
Metastatic tumors	1.5 × 2 cm	no morbidity
Intramedullary tumors	—	no morbidity
Intradural spinal cord tumors	—	no morbidity
Extradural spinal cord tumors	—	14% of cases

The results of the treatment of brain stem tumors are more widely discussed. Our series includes 7 tumors infiltrating the brain stem (6 solid, 1 cystic) and 4 tumors arising from the brain stem and protruding into the cerebello-pontine angle (2 cases) or 4th ventricle (2 cases). Histological examination revealed a pylocitic astrocytoma in 6 cases (4 of the first group and 2 of the second: 5 children and 1 adult); an anaplastic astrocytoma in 4 cases (2 of the first group and 2 of the second: 3 adults and 1 child); a metastases in 1 case (adult; of the first group). A transitory ataxia was a common postoperative symptom. Postoperative worsening of the neurological status never appeared. In 4 cases an immediate clinical improvement was noticed. One patient with anaplastic astrocytoma died 2 weeks after surgery since postoperative extracerebral complications occurred. Other patients were submitted to X-ray therapy. Survival in cases of high grade malignant tumor ranged from 5 to 12 months. All cases of pylocitic astrocytoma are still alive and have useful life. The longest follow-up shows a survival time of 60 (1 case) and 36 (1 case) months.

7. Conclusive Considerations

We think that laser and ultrasonic aspirator are both effective in the treatment of the cerebral tumors. CUSA only, associated to bipolar coagulation, is used in poorly vascularized tumors. Laser only is used in the dissection of the tumor from the surrounding structures by progressive vaporization. A recent innovation is the laser scalpel consenting, by direct contact, dissecting or cutting maneuvers. Advantage consists in the tactile feedback which consents a direct control of the maneuver. Laser and CUSA are used associated in:

a) high vascularized tumors; Nd : YAG laser is used to produce a fair devascularization of the mass consenting a relatively bloodless suction,

b) tumors of base of the skull, parasagittal meningiomas, infratentorial tumors; in these cases a rapid debulking by suction and a sharp dissection by CO_2 or argon laser are attained.

A problem of the laser in the treatment of the nervous system tumors arises from the forecast of the effects of the interaction between light and neoplastic tissues. Moreover penetration depth may vary in relation to the regressive changes encountered (necrosis, calcification, hemorrhage etc.). Operating parameters currently used are therefore rough, energy being delivered according to the direct experience of the surgeon. Studies on this subject will provide in the future sufficient data for a correct use of these instruments.

Malis has recently proposed the use of the Bipolar cutting as rival of the CUSA to remove blocks of tumor up to 1 cm; main indications are in fleshy meningiomas but even solid or heavily calcified tissue can be treated. Technique is quite hemostatic and therefore particularly useful in highly vascular tumors.

Continuous saline irrigation is required to assure maximal conductivity and to prevent heating. If tissue is totally avascular conductivity is very little and it may be difficult to use this technique. Maneuver is poorly controlled since forceps is directly sent to the bottom; moreover the fragments of tissue must be removed by suction with consequent encumbrance of the operating field. Technique seems to be useful for removing tumor plaques adherent to the dura, especially in parasagittal region, and remnants in restricted areas directly controllable.

Laser Surgery of the Cerebral Vascular Malformations

1. Arteriovenous Malformations

1.1. General Considerations

Experiments on the effects of the Nd : YAG on blood vessels have demonstrated that laser can occlude instantaneously small arteries (up to 0.5–1 mm) because of the thin wall and the reduced volume of flow; larger arteries with thicker walls and high volume of flow (rabbit carotid) cannot be obliterated immediately; complete exlusion however can be obtained within few days by endoluminal thrombosis. Veins despite their size, are very easily coagulated because of the thin wall and the low blood flow. These data suggest that a complete coagulation can be achieved in low flow arteriovenous malformations (AVMs) fed through a single main artery and few feeding channels.

In other investigations Wharen et al.[35] have studied the thermal response of normal cat brain to Nd : YAG laser. After irradiation blood temperature rose rapidly and reached 90% of the maximum value in 2–3 seconds; on the contrary brain temperature increased more slowly. In both cases temperature dropped rapidly within few seconds especially after pulses of short duration. To limit thermal spreading to brain, coagulation should be, therefore, achieved within approximately 3 seconds. If coagulation is not complete higher powers produce complete occlusion of the vessel without increasing brain temperature. Further prolonged irradiation, however, is not likely to be helpful and will only serve to increase brain damage. These data indicate that short intermittent laser pulses focused upon blood vessels can be used safely to coagulate within brain since damage of the surrounding tissues is very limited.

1.2. Operative Technique

Traditional technique consists in isolation and coagulation of vessels entering the malformation to interrupt flow to the nidus, dissection and resection of the nidus with reduced blood loss. Feeding arteries, located subcortically and usually in depth, require a deep dissection in the healthy tissue and since they always supply blood to normal brain, only the shunting arterioles arising from the feeding channels should be interrupted.

Surgical procedure with Nd : YAG laser consists in intraoperative localization of the shunt with doppler flowmeter and irradiation of the entire area of the nidus to coagulate it.

The beam is defocused until spot size is three times larger than the vessel to be irradiated; short intermittent pulses of less than 3 seconds at incident power of 40 to 80 watts are used. The maneuvre can be facilitated by intraoperative hypotension (80–90 mm Hg).

The disappearance of the shunt is checked by echodoppler flowmeter and then the nidus is resected with minimal blood loss.

1.3. Surgical Results

All authors agree on the usefulness of the laser in coagulating small arteriovenous malformations.

Hara et al.[14] used the CO_2 laser, defocused, in one arteriovenous malformation, but perforation of the vessel wall occurred during coagulation.

An open stereotactic approach for the treatment of a deep-seated arteriovenous malformation with CO_2 laser was utilized by Kelly with excellent result [18].

Beck obtained good results with Nd : YAG laser in 2 arteriovenous malformations whose feeding vessels up to 2.5 mm were easily coagulated [2].

Edwards et al. [8] reported that argon laser was helpful for the removal of a low flow small arteriovenous malformation but no effective in the resection of a large high-flow lesion because of the loss of heat in blood.

Wharen et al. [36] described the results of the treatment of arteriovenous malformations with Nd : YAG laser in 10 cases. The laser was helpful for defining the plane between the arteriovenous malformation and the brain, coagulating any dural component of the arteriovenous malformation, achieving hemostasis in the bed following resection of the lesion. Laser however has not reduced appreciably the operating time or the blood loss. Moreover the laser has not solved the problem of the control of the small high-flow vessels on the deep surface of the malformation. These vessels would only be controlled with bipolar coagulation. Surgical results showed a worsening in 2 cases but neurologic deficits were considered secondary to the location of the lesion and not to the use of the laser. Hyperperfusion consequent to resection of the malformation was described in 2 cases. 2 arteriovenous malformations were located in the region of the motor strip and were resected without impairment of the neurologic status.

Our series is of 15 cases treated with Nd : YAG laser: 9 were supratentorial arteriovenous malformations located in the right temporo-parietal region (5 cases), left temporo-parietal region (2 cases) and right frontal region (2 cases). 3 were deep-seated arteriovenous malformations (2 intraventricular and 1 fed by the anterior perforating arteries on the left). 3 were infratentorial arteriovenous malformations located in the cerebellar region (1 case) and in brain stem (2 cases). According to angiographic and

Table 3. *Surgical Results in 15 Arteriovenous Malformations Operated with ND : YAG Laser*

	Number of patients with AVMs—15 cases*
Postoperative morbidity	
worsened	1
improved	6
Follow-up	
further partial or total recovery	7

* 8 patients were neurologically normal preoperatively and had no deficit after surgery.

operative findings extension of the nidus was estimated to be from 1 to 3 cm. Total removal of the malformation was achieved in all cases. Surgical results are reported in Table 3.

1.4. Conclusive Considerations

In our experience Nd:YAG laser was helpful in small arteriovenous malformations where total irradiation of the nidus is easy. The main indications are in critical areas of the brain.

Contrary to the traditional technique laser acts directly on pathological vessels of the nidus coagulating them without blood loss; isolation and coagulation of feeding arteries is avoided and there is no manipulation of the healthy tissue (Fig. 11).

The progressive conversion of the shunt flow in perfusion flow reduces the complication related to the hyperfusion as swelling, hyperemia, edema and sometimes hemorrhage.

In comparison with radiosurgery, producing delayed thrombosis of the nidus, the latency period for complete exclusion is shorter and side effects more predictable and limited to few mm.

In case of large arteriovenous malformations the problem is more complex because of the high flow and the alimentation by 2 or more main arteries and multiple feeding channels. In these cases the nidus cannot be entirely coagulated. Delayed thrombosis could be expected on the basis of the experimental data but, at present, there are no experiences to demonstrate the effectiveness of this.

2. Arterial Aneurysms

The reports in literature on the laser treatment of arterial aneurysms consist in the experimental study of Maira *et al.*[20] and in our clinical and experimental research[10–12]. We studied the effects of the laser light on the vessel wall in rabbit carotid arteries irradiated with CO_2, argon and Nd:YAG. As has been reported (see chapter: laser effect on normal vessels. Histological data) instantaneous shrinkage of the wall resulting in a diameter reduction of about 20% was noticed. Immediate occlusion was never observed. The most important results consisted in the increase of the elastic resistance of the wall (more than 50%) as demonstrated by the evaluation of tension/strain curves (Fig. 12). The vessel did not overstretch nor break when loaded at more than 600 mm Hg. These modifications of the elastic behaviour of the irradiated arteries persisted even after 2 months[11, 12]. The changes of the collagen fibers observed under electron microscope supported, from a morphological point of view the increase of the wall tension.

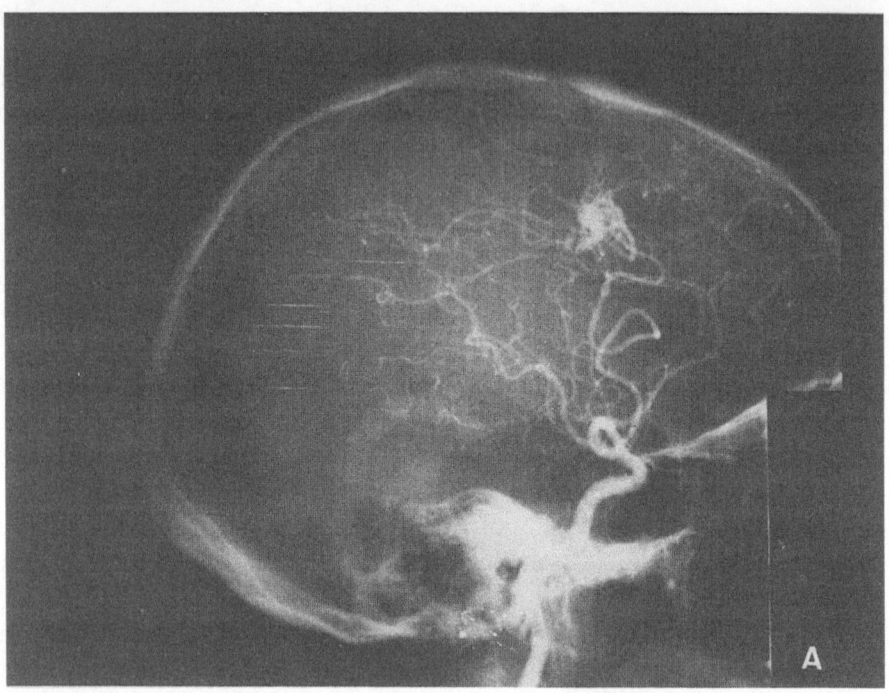

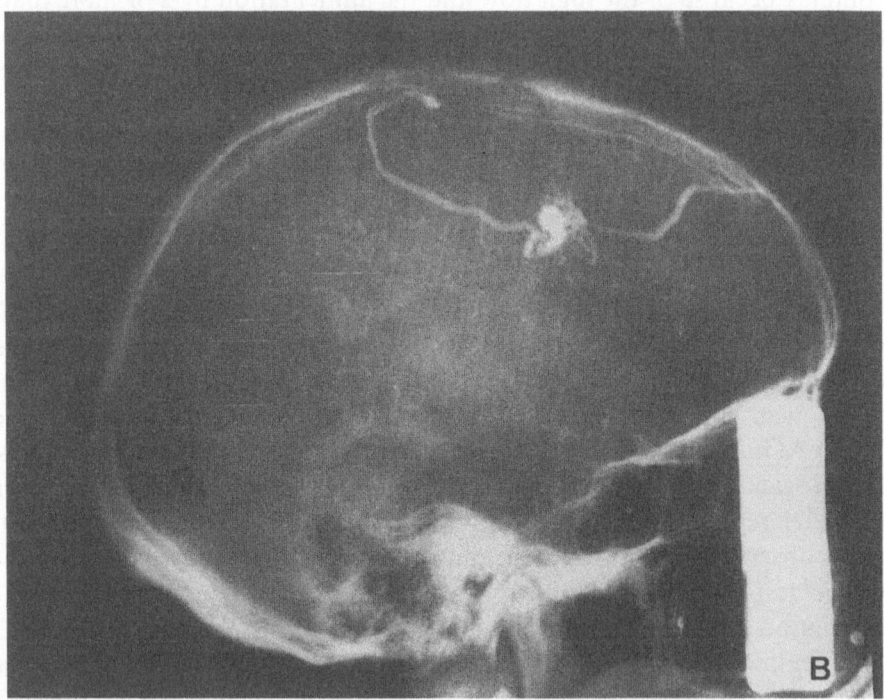

Fig. 11. Frontal arteriovenous malformation operated with Nd:YAG laser. Preoperative angiography: feeding channels (A) and venous outflow (B). Postoperative angiography: arterial (C) and venous (D) phase

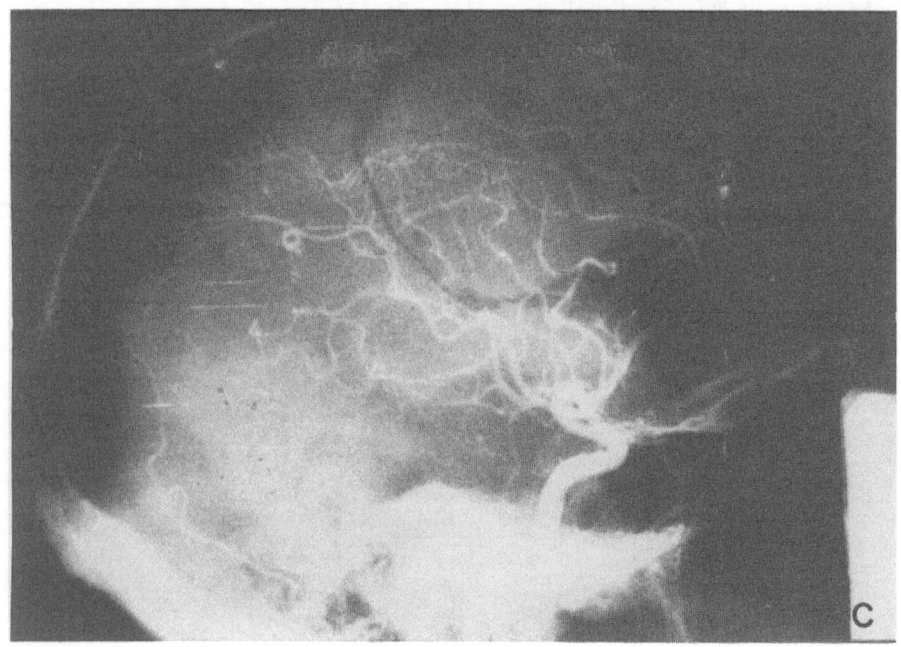

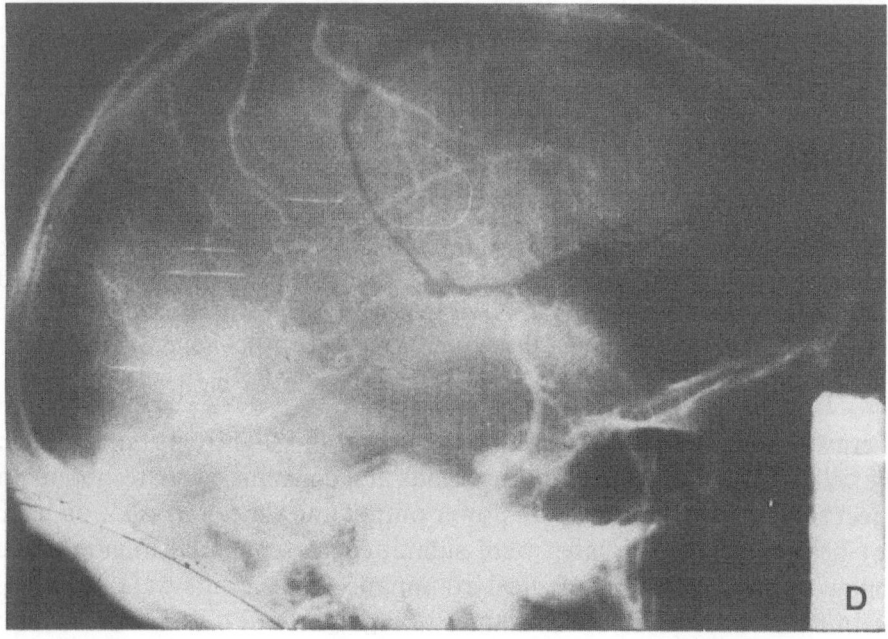

Figs. 11 C and D

Maira *et al.* [20] treated with argon laser 25 autologous aneurysms created on the carotid artery in rabbits by venous and arterial pouch grafts using microsurgical techniques. Aneurysm size ranged from 2×2 to 4×5 mm.

Continuous beam was used. Energy was 1.5 watts and spot diameter was set at 1 mm. Irradiation was applied to part or all of the aneurysm sac and

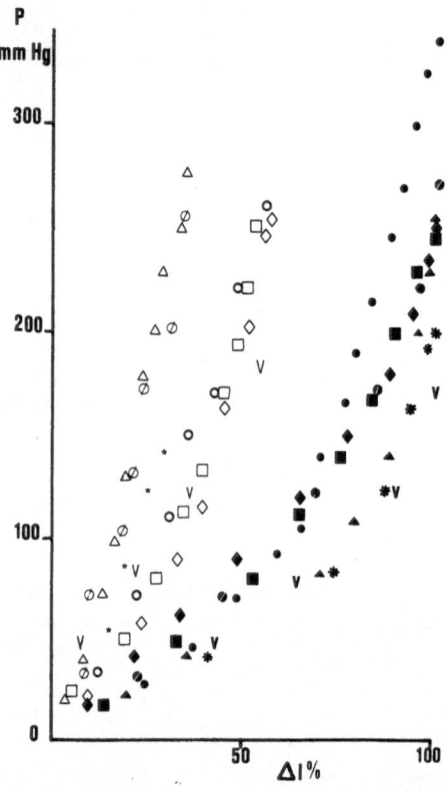

Fig. 12. Pressure versus percentage strain (seven experiments). On the right curve before laser, on the left curve after laser. The strain degree occurring for a fixed intraluminal pressure diminishes to $51 \pm 15\%$ after laser irradiation and therefore the stress opposing the strain increases correspondingly

energy was delivered until the wall became pale and slightly shrunken. Then the wall was irradiated for longer periods at a constant level "to obtain an effect similar to carbonization"; power output and time of irradiation have not been precised. All cases were submitted to sequential angiographic follow-up studies and histological examination and results were reported.

In 12 small aneurysms with diameter ranging from 2×2 to 2.5×3.5 mm: *total irradiation* of the sac (7 cases) produced complete exlusion in 4 cases (immediate in 2 cases, delayed in the others), incomplete occlusion in 3 cases (immediate in 1 case, delayed in the others);

	Symptoms of subarachnoid hemorrhage	CT scan	Multiple aneurysms	Approximate size at surgery	Perivascular hemorrhage infiltration of the wall	Results of the treatment
1st case: saccular aneurysm of the ACoA	present	blood in subarachnoid space: hemorrhage in both lateral ventricles	no	4 mm	present	exclusion demonstrated at angiography within 2 months
2nd case: saccular aneurysm of the ICA	present	blood in subarachnoid space: tetraventricular hemorrhage	no	4 mm	present	exclusion demonstrated at histologic control 45 days later
3rd case: junction aneurysm of the ICA	present	negative	no	3 mm	absent	exclusion demonstrated at angiography 7 days later
4th case: junction aneurysm of the ICA	present	blood in subarachnoid space	saccular aneurysm of the MCA	3 mm	absent	exclusion demonstrated at angiography 10 days later
5th case: junction aneurysm of the ICA	present	negative	saccular aneurysm of the vertebral artery	< 3 mm	absent	incomplete occlusion demonstrated at angiography 10 days later
6th case: saccular aneurysm of the ICA	present	blood in subarachnoid space	no	> 5 mm	present	incomplete occlusion demonstrated at angiography 13 days later
7th case: saccular aneurysm of the ICA	present	negative	no	2 mm	absent	no changes at angiography 15 days later
8th case: saccular aneurysm of the ACA	present	blood in subarachnoid space	no	4 mm	present	no changes at angiography 7 days later

partial irradiation of the sac to one side only (2 cases) produced immediate exclusion in 1 case and immediate incomplete occlusion in 1 case;

focal coagulation of the basis of the aneurysm (3 cases) produced exclusion in 2 cases (immediate in 1 case and delayed in the other) and immediate incomplete occlusion in 1 case.

In 13 large aneurysms with diameter ranging from 2.5 × 4.5 to 4 × 5 mm:

total irradiation of the sac (6 cases) produced delayed exclusion in 2 cases, delayed incomplete occlusion in 3 cases and 1 aneurysm was unchanged;

partial irradiation to one side only of the sac (3 cases) produced delayed exclusion in 2 cases and immediate incomplete occlusion in 1 case;

focal coagulation of the basis of the aneurysm (4 cases) produced exclusion in no case, immediate incomplete occlusion in 1 case and 3 cases were unchanged.

Better results were therefore obtained in small aneurysms (exclusion in 58% of cases, incomplete occlusion in 42% of cases) than in larger ones (exclusion in 31% of cases, incomplete occlusion in 38% of cases, no change in 31% of cases).

Authors conclude that in aneurysms treated by total irradiation of the sac almost 90% were either completely thrombosed or markedly reduced as consequence of intense fibrotic intramural reaction and endothelial hyperplasia. Even the limited application of the laser beam induced a dramatic fibrotic reaction in virtually all cases. Although fibrosis was found to involve histologically a limited segment of the parent artery a significant narrowing of the vessel, even after a delay as long as three months was never observed.

Our surgical experience is referred to 8 cases of arterial aneurysms treated with argon laser (Table 4). Laser beam was defocused to a spot size of 2–3 mm and irradiation of the exposed areas of the sac was delivered in a continuous mode for 10–15 seconds at power from 2 to 5 watts. To reduce the internal pressure on the wall intraoperative hypotension (80–90 mm Hg) was used. The immediate effect of the irradiation consisted in whitening and slight shrinkage of the wall; in one case carbonization of the sac and neck was produced; in no case instantaneous exclusion was obtained. Postoperative angiography was performed after 6 days and 2 months in 1 patient (case 1) and from the 7th to 15th day in the other patients (case 2–8) (Table 4). Complete exclusion was noticed in 3 cases (cases 1, 3, and 4); partial exclusion in 3 cases (cases 2, 5, and 6) and no change in 2 cases (cases 7 and 8) (Fig. 13). Patency of the parent artery was preserved in all cases.

Case 2 was admitted in deep coma with tetraventricular hemorrhage. Angiography 15 days after surgery showed a slight reduction in volume of the dome. Patient died 45 days later and histological examen demonstrated complete exclusion of the aneurysm (Figs. 14 and 15); parent artery was preserved. In this case, as in case 1, exclusion was demonstrated after a delay

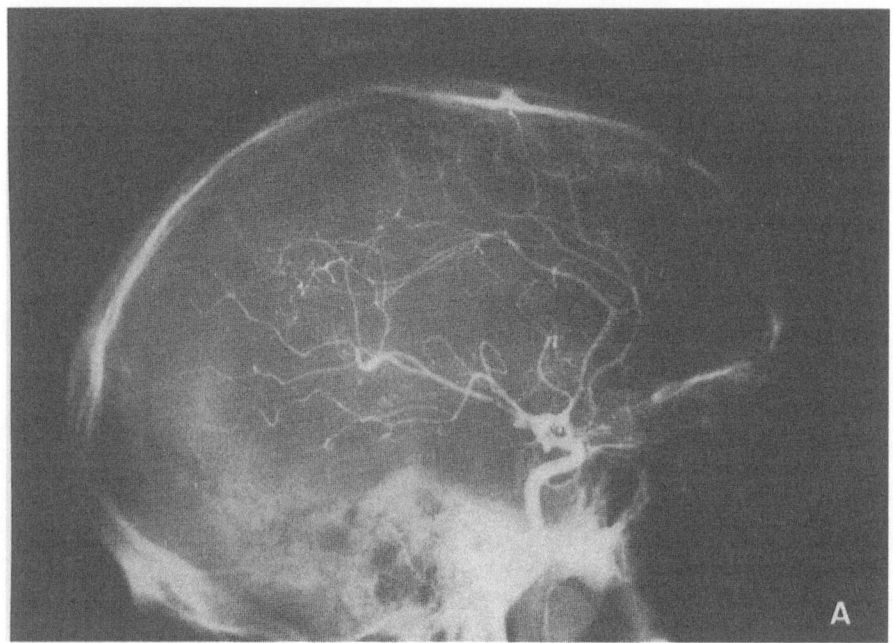

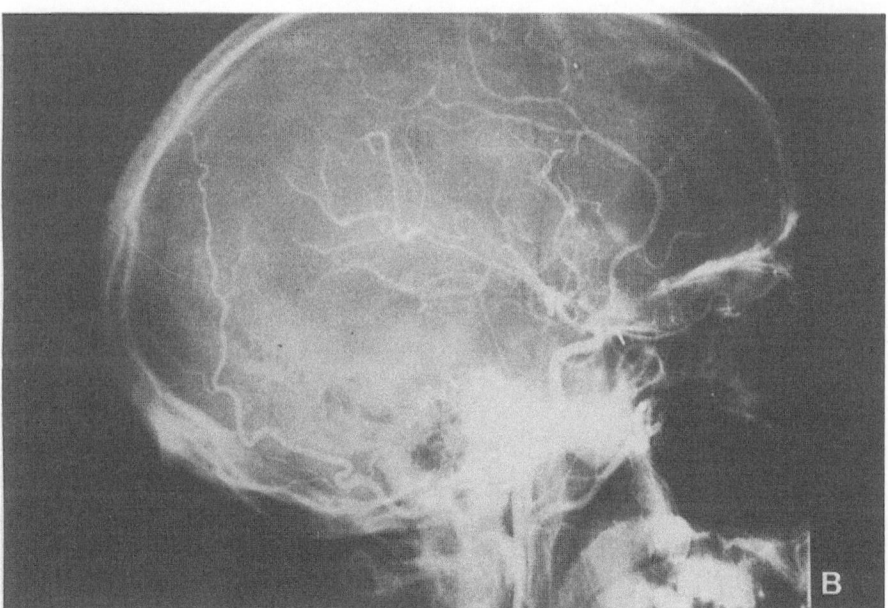

Fig. 13. Multiple saccular arterial aneurysms: aneurysmal dilatation of the internal carotid artery irradiated with argon laser; saccular aneurysm of the middle cerebral artery treated in the traditional way. (A preoperative angiography; B postoperative angiography)

V. A. Fasano:

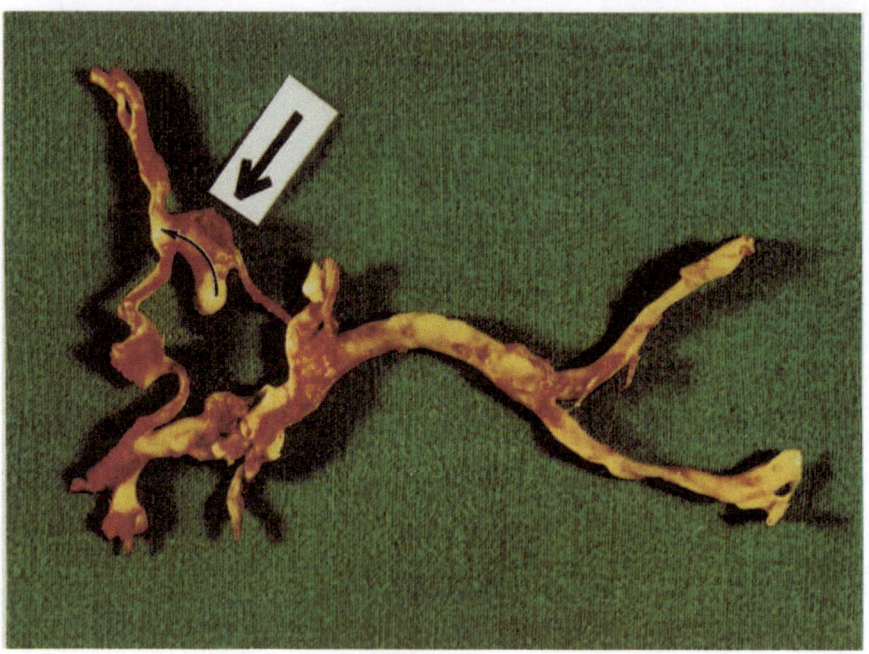

Fig. 14. Autoptic examen: circle of Willis. Arrow indicates the saccular aneurysm irradiated with argon laser

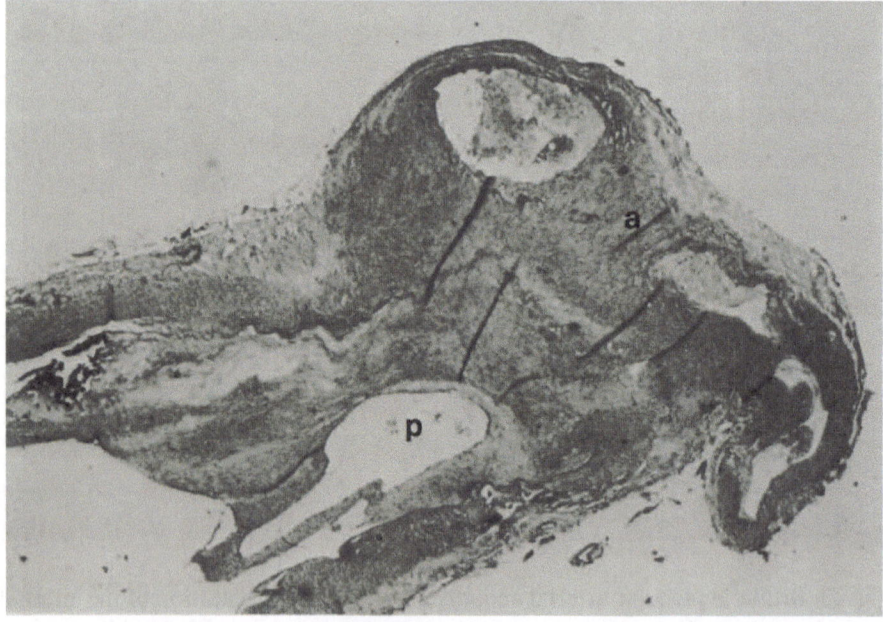

Fig. 15. Saccular aneurysm irradiated with argon laser. Histological finding. Hematos. Eos (*p* parent artery; *a* aneurysm)

as long as 1 month and therefore results are not conclusive in the other 4 cases submitted to early angiography only.

Our results show that:

a) A delayed exclusion can be achieved within 2 months in both bled and junction aneurysms.

b) The technique does not produce postoperative complications (in no case worsening has been noticed).

c) Laser, increasing elastic resistance of the wall, reduces the risk of rupture of the aneurysm. Symptoms of recurrence of the subarachnoid hemorrhage have not been observed in any case after a 4-year follow-up.

d) There are not differences between small and large aneurysms; in both exclusion has been noticed in 50% of cases, incomplete occlusion in 25% of cases and no change in 25% of cases.

The histological characteristics of the aneurysm wall and the hemodynamic pattern play an important role in the laser treatment. In junction aneurysms and small saccular aneurysms the wall is composed of loose fibrous tissue similar to the adventitia of the parent artery; when aneurysm grow larger than 4 mm, the walls become collagenous with few cells and thin portions develop in their domes. After aneurysmal rupture, surrounding the clot a fals sac may be formed which becomes progressively transformed into a hyalinized, fairly acellular collagenous wall[26, 28].

The relationship between volume and size of the orifice of small saccular aneurysms plays an important part in intraaneurysmal hemodynamic and can therefore influence the natural evolution; Black and German showed in experimental saccular aneurysms that when the ratio of the neck to sac volume was reduced to 1:25, spontaneous thrombosis could occur[3].

Because wall of most aneurysms is collagenous[26–28] and can therefore undergo heat induced contraction by tightening of collagen fibers, independently from the complete exclusion, laser irradiation may produce a strengthening of the wall thus avoiding further growth and rupture.

Miscellaneous Indications for Laser Surgery

1. Syringohydromyelia: Laser Fenestration

The CO_2 laser produces a precise and theoretically permanent fenestration into the syrinx, while minimizing adjacent tissue damage.

The surgical technique consists in coagulation of the cordal surface at dorsal root entry zone with argon laser and then laser fenestration is made with defocused CO_2 laser of the syrinx through the dorsolateral fasciculus.

Brown[5] reports an intraoperative improvement in somatosensory evoked potentials in 9 cases. In addition, clinical and physiologic improvement have persisted postoperatively with the longest period of follow-up being 33 months, the effectiveness of laser fenestration coming from vaporizing, removing tissue and sealing the edges of the fenestration to prevent scarring and maintain patency rather than cutting.

Our series is of 6 cases operated with CO_2 laser; results after 3 years of follow-up are good.

2. Chronic Pain of Spinal Origin: Dorsal Root Entry Zone Lesions

The laser is used to make lesions in the dorsal root entry zone (DREZ) in patients with chronic pain of spinal origin.

Powers et al.[24] have used argon laser, attached to an operating microscope to produce a series of punctate lesions in DREZ on the affected side. The beam was angled at 30° with respect to a perpendicular from the midline of the spinal cord and used at 6–7 watts for 1 second with a spot size of 150 microns.

In 13 patients treated in this way results were encouraging at follow-up ranging between 1 and 8 months. The authors report the advantages of the laser over the use of radiofrequency probe, as follows:

a) Very little tissue injury surrounding the lesion (not exceeding 0.15 mm).

b) Lesions more accurately placed.

Similar results have been reported by Levy and coworkers with CO_2 laser in three patients[19]. They used a laser pulsed duration of 0.1 second at approximately 20 watts. The beam was angled at about a 25° to the vertical midline of the cord. The authors concluded that the technique does result in highly reproducible lesions with very low morbidity due to lesion spillover.

The preliminary results reported by Nashold and Walker[22] on the effects of the laser on the normal DREZ of cats are important. In one series of cats the use of the laser on the spinal cord in 62.5% of cases resulted in development of a syrinx in the central part of the cord after a 1 to 4 week survival period. This pathology has not been noted in similar studies with the radionics thermal electrode system.

3. Discectomy

Nucleus pulposus can be vaporized with CO_2 laser defocused at low power. The advantages and disadvantages of the method are:

a) Lack of tugging or pulling on loose fragments of nucleus pulposus.

b) Less danger of perforating the anulus and damaging the structures anterior to the vertebral column.

c) Less chance of regeneration of the disc.

d) Interference with the fusion process after the graft is inserted; laser technique should therefore not be used in cases of interbody fusion.

References

1. Bartal, A. D., Heilbronn, Y. D., Avran, J., Razon, N., 1982: Carbon dioxide laser surgery of basal meningiomas. Surg. Neurol. *17*, 90–95.
2. Beck, O. J., 1980: The use of the Nd : YAG and the CO_2 laser in neurosurgery. Neurosurg. Rev. *3*, 261–266.
3. Black, S., German, W. J., 1960: Observations on the relationship between the volume and the size of the orifice of experimental aneurysms. J. Neurosurg. *17*, 894–899.
4. Bleehan, N. M., 1982: Hyperthermia in the treatment of cancer. Br. J. Cancer *45* (suppl. V), 96–100.
5. Brown, J. T., 1982: Laser fenestration for syringohydromyelia. In: Proceedings of the Congress on Laser Neurosurgery II, p. 237. Chicago.
6. Cerullo, L. J., 1981: CO_2 laser for extraaxial neoplasms: technique. In: Proceedings of the I American Congress on Laser Neurosurgery, p. 66. Chicago.
7. Edwards, M. S., Boggan, J. E., Bolger, C. A., Davis, R. L., 1984: Effect of microsurgical and CO_2 laser and argon laser resection on recurrence of the intracerebral 9 L rat gliosarcoma. Neurosurg. *14*, 52–56.
8. Edwards, M. S. B., Boggan, J. E., Fuller, T. A., 1983: The laser in neurological surgery. J. Neurosurg. *59*, 555–566.
9. Fasano, V. A., Benech, F., Ponzio, R. M., 1982: Observations on the simultaneous use of CO_2 and Nd : YAG lasers in neurosurgery. Lasers Surg. Med. *2*, 155–161.
10. Fasano, V. A., Urciuoli, R., Ponzio, R. M., 1982: Photocoagulation of cerebral arteriovenous malformations and arterial aneurysms with the Nd : YAG or argon laser: Preliminary results in twelve patients. Neurosurg. *11*, 754–760.
11. Fasano, V. A., Ponzio, R. M., Benech, F., Sicuro, M., 1983: Effects of laser sources (Argon, Nd : YAG, CO_2) on the elastic resistance of the vessel wall: histological and physical study. Lasers Surg. Med. *2*, 45–54.
12. Fasano, V. A., Ponzio, R. M., Benech, F., 1983: Effects of laser sources on the elastic resistance of the vessel walls. In: Neodymium-YAG Laser in Medicine and Surgery (Joffe, S., ed.), pp. 266–270. New York-Amsterdam-Oxford: Elsevier.
13. Handa, H., Takeuchi, J., 1983: Experiences with CO_2 and Nd : YAG lasers in neurosurgery. In: New Frontiers in Laser Medicine and Surgery (Atsumi, K., ed.), pp. 196–206. Amsterdam-Oxford-Princeton: Excerpta Medica.
14. Hara, M., Okada, J., Takeuchi, K., Takizawa, T., Matsumoto, M., 1979: Evaluation of brain laser surgery. In: Laser Surgery III, part one (Kaplan, I., ed.), pp. 158–165. Tel-Aviv: OT-PAZ.
15. Heppner, F., Ascher, P. W., 1979: CO_2 laser surgery of the spinal cord. In: Laser Surgery III, part one (Kaplan, I., ed.), pp. 57–59. Tel-Aviv: OT-PAZ.
16. Inaba, Y., Fujimoto, T., Kuroiwa, T., Fujiwara, K., 1979: CO_2 laser microsurgery for brain tumor. In: Laser Surgery III, part one (Kaplan, I., ed.), pp. 119–127. Tel-Aviv: OT-PAZ.
17. Kelly, P. J., Alker, G. I., Jr., Goerss, S., 1982: Computer-assisted stereotactic laser microsurgery for the treatment of intracranial neoplasms. Neurosurg. *11*, 324–331.

18. Kelly, P. J., Alker, G. I., Jr., Zoll, J. G., 1982: A microstereotactic approach to deep-seated arteriovenous malformations. Surg. Neurol. 7, 260–262.

19. Levy, W. J., Nutkiewicz, A., Ditmore, M., Watts, C., 1983: Laser-induced dorsal root entry zone lesions for pain control. J. Neurosurg. 59, 884–886.

20. Maira, G., Mohr, G., Panisset, K., Hardy, J., 1979: Laser photocoagulation for treatment of experimental aneurysms. J. Microsurg. 1, 137–147.

21. Mattos Pimenta, L. H., Mattos Pimenta, A., 1979: Evaluation of difficult placed meningiomas operated with CO_2 laser. In: Laser Surgery III, part one (Kaplan, I., ed.), pp. 145–146. Tel-Aviv: OT-PAZ.

22. Nashold, B. S., Jr., Walker, J. S., 1984: Laser effect on spinal cord. J. Neurosurg. 60, 870.

23. Perria, C., Francaviglia, N., Borzone, M., Chinnici, A., Piano, E., Pacini, P., 1983: The value and limitations of the CO_2 laser in neurosurgery. Neurochirurgia 26, 6–11.

24. Powers, S. K., Edwards, M. S. B., Boggan, J. E., Pitts, L. H., Gutin, P. H., Hosobuchi, Y., Adams, J. E., Wilson, L. B., 1984: Use of the argon surgical laser in neurosurgery. J. Neurosurg. 60, 523–530.

25. Robertson, J. H., Clark, W., Robertson, J. T., Gardner, L., Shea, M., 1983: Use of the carbon dioxide laser for acoustic tumor surgery. Neurosurg. 12, 286–290.

26. Sekhar, L. N., Heros, R. C., 1981: Origin, growth, and rupture of saccular aneurysms: A review. Neurosurg. 8, 248–260.

27. Strait, T. A., Robertson, J. H., Clark, W., 1982: Use of carbon dioxide laser in the operative management of intracranial meningiomas: a report of twenty cases. Neurosurg. 10, 464–467.

28. Suzuki, J., Ohara, H., 1978: Clinicopathological study of cerebral aneurysms. J. Neurosurg. 48, 505–514.

29. Svaasand, L. O., Ellingsen, R., 1983: Penetration of laser irradiation in neoplastic and normal human brain tissue. In: Proceedings of the Congresso Nazionale Società Italiana di Laser Chirurgia e Applicazioni Biomediche, p. 41. Milano.

30. Takizawa, T., Yamazaki, T., Matsumoto, M., Sano, K., 1979: Laser surgery of brain tumors which were difficult to extirpate with the conventional modalities. Laser Surgery III, part one (Kaplan, I., ed.), pp. 133–144. Tel-Aviv: OT-PAZ.

31. Takizawa, T., 1978: Laser surgery of brain tumors. No Shinkei geka 9, 743.

32. De Tommasi, A., Occhiogrosso, M., Vailati, G., Bladassarre, G., Cingolani, A., 1983: Previsione dell'effetto di interazione laser-neoplasia cerebrale mediante studio foto-acustico dei coefficienti di assorbimento ottico di vari oncotipi alla lunghezza d'onda Ar + laser. In: Proceedings of the Congresso Nazionale Società Italiana di Laser Chirurgia e Applicazioni Biomediche, p. 37. Milano.

33. Whakaki, M., Yokoto, H., Tamino, H., Nimsakul, N., Osada, M., Ishizuki, M., Izn, S., 1979: Thermal effect of the CO_2 laser and our technic in dealing with it. In: Laser Surgery III, part one (Kaplan, I., ed.), pp. 27–42. Tel-Aviv: OT-PAZ.

34. Welch, A. J., Motamedi, M., Gonzales, A., 1983: Evaluation of cooling techniques for the protection of the epidermis during Nd-YAG laser

irradiation of the skin. In: Neodymium-YAG Laser in Medicine and Surgery (Joffe, S., ed.), pp. 195–204. New York-Amsterdam-Oxford: Elsevier.

35. Wharen, R. E., Jr., Anderson, R. E., Scheithauer, B., Sundt, T. E., Jr., 1984: The Nd : YAG laser in neurosurgery. Part 1. Laboratory investigations: dose-related biological response of neural tissue. J. Neurosurg. 60, 531–539.

36. Wharen, R. E., Jr., Anderson, R. E., Sundt, T. E., Jr., 1984: The Nd : YAG laser in neurosurgery. J. Neurosurg. 60, 540–547.

37. Yamagami, T., Handa, H., Takeuchi, J., Hashimoto, N., Taki, W., Yonekawa, Y., Otsuki, H., 1984: Extent of thermal penetration of Nd-YAG laser. Histological considerations. Neurosurg. Rev. 7, 165–170.

Contact Laser

Victor A. Fasano

Institute of Neurosurgery, University of Turin (Italy)

Contents

Introduction 140
Contact Delivery Systems 140
Results 142
    1. Experimental Data 142
    2. Preliminary Applications in Neurosurgery 142
Conclusion 143
References 144

Introduction

The possibility to operate within brain without any contact with the tissue is generally considered one of the main advantages of the laser which is particularly important in small deep-seated lesions to limit side effects on adjacent healthy tissue.

Conventional focused noncontact lasers require, however, high power levels to be effective with significant backscatter and thermal conductivity; most of all tactile feedback is lost. For these reasons contact artificial delivery systems have been developed in the last months and recently introduced in surgery. The scalpel laser is the first tool of contact laser surgery which has already replaced the radiofrequency unit. The precision of the surgical maneuver, together with the minimal tissue damage and the excellent hemostatic and cutting properties make this instrument, taking over the main characteristics of laser sources keeping the tactile feedback, a new instrument for neurosurgery.

Contact Delivery Systems

The ideal material for a contact laser should transmit the laser beam, avoid tissue adhesion and have a low thermal conductivity. Recent experiments showed that a single artificial sapphire crystal of Al_2O_3 transmits laser beam well, provided that air bubbles are absent from the crystal.

The characteristics of this highly transmissible sapphire, when compared with quartz crystal, show an higher melting point (2,050 °C versus 1,600 °C), elastic coefficient ($5.0 \cdot 10^{-6}$ kg/cm² versus 0.76), hardness (9 MOHS versus

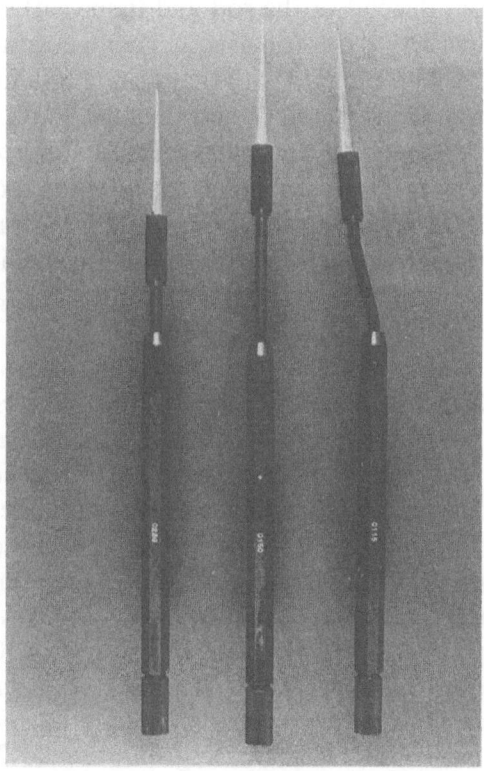

Fig. 1. Laser rod showing handle and sapphire tip

7), and a reduced thermal conductivity (0.0016 g · cal · cm² · sec at 40 °C versus 9.0158).

Sapphire conoids of different size and diameter (0.2; 0.4; 0.6) are disposable. A holder is required to connect the rod to the optical quartz fiber (Fig. 1). For cooling, the end of the quartz fiber gas is delivered to the end of the holder removing at the same time the smoke from the field of vision. Laser guiding beam allows the operator to direct the incision.

Procedure requires only to keep the end of the rod in contact with the tissue during incision. The incisional capability depends on the laser power input and the diameter of the distal end of the rod.

Results

1. Experimental Data

Comparisons were made between the laser beam emitting from the quartz fiber and from the laser rod (Daikuzono et al.)[1].

The laser beam emitting from the laser rod had a greater divergence than the beam emitting from the quartz fiber with a concentric circular pattern. Due to the large divergence of the beam, power density decreased rapidly as the distance between the end of the rod and tissue surface increased. The damage to the liver with the laser rod used as a contact cutting instrument at a power of 20 watts was compared with that caused by a noncontact quartz fiber held 1 cm from the tissue at a power of 60 watts. Contact cutting decreased the deep tissue damage in both vertical and horizontal directions. Furthermore, the power density at the distal tip of the rod was sufficiently high that the resulting rapid vaporization of the tissue facilitated incision with less production of smoke. The degree of divergence calculated by geometric optics revealed that noncontact laser beam irradiation from an optical quartz fiber involves considerable backscattering. The laser rod has no sideward irradiation from the surface of the tapered conical portions and all of the irradiation is from the distal end. Because of this characteristics the useful energy of contact irradiation is much greater decreasing most of the backscattering of laser beam. For these reasons the energy required to produce a cut is considerably reduced. For example the Nd : YAG laser power settings are approximately 25 to 33 percent of those required with a noncontact quartz fiber. Preliminary histological data on canine stomach mucosa changes after incision of the mucosa with Nc : YAG laser rod have shown that at low power (8–10 watts) and short duration (0.5 sec) only mild localized epithelial destruction occurs. At power of 24 watts depth of the lesion *increased passed to the muscolaris mucosae to the muscle*. A similar increase in depth was observed increasing duration to 2 sec keeping the power at 8 watts[1].

This means that as in a normal scalpel lesion depth can be changed easily.

2. Preliminary Applications in Neurosurgery

Our preliminary experience is related to 10 cases operated with Argon or Nd : YAG laser scalpel: 4 basal meningiomas and 6 invasive gliomas involving vessels and nerves. Tumor remnants, after debulking of the mass by ultrasonic aspirator, and small neoplasms are first vaporized with CO_2 laser to produce shrinkage of the tissue and hemostasis of the smaller vessels. Dissection is then made with laser scalpel:

In highly vascularized tumors the Nd : YAG laser is used to ensure a rapid maneuver without carbonization and thermal extension to the adjacent healthy tissue and reduced blood loss. Power changes from 5 to 10 watts and radiation is delivered in continuous wave (Fig. 2).

Argon is used at 5 watts of power in continuous to dissect safely tumoral tissue from vessels and nerves.

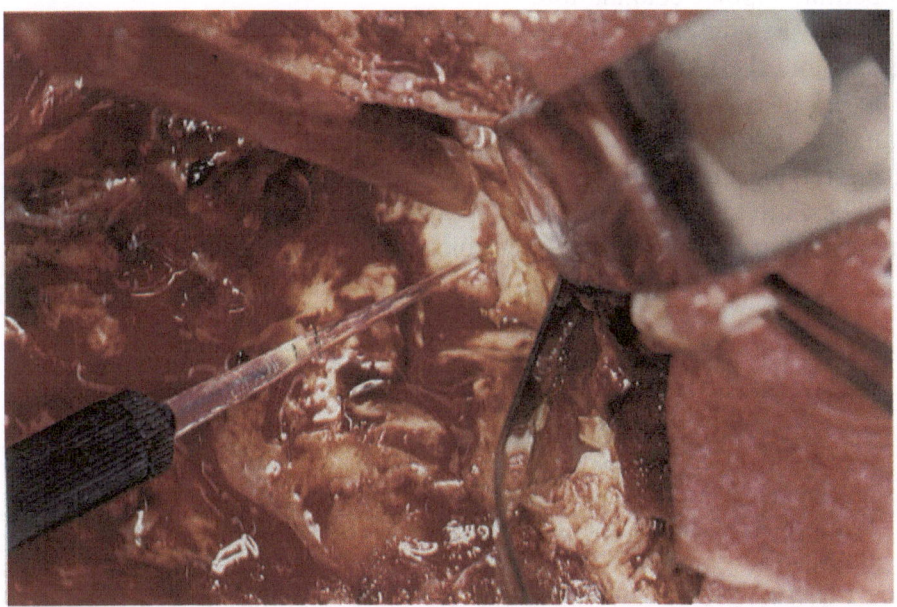

Fig. 2. Removal of a brain tumor with the laser rod

Both Argon and Nd : YAG scalpels can be used for vessel coagulation by a direct contact of the tip[2].

Conclusion

Scalpel laser is a real new development of the laser surgery. In comparison with conventional noncontact lasers it allows greather sharpness and rapidity of surgical maneuvers and reduced thermal damage. Nd : YAG in particular turns into a cutting tool associating a sharp incision similar to that produced by CO_2 to a more complete hemostasis.

Because of the homogeneous coagulation around the incised part there are no carbonized debris and smoke. Tissue damage is minimal and adhesion never occurs, due to the high temperature at the end of the rod.

Finally the reduced backscattering of the beam and the low thermal conductivity increase the thermal efficiency, reducing the need of high power irradiation.

At present only lasers delivered by optic fibers are available for contact laser surgery, the new development of optic fibers suitable for CO_2 will make the use of this source possible in the future.

A future application of the contact laser is the laser coagulator which will substitute bipolar coagulation.

Main advantages are the lack of sticking, carbonization of surrounding tissues and the control of the uniformity and amount of energy delivered. The risk of vessel perforation is moreover reduced because a similar effect can be obtained with less energy in comparison with traditional coagulators using radiofrequencies.

These advantages could make an application of this instrument in the surgery of arterial aneurysms possible.

References

1. Daikuzono, N., Joffe, S. N.: Artificial Sapphire Probe for Contact Photocoagu-lation and Tissue Vaporization with the Nd:YAG Laser. Medicine Instru-mentation (in press) 1985.
2. Fasano, V. A., Ponzio, R. M., Lanotte, M. M., Gawlik, J.: Prime osservazioni preliminari sull'uso del laser scalpel ad Argon ed a Nd:YAG in neurochirurgia. Proceedings of the International Congress on Laser in Medicine and Surgery. Bologna, June 26–28, 1985 (in press).

The Argon Laser and Its Application in Neurological Surgery

MICHAEL S. B. EDWARDS[1] and JAMES E. BOGGAN[2]

[1] Departments of Neurological Surgery and Pediatrics, University of California,
San Francisco, California, and
[2] The Department of Neurosurgery, University of California, Davis, California
(U.S.A.)

Contents

Introduction 145
Technique and Operative Results 147
    Intracranial Extraaxial Tumors 147
    Intracranial Intraaxial Lesions 149
    Intraspinal Lesions 150
    Pain Procedures 150
    Syringomyelia 151
Discussion 151
Acknowledgments 152
References 152

Introduction

Although the argon (Ar) ion laser has been available for many years and has been widely used in ophthalmology and dermatology, its use in neurological surgery has been limited. The recent availability of high powered Ar lasers that can rapidly vaporize tissue, transmit light through fiberoptic delivery systems, and have variable and small spot diameters has allowed us to use the laser beneficially for a variety of neurosurgical procedures.

The Ar ion laser operates in the blue-green portion of the visual spectrum. Its efficiency is low (0.1%), and 1,000 watts of electrical energy are needed to produce one watt of laser energy output. The unit must be water-cooled (approximately 10 l/minute) to dissipate heat generated by the conversion of electrical to light energy. Because the high power units require a 208 volt, triple phase, 00 amp line and must be water-cooled, these Ar lasers are not portable. Modern Ar lasers can produce 20 watts of power at the laser tube and deliver 12–14 watts to tissue. We used a 16 watt continuous wave Ar ion surgical laser system (Cooper Laseronics model 770 AMPL) for clinical and laboratory work. This model operates between 488 to 514.5 nm; approximately 80% of the power output is available at these wavelengths. The laser is coupled to the operating microscope via a fiberoptic micromanipulator delivery system. The beam is a combination of TEM_{00} and TEM_{01} mode structures. The direction and spot size of the laser beam are controlled, respectively, by a joystick and a focus knob on the micromanipulator. The joystick has the ability to decrease physiologic tremor by a factor of 20:1. The laser beam spot diameter can be continuously varied between 0.15 and 1.5 mm. The power output, pulse duration, and repetition rate of the laser are controlled from the laser console. Because light from an Ar laser is transmitted through the cornea and lens of the eye and is rapidly absorbed by the pigment in the retina, protective eyewear or integral eye filters in the micromanipulator are required during its use.

The effect of the interaction between the Ar laser and tissue is intermediate between that of the carbon dioxide (CO_2) and neodyium:YAG (Nd:YAG) lasers; both absorption by tissue chromophores and scattering play important roles. In this case, the photobiological "sieve effect", which occurs when any significant chromophore is compartmentalized as is hemoglobin in red blood cells, leads to an underestimation of the tissue absorption coefficient and extinction length. The measured transmission of the Ar laser into human brain is less than 0.5 mm[8].

The depth of lesions produced in rat brain by CO_2 and Ar laser beams with equal high-energy density (5,000 joules/cm^2) is the same. The CO_2 laser can vaporize more tissue, however, and produces a thinner layer of homogeneous coagulation. The Ar laser beam is highly absorbed by hemoglobin, melanin, and cytochromes, and absorption coefficients approach that of the CO_2 laser in tissue water. The Ar laser is more hemostatic than the CO_2 laser but less so than the Nd:YAG laser. Because of selective absorption in hemoglobin, however, at low power densities a selective coagulation of vessels can occur with minimal direct effect on surrounding tissue[5].

Based on our laboratory experience and the benefit of increased hemostasis and fiberoptic delivery afforded by the Ar laser, we began using an Ar surgical laser in June of 1981. Our experience obtained in 93 surgical procedures (June 1984) is listed in Table 1.

Table 1. *Experience with the Ar Laser in 93 Neurosurgical Procedures*

Procedure	Very helpful (72)	Helpful (16)	Not helpful (5)
Craniotomy			
Intraaxial tumors			
Glioma	4	3	—
Metastatic	3	1	1
Hemangioblastoma	1	2	—
Medullablastoma/ependymoma	4	2	1*
Cerebellar astrocytoma	4	–	—
Brain stem astrocytoma	—	1	—
Miscellaneous	3	—	—
Arteriovenous malformation	3	—	1
Hydrocephalus	1	1	—
Extraaxial tumors			
Acoustic neuroma	5	—	—
Meningioma	7	1	—
Craniopharyngioma	2	—	—
Miscellaneous	1	—	—
Laminectomy			
Spinal cord tumors	11	—	—
Pain procedures			
Dorsal root entry zone	17	3	2*
Comissural myelotomy	1	—	—
Syringomelia	3	2	—
Transsphenoidal			
Tumor	2	—	—

Very helpful: surgical procedure performed better than with standard microsurgical techniques. *Helpful:* surgical procedure performed as well as with standard microsurgical techniques. Some aspects of the procedure, however, were improved by used of the laser. *Not helpful:* no advantage over standard microsurgical procedure, or equipment failure*.

Technique and Operative Results

Intracranial Extraaxial Tumors

The Ar laser was used for the resection of 18 extraaxial supra- and infratentorial lesions for which proximity or attachment to important neural structures necessitated a particularly gentle surgical technique. For some larger tumors, the Ar laser was used only for resection of the portion of the tumor involving critical structures. In most cases the laser produced essentially hemostatic vaporization of tumor, which allowed resection in cerebrospinal fluid (CSF)-containing spaces, minimized brain retraction, and decreased manipulation of vital structures.

The first step in laser-aided resection of an extraaxial tumor is the coagulation of the tumor surface with a defocused low power density beam. This technique produces thrombosis (coagulation) of superficial blood vessels and shrinkage and retraction of the tumor capsule away from adjacent structures. Vaporization (debulking) of the tumor is then performed using a high power density-large spot diameter beam. In some large tumors a high power density (small spot diameter) beam was used to incise tumor in a piecemeal fashion. By gutting the central portion of the tumor, the thin rind of tumor capsule can be delivered into the operative field and dissected from surrounding neural structures, after which the capsule can be vaporized or excised. This technique allows minimal manipulation of surrounding structures. Residual tumor attached to cranial nerves or vessels is vaporized using short duration pulses (less than 250 msec) and small spot diameters, thereby avoiding manipulation and traction injury.

Neurilemomas of the 8th and 5th cranial nerves were vaporized off the nerve of origin without traction. Five acoustic neurilemomas were totally removed without injury to the facial nerve in any patient. During vaporization of tumor, a suction device to aspirate smoke is usually the only instrument necessary in the operative field. Thus, wide exposures and excessive brain retraction are generally avoided. Decreased manipulation of tumor tissue is aided by the coagulation effect of the laser that produces retraction of tissue, which tends to deliver tumor into the operative field. For 18 extraaxial tumors (Table 1), the laser was judged to be very helpful (a better surgical result than could have been obtained by standard microneurosurgical techniques) in seventeen procedures, and in one patient the laser was judged to be useful (equal to standard microneurosurgical techniques).

Two children with craniopharyngiomas extending into the third ventricle were operated on through a transcallosal approach. A fine spot diameter beam was used to incise the corpus callosum and to coagulate and vaporize the intraventricular portion of the tumor. A segment of the septum pellucidum was vaporized to allow flow of CSF between the two lateral ventricles. Because of the high transmission through water of light from the Ar laser, the presence of CSF does not alter the effect of Ar laser on tumor removal.

The laser was used in conjunction with the cavitron ultrasonic aspirator (Cooper Laseronics) for the excision of 8 meningiomas that were in critical locations. In seven of these tumors a complete removal was obtaining using techniques described above. One tentorial meningioma that extended into the cerebellopontine angle, however, was extremely vascular and difficult to remove because of bleeding. This "sinusoidal type" of tumor was the only extraaxial lesion for which the laser was felt to be only "helpful". Large or calcified lesions can be removed only slowly using the Ar laser. Spot sizes of more than 2 mm in diameter produce low power densities and do not provide rapid vaporization. Small spot diameters, however, may be used with a technique in which pieces of tumor tissue are excised rather than vaporizing the tumor bed.

Intracranial Intraaxial Lesions

Thirty-six patients were operated upon for intracranial intraaxial lesions (Table 1). In 23 patients the laser was judged to be very helpful, in ten patients helpful, and in 3 patients not helpful (this includes one instance of equipment failure).

Seven gliomas were resected with the argon laser because they appeared to be hypervascular on preoperative angiograms. The pial surface vessels were selectively coagulated under low power (1–2 watts) and then a cortical incision was made with a 150 μ spot diameter. Because of the large tumor size, the limited power output (approximately 10 watts at the tissue surface), and the relative small size of the largest Ar laser spot (1.5 mm), tumor excision by vaporization alone is impractical. Friable tumor is suctioned away or removed using the ultrasonic aspirator and the Ar laser is used to coagulate small bleeding vessels in the tumor bed, and to cut firm, fibrous portions of tumor. Using this technique, relatively rapid tumor excision with minimal blood loss is possible. Hemostasis of the tumor bed is accomplished by using a large defocused laser spot size and low power density to coagulate tumor vessels under constant saline irrigation. In general, only blood vessels less than 2 mm in diameter can be coagulated readily with the Ar laser. Despite this decreased manipulation of surrounding brain during laser resection, we found the laser provided no particular advantage for use in the excision of gliomas, nor did the laser affect long-term prognosis.

The Ar laser was used to excise 13 intraaxial infratentorial lesions that either extended into the brain stem or bordered on the 4th ventricle. The Ar laser allowed hemostatic tumor removal with decreased manipulation and tissue dissection within the brainstem without changes in vital signs or increased neurologic deficit. Laser resection was most helpful for lesions that extended into the brain stem.

The Ar laser was used for 4 arteriovenous malformations (AVMs). The laser was helpful for the removal of three low-flow, partially calcified AVMs, but was of no benefit for the removal of a large, high-flow AVM of the temporal lobe. Another patient with a solid hemangioblastoma of the right sylvian fissure was successfully treated by coagulation of the external surface of the tumor under iced saline irrigation, which caused the tumor to shrink and allowed nonmanipulative dissection of the tumor away from surrounding brain.

In one instance the Ar laser was used to treat an infant with loculated ventricles secondary to ventriculitis. In this patient a rigid 1.2 mm fiberoptic endoscope was placed into the atrium of the lateral ventricle and the laser fiber passed through a side-port in the endoscope. The septae within the ventricles were fenestrated and the choroid plexus coagulated. This allowed the removal of 3 ventricular catheters that were replaced by a single catheter inserted through the fenestrations.

Intraspinal Lesions

Eleven patients underwent myelotomy and removal of an intramedullary spinal cord tumor. All but one patient with a metastatic spinal cord tumor had a gross total removal of tumor. Somatosensory evoked potentials (SEPs) were used to monitor dorsal column function during these procedures. The Ar laser with a $150\,\mu$ spot size (at 1–2 watts) was used for the midline myelotomy. No change in SEPs were seen, suggesting that use of the Ar laser spared the posterior columns. In all eleven patients the laser was judged to be better than standard microsurgical techniques.

Pain Procedures

The argon laser was used to relieve pain in 23 patients [22 dorsal root entry zone (DREZ) lesions and one commissural myelotomy]. For DREZ lesions, the laser was used slightly defocused at 1–2 watts to coagulate the pial vessels overlying the DREZ on the side of the patients pain after a standard laminectomy. Pial traction sutures were placed and/or the table rotated to allow the laser to enter the DREZ at a 45° angle. To assure that the patient remained still during the period lesions were being made, ventilation was stopped for 30 seconds, and five consecutive adjacent lesions were made such that the circumferences of each lesion touched. The patient was then ventilated for 1–2 minutes, and the procedure was repeated until the appropriate number of lesions had been made in the DREZ. Lesions were probed with a microinstrument marked at 1 mm increments to assure that the depth of the lesion was adequate (1–2 mm). In some patients with pain secondary to paraplegia, brachial plexus avulsion, or previous dorsal rhizotomy, lesions were made primarily in cord segments in which dorsal rootlets were absent or distorted. In patients in whom there were root avulsions, the laminectomy was extended cephalad and caudad to identify normal dorsal roots and the DREZ. It is imperative that this precaution be taken to avoid injury to the dorsal and/or lateral columns. After the dura had been opened and the spinal cord had been rotated, lesions could be made in 3–5 minutes. In one other patient a commisural myelotomy for midline pain was performed with excellent results.

Syringomyelia

Based on our experience with laser myelotomy for spinal cord tumors and the use of the laser for DREZ lesions, we used the Ar laser to fenestrate a syrinx in five patients. Fenestration was performed using a 150 µ spot diameter and 1–5 watts of power over a distance of 1.0 cm through the DREZ on the side of the patient's worse symptoms (the thinnest portion of the syrinx was confirmed by metrizamide CT scans). All patients then underwent placement of a syrinx to subarachnoid or peritoneal shunt. We have not performed laser syringotomy without the placement of a shunt tube. The use of the laser for syringomyelia seems to be of value only for the myelotomy, but is not a means of treatment in its own right.

Discussion

The blue-green light of the Ar laser is in the visible portion of the spectrum and is transmitted through water and aqueous media such as CSF without much loss of power, which allows the use of iced saline irrigation to cool delicate tissues such as the spinal cord during vaporization of tumor. The ability to transmit Ar laser light down thin fiber optic bundles makes use of the laser in endoscopic procedures possible such as choroid plexus coagulation[3,4]. Neither is feasible with the CO_2 laser. Moreover, because the beam is visible, a separate aiming device such as the visible helium-neon laser beam used with the invisible CO_2 laser beam is unnecessary. This factor greatly improves the precision of the laser as a microsurgical instrument. Pigments such as melanin, hemoglobin and cytochromes readily absorb Ar light energy and convert it into thermal energy. Because all tumors contain these pigments, the Ar laser can be used to vaporize these lesions.

Changes that occur in absorption coefficients of biologic tissues as the result of thermal injury will affect the reaction of tissues to continuous laser irradiation[2]. This may explain the discrepancy we have observed between the predicted and actual biological effects that are seen after laser applications in vivo.

At very low power densities (50–500 mwatts/cm²), the Ar laser acts as a photocoagulator. Coagulation of tissue, especially blood vessels, is the result of the combination of the selective absorption of Ar light by hemoglobin and of scattering of light within tissue, which decreases the power density per volume of tissue and thereby disperses the thermal effects of laser light over a larger volume of tissue. Because the energy absorption of tissue becomes increasingly independent of the absorption coefficient and the beam wavelength at high power densities[1], however, application of the same beam spot size at high power densities rapidly vaporizes tissue at the point of impact and, because absorption characteristics of the adjacent tissues are changed, the amount of scattering is reduced. This effect may explain the similarity of lesions produced by Ar and CO_2 lasers with respect to the depth of thermal effects in bordering neural tissue at high power densities[2].

Our clinical experience with the Ar laser is similar to the experience with the CO_2 laser reported by others[7]. In addition we have found that the Ar laser particularly is suited for making fine precise incisions in critical neural tissue (myelotomy) and for making discret, reproducible lesions in the DREZ of the spinal cord[7].

Our parallel experience with the CO_2 laser suggests that it is easier to learn how to use, is superior for resection of nonpigmental avascular lesions such as lipomyelomengocele, and, because of its higher power densities, debulks large, fibrous relatively avascular tumors better than the Ar laser. However, for fine microsurgical procedures that do not require high power densities and where extreme precision is desirable, the Ar laser has a slight advantage over the CO_2 laser because of its maneuverability (fiber optic delivery system), smaller spot size, direct visual control of the beam, hemostasis and transmissibility through CSF[6].

Because technological advantages are being made rapidly in medical laser research, it is likely that new visible wavelengths will be available for use in the future. Laser systems with different wavelength lasers have specific advantages and disadvantages that can be exploited for clinical use. More experimental work and clinical experience will dictate the part these laser systems will play for the surgical treatment of neurologic disorders.

Acknowledgments

We thank Jain Smith and Tania Retivov for typing the manuscript in draft, and Neil Buckley for editorial assistance.

References

1. Bartal, A. D., Heilbronn, Y. D., Auram, J., Razon, N., 1982: Carbon dioxide laser surgery of basal meningiomas. Surg. Neurol. *17*, 90–95.
2. Boggan, J. E., Edwards, M. S. B., Davis, R. L., Bolger, C. A., Martin, N., 1982: Comparison of the brain tissue response in rats to injury by argon and carbon dioxide lasers. Neurosurgery *11*, 609–616.
3. Edwards, M. S. B., Boggan, J. E., Fuller, T. A., 1983: The laser in neurological surgery. Review article. J. Neurosurg. *59*, 555–566.

4. Edwards, M. S. B., Boggan, J. E., 1984: Argon laser surgery of pediatric neoplasms. Child's Brain *11*, 171–175.
5. O'Reilly, G. V., Colucci, V. M., Astorian, D. G., Schoene, W. C., Clarke, R. H., Hammerschlag, S. B., 1982: Transcatheter fiberoptic laser coagulation of blood vessels. Radiology *142*, 777–780.
6. Powers, S. K., Edwards, M. S. B., Boggan, J. E., Pitts, L. H., Gutin, P. H., Hosobuchi, Y., Adams, J. E., Wilson, C. B., 1984: Use of the argon laser in neurosurgery. J. Neurosurg. *60*, 523–530.
7. Powers, S. K., Adams, J. E., Edwards, M. S. B., Boggan, J. E., Hosobuchi, Y., 1984: Pain relief from dorsal root entry zone lesions made with argon and carbon dioxide microsurgical lasers. J. Neurosurg. *61*, 841–847.
8. Svaasand, L. O., Ellingson, R., 1983: Optical properties of human brain. Photochem. Photobiol. *38*, 293–299.

Laser in the Removal of Extraaxial Tumors of the Brain and Spinal Cord

Leonard J. Cerullo

Neurological Surgery, University Neurosurgeons, S.C., Chicago, Illinois (U.S.A.)

Most neurosurgeons who have had the opportunity to use a laser or see laser removal of extraaxial tumors have been impressed, if not convinced, of the usefulness of the instrument in this application. One can speculate that had meningiomas rather that gliomas been chosen for the initial clinical applications of carbon dioxide laser in the early 60s, the subsequent history of laser in neurosurgery would have been drastically different. At present, it appears that the most widely accepted and uniformly appreciated use of laser in neurosurgery is in the removal of extraaxial tumors of the central nervous system. These neoplasms offer the surgeon the opportunity to capitalize on the inherent gentleness and precision of laser. These diseases histologically benign, but frequently malignant by location should be gratifying but frequently because of unsuspectedly poor results leave surgeon and patient frustrated and angry. On the other hand, several series have now demonstrated that the use of laser for this group of patients has been rewarding and appreciated. Statistically, patients do better immediately, are released from the hospital sooner, and enjoy a more neurologically normal life. When one considers that this group is expected to have a full life expectancy, the neurological status of the patient becomes all the more important both from a personal as well as a societal point of view.

The basic technique of removal of extraaxial tumors of the brain and spinal cord is similar regardless of histologic variation or location of the tumor. There are, however, several nuances which relate to the type of tumor and its location as well as several surgical variations, both in terms of wavelength and technique. Both will be discussed after the initial principles have been elucidated.

The tumor is exposed through a modest craniotomy or laminectomy directly over the neoplasm if this is possible. Ideally the surface of tumor, albeit minimal, can be appreciated from the surgical exposure without retraction of central nervous tissue. At this point, the arachnoidal plane between tumor and brain is identified and opened. It is critical to maintain this plane in order to avoid damage to surrounding neural and vascular structures and in order to completely follow the tumor through its, often irregular course. The arachnoidal plane can be maintained open using moist cotton insinuated between the arachnoid on the outside and the tumor on the inside. During this phase of tumor preparation careful attention should be paid to hemostasis and to avoiding mechanical trauma to the already severely compromised nervous tissue.

Carbon dioxide laser has been most widely used for the vaporization of extraaxial neoplasms and will be considered synonymous with "laser" during this discussion. Other wavelengths will be treated separately, regarding their peculiar applications and indications. A site on the surface of exposed tumor is ascertained to be free from transversing neural and vascular structures. This site is chosen as the point of capsule entry. When the capsule of the tumor has been entered the laser is used at low power to begin to vaporize tumorous tissue in an intracapsular fashion. Initially low powers, either intermittent or continuous, with a slightly defocused spot are used. This allows appreciation of the particular consistency and vascularity of the individual tumor. Each neoplasm is different in this regard, and further modifications of power density and radiant exposure are a function of the biophysical reaction of the particular tissue to this wavelength. The beam should be moved continuously in order to avoid drilling a hole into the tumor, perhaps precipitating bleeding in a location inaccessible without significant mechanical distortion of the tissues. Venous ooze can be controlled with suction while the laser is used to vaporize beyond the bleeding point. This will frequently result in excellent hemostasis without the use of other lasers or other tools for coagulation. Normally, the area closer to the capsule is more vascular, and bipolar cautery may be necessary to control the more active venous or arterial hemorrhage. Characteristically, extraaxial tumors are variegated in consistency. Naturally, the particular area of tumor being dealt with will mandate the technical variations which are necessary for its vaporization. An attempt should be made to vaporize intracapsular tumor in a cylindrical or reverse conical fashion in order to keep the interior as open as possible while allowing the tumor itself to fall into the evacuated area. For large tumors, the laser may be used as a cutting loop with higher power at a more tightly focused spot in order to morsilate chunks of tumor in an atraumatic and hemostatic fashion. Naturally, the geometry and size of the tumor will dictate the extent to which the intracapsular removal in this fashion is performed.

When an appreciable portion of the neoplasm has been so removed, attention is paid to the capsule. Using highly defocused energy at relatively low power, the capsule is radiated. Depending on the collagen content of the particular tumor, the capsule will shrink to a greater or less degree. Shrinkage can be assisted by gentle massaging of the arachnoid over the surface of the tumor using moist cotton pressing against the capsule of the tumor rather than against the surrounding neural structure. The vessels which have been "swept away" by this procedure are normal vessels, while those which actually nourish the capsule can be either coagulated with the defocused laser or with the bipolar cautery. While the capsule is being irradiated and shrunken, the constriction of tumor will refill the previously evacuated intracapsular compartment. Occasionally, a nontumor vessel will be encased by neoplasm and can be appreciated at the surface. Meticulous dissection around the vessel, either with laser or with conventional technique is necessary to protect that structure. Upon dissection, the vessel is flipped over or under the capsule if possible or protected with moist cotton if mobilization is difficult or dangerous. The location of vessels such as this can usually be appreciated with preoperative angiography. The plane, having been open up between tumor and surrounding neural structure, is maintained using pledgets of cotton soaked in saline. This prevents neural tissue from falling into the working space, generally without relying on mechanical retractors. It also allows preservation and maintenance of the arachnoidal plane over the surface of the tumor. Finally, it prevents excessively deep penetration by allowing the surgeon to appreciate the limit to which he can safely vaporize tumor.

By alternating between intracapsular vaporization (or morsilation) and capsule shrinkage, the mass is eventually reduced in size. As the lesion becomes smaller and smaller, greater appreciation of the circumference, whether regular or lobulated, can be attained. As greater familarity with the biophysical reaction of the particular tumor is achieved, higher output energy can be utilized in order to expedite the process. When sufficient space has been purchased to allow mobilization of tumor without mechanical distortion of surrounding neural structures, the vascular pedicle should be searched and devitalized. This may be possible with laser of the same or a different wavelength or with bipolar cautery. The devascularization of the pedicle of the tumor will frequently allow further shrinkage because of decrease in vascular engorement and will make the laser vaporization more effective because of the loss of intratumoral fluid. On the other hand, the heat sink's beneficial effect of blood flowing through tumor is minimized, and care must be utilized to avoid more deep and rapid penetration than had been previously noted.

The steps, then, of extraaxial tumor removal can be summarized as follows:

1. Exposure of tumor surface through a relatively limited craniotomy or

laminectomy, centered over the most superficial and accessible portion of the neoplasm. Obviously, there are situations in which this is not possible.

2. Meticulous dissection of the arachnoidal plane between tumor and surrounding neural and vascular structures. Maintenance of this plane is essential in order to avoid damage to nontumorous vessels and structures and to allow complete removal of neoplasm.

3. Entrance into the tumor through the capsule at a safe area, free from traversing neural and vascular tissue.

4. Evacuation of the interior of the neoplasm (intracapsullary removal) either by vaporization or morsilation of tumor. Maintenance of hemostasis during this phase using either a YAG laser or bipolar cautery is essential.

5. Shrinkage of capsule with defocused energy and continued preservation of the arachnoidal plane using moist cotton pledgets.

6. Continued alternation between points four and five.

7. Devitalization through vaporization or coagulation of the vascular pedicle and/or site of attachment.

Although the foregoing supplies a general rationale for extraaxial tumor removal, several specific variations may alter technique. Most notable among these is the specific location of the tumor.

Medial sphenoid wing tumors, particularly meningiomas, often encase the carotid artery and invade the cavernous sinus. While the approach to these lesions follows the same general outline as detailed above, as the medial extent of the tumor is approached, manual microdissection is recommended to initially identify the carotid adventitia. The manual dissection is not deleterious to surrounding neural structures because significant space for dissection has already been achieved through tumor vaporization. Once the adventitial plane has been identified, it is dissected open using moist cotton. This allows tumor removal through low power vaporization rather than mechanical tugging while simultaneously protecting the vessel from inadvertent puncture by laser. At the cavernous sinus, a decision must eventually be made regarding extent of removal. Unless the sinus is known to be occluded and the cranial nerves are known to be irreversibly damaged, vaporization up to the dura is recommended. Transdural denaturation using Nd : YAG laser has been recommended but is felt by this author to be at least theoretically dangerous. A practical guide in knowing when sufficient tumor has been removed is the appreciation of pulsations of the dura reflecting underlying blood flow. When the tumor invaded dura has been sufficiently thinned to appreciate these pulsations, it can be assumed that little if any neoplasm remains.

In the medial parasellar region, tumor is often seen extending under and lateral to the optic nerves with insinuation between the optic nerve and carotid artery. In these situations, inward collapse of the tumor is difficult because the lesion remains relatively stationary at its fixation on the planum of sphenoidale and greater wing. Tumor can be shrunken in volume by vaporization until the arachnoidal plane between tumor and carotid artery or optic nerve has been opened. At this point, protection of these structures is possible and vaporization can proceed.

Tumors of the clivus will frequently extend to the opposite side, and a similar technique of tumor shrinkage with opening of planes followed by protection is recommended. It should be remembered that the laser cannot travel around corners unless deflected by mirrors, a practice which requires considerable skill and experience. Pulling on the tumor with a pituitary forceps is just as dangerous, if not more so, and is not considered a suitable alternative for vaporization after protection.

The frequent encasement of the vertebral artery by tumors of the foramen magnum make preoperative angiography mandatory and gentle palpation or Doppler sonography very helpful during removal. The same technique of major vessel protection as discussed under carotid artery protection in medial sphenoid tumors is recommended. These tumors do not actually invade the adventitia and, therefore, this plane should be able to be opened. Too intense heat, however, will cause shrinkage of the adventitia and the eventual occlusion of the vessel, even in the absence of spasm. Short exposure times help to reduce spread of thermal damage and should be used in this situation.

It is the feeling of this author that acoustic nerve tumors should be debulked medially and laterally prior to opening the internal auditory canal. While the laser is very effective in vaporizing dura from the posterior aspect of the canal, it is not recommended that the instrument be used to vaporize bone, as the intense heat may cause both neural and vascular damage to the structures within. Vaporization of tumor fragments off cranial nerves can be accomplished using very low power and short exposure times. Surrounding structures are protected with wet cotton. A small spot is ideal.

Extraaxial tumors vary in consistency and vascularity. While as a general rule the laser is the single most effective instrument for removing these neoplasms, each case is individual. Often, a very gelatinous tumor is just as well, if not preferably, debulked through suction or ultrasonic aspiration. The more sensitive the area, the more fibrous the attachment, and the more firm the consistency, the better carbon dioxide laser will function. Fatty tumors are particularly well vaporized because of the differential heat of melting of fat vis à vis neural tissue. In addition, the melted fat assumes a very low temperature because of energy absorption and will not cause further damage. It can be easily aspirated.

While carbon dioxide has remained the mainstay of extraaxial tumor surgery, because of its immediate absorption in water and minimal scatter, other wavelengths have been used adjunctively. The Nd : YAG laser is most valuable in the devascularization of extraaxial tumors prior to their vaporization or morsilation with carbon dioxide. Several aspects of the biophysical reactions of this wavelength of light on tissue deserve notice. As demonstrated by Burke *et al.,* the maximal thermal conversion occurs beneath the surface. This has been used by Beck and Ascher in denaturing tissue beyond and intact structure, such as the dura of the sella or the superior saggital and transverse sinuses. Because of this gradient in temperature elevation, however, an intra tumor explosion, the "popcorn effect" described by Jain, can occur. Also described by Burke was the extension of damage, presumably thermal, to tissues beyond the margins of change demonstrated by histology. This zone of reversible altered metabolism, visible on histofluorescent techniques, widens the effective zone of YAG damage. This must be considered when using the laser any where near the interface between tumor and normal structures. It is contraindicated, then, to employ the YAG wavelength near the midbrain, the floor of the fourth ventricle, and the cranial nerves. The heat sink effect of tissue is compromised when Nd : YAG is used. The elevated temperature dissipates more slowly, and temperature build up is common. The applications of energy must, therefore, be relatively short in duration and of modest power. This becomes more critical in dealing with tumors located in more sensitive areas.

It appears that the primary use of the Nd : YAG laser in the removal of extraaxial tumors is in the devascularization of the particularly bloody neoplasms both in their center and at their vascular pedicle. This assumes, of course, that the vascular pedicle is not adherent to or immediately adjacent to sensitive and functioning neural structures.

The argon laser has been used for the devascularization and vaporization of relatively small extraaxial tumors. The low power of most available systems makes this wavelength, although theoretically very desirable, practically handicapped. The small spot size and coincidence of aiming beam with treating beam allow great precision and can be used to advantage in sensitive areas. It should be remembered, however, that the depth of penetration and degree of scatter are greater with argon than carbon dioxide. The net result, as demonstrated by Edwards and Boggan, is a lesion comparable in size to that of the larger spot carbon dioxide. The availability of optical fibers to carry this wavelength and the ability of the argon laser to pass through clear media may make it ideal for extraaxial tumors in spinal fluid compartments such as meningiomas within the ventricular system. Again, however, the low power output of this relatively inefficient laser makes debulking through vaporization a relatively slow process. The frequency doubled YAG laser, emitting near the argon green wavelength may compensate for this shortcoming.

The surgical approach to extraaxial tumors should offer the following advantages: 1. immediate access to tumor with minimal retraction of already compromised neurologic tissue. 2. Minimal thermal and mechanical trauma coincident with tumor removal. 3. Preservation of normal arterial and venous anatomy to avoid vascular compromise at the site of the lesion or distal to it. 4. Avoidance of cranial nerve sacrifice. 5. Complete removal. Laser is the local tool to achieve these ends.

References

1. Ascher, P. W., Cerullo, L. J.: The laser in neurosurgery. In: Surgical Applications of Lasers (Dixon, J. W., ed.), pp. 163–174. Chicago-London: Yearbook Medical Publishers.
2. Bartal, A. D., et al., 1983: Carbon dioxide laser surgery of basal meningiomas. Surg. Neurol. 17 (2), 90–95.
3. Beck, O. J., 1980: The use of the Nd : YAG and the CO_2 laser in neurosurgery. Neurosurgical Review 2, 261–266.
4. Boggan, J. E., et al., 1982: Comparison of the brain tissue response on cerebral cortex. Neurosurgery 11 (5), 609–616.
5. Burke, L. P., Rovin, R. A., Cerullo, L. J., Brown, J. T., Petronio, J., 1983: Yag laser in neurosurgery. In: Nd : YAG Lasers in Medicine and Surgery (Joffe, ed.). New York: Elsevier Science Publishing Co., Inc.
6. Cerullo, L. J., Burke, L., 1984: Use of laser in neurosurgery. In: Surgical Clinics of North America, 64 : 5, pp. 995–1000. Philadelphia: W. B. Saunders Company.
7. Cerullo, L. J., Mkrdichian, E. H.: Acoustic nerve tumor surgery before and since laser—comparison of results (Submitted—Journal of American Medical Association).
8. Cozzens, J., Cerullo, L. J., 1985: A comparison of the effect of CO_2 laser and bipolar coagulator on the cat brain. Neurosurgery 16, No. 4, 449–453.
9. Fasano, V. A., et al., 1982: Observation on the simultaneous use of CO_2 and Nd-YAG lasers in neurosurgery. Lasers in Surgery and Medicine 1, 155–161.
10. Fox, J. L., et al., 1966: Lasers and their neurosurgical application. Military Medicine 31, 493–498.
11. Hara, M., et al., 1980: Evaluation of brain tumor laser surgery. Acta Neurochir. (Wien) 53, 141–149.
12. Hudgins, W. R., 1980: Use of the CO_2 laser in neurological surgery. In: Laser Surgery Seminar. A Manual on the Carbon Dioxide Laser in Surgery (Snider, W. R., ed.). Kansas City: Biomedical Lasers, Inc., Truman Medical Center.
13. Hudgins, W. R., et al., 1981: Microsurgical laser vaporization of inaccessible tumors of the central nervous system. Dallas Med. J. 76, 245–250.
14. Jain, K. K., 1985: Complications of use of the neodymium : Yttrium-alumnium-garnet laser in neurosurgery. Neurosurgery 16, No. 6, 759–761.
15. Kamikawa, K., et al., 1976: Application of laser surgical unit in neurosurgery. Surg. Therapy 35 (6), 626.
16. Khromov, B. M., et al., 1974: Use of the laser in neurosurgery. (Literature survey.) Vopr Neiokhir 6, 50.
17. Nishiura, I., et al., 1981: Successful removal of a huge falcotentorial meningioma by use of the laser. Surg. Neurol. 16 (5), 380–385.

18. Perria, C., *et al.,* 1979: The CO_2 laser beam in the surgical treatment of cerebral tumors. J. Neurosurg. Sci. *23* (2), 125–128.
19. Pimenta, L. H. M., *et al.,* 1981: The use of the CO_2 laser for the removal of awkardly situated meningiomas. Neurosurg. Rev. *4*, 53–55.
20. Pimenta, L. H. M., Pimenta, A. M.: Evaluation of difficult placed meningiomas operated with CO_2 laser. In: Laser Surgery, Proceedings of the International Society for Laser Surgery, Israel, November 1975; Dallas, October 1977 (Kaplan, I., ed.), pp. 147–148. Tel-Aviv: OT-PAZ Press.
21. Rosomoff, H. L., Carroll, R., 1965: Effect of laser on brain and neoplasm. Surg. Forum *16*, 431.
22. Saunders, M. L., Young, H. F., Becker, D. P., *et al.,* 1980: The use of the laser in neurological surgery. Surg. Neurol. *14*, 1–10.
23. Stellar, S., 1972: Application of CO_2 laser to neurosurgical and other surgical problems. Proc. 4th European Congress of Neurosurgery, 1971; Prague: Avicenum, Czech Med Press.
24. Strait, T. A., Robertson, J. H., Clark, W. C., 1982: Use of the carbon dioxide laser in the operative management of intracranial meningiomas: a report of twenty cases. Neurosurgery *10*, 464–467.
25. Takizawa, T., *et al.,* 1980: Laser surgery of basal, orbital and ventricular meningiomas which are difficult to extirpate by conventional methods. Neurol. Med. Chir. (Tokyo) *20*, 729–737.

The Stereotactic CO$_2$ Laser: Instrumentation, Methodology and Clinical Results

PATRICK J. KELLY

Department of Neurosurgery, Mayo Clinic,
Rochester, Minnesota (U.S.A.)

Contents

Summary.. 162
Introduction... 162
Surgical Instrumentation 163
Data Base Acquisition.. 166
Surgical Procedure... 167
Clinical Material.. 170
Discussion.. 173
References.. 174

Summary

The carbon dioxide laser has been incorporated into a computer-assisted stereotactic system for precision resection of deep-seated intraaxial neoplasms. Stereotactic CT scanning provides a precise three dimensional tumor volumetric data base in relationship to a custom arc-quadrant stereotactic frame. A carbon dioxide laser beam is directed by the stereotactic instrument. It is monitored by an interactive computer graphic system in relation to boundaries of the tumor volume which has been sliced orthogonal to the surgical viewline. Theoretically, the procedure allows removal of all tumor identified by CT scanning. Thirty-five of these procedures have been performed on thirty-three patients having a variety of neoplasms in various deep-seated locations with satisfactory postoperative results.

Keywords: Brain neoplasm; Carbon dioxide laser; Computers; CT scanning; Stereotactic techniques; Thalamus.

Introduction

Neurosurgeons have long depended on hand-eye coordination in the performance of intracranial surgical procedures. It is not surprising, therefore, that little progress has been made in the treatment of intraaxial neoplasms since the description of the internal decompression of malignant gliomas over 50 years ago. A surgeon's three dimensional spatial orientation decreases the deeper a procedure extends below the cortical surface.

Furthermore, at surgery the gross distinction between primary neoplasm, edematous brain tissue and normal brain is frequently unclear. Precise three dimensional proprioception is required in order to remove significant portions of these neoplasms while damage to surrounding healthy brain tissue is avoided.

Stereotactic technique has been employed in humans for the accurate placement of subcortical probes for the treatment of movement disorders and chronic pain for 35 years. Modifications of classical stereotactic methods can provide the precise three dimensional proprioception required by contemporary neurosurgeons for the treatment of intraaxial lesions. Here, incorporation of the surgical laser into stereotactic methodology is most appropriate.

The carbon dioxide laser has been used in neurosurgery since its application was first described by Stellar et al.[10]. It is a precise cutting and vaporizing tool and can be controlled and monitored in three dimensional space. The CO$_2$ laser is a convenient means for removing tissue from the depths of a deep cavity, which is a distinct advantage when vaporizing a deep-seated tumor stereotactically. In addition, the zone of thermal necrosis adjacent to an area subjected to CO$_2$ laser cutting or vaporization is on the order of a few hundred microns[10]. This precision is necessary when vaporizing the edge of an intraaxial tumor located in a neurologically important subcortical area. Because of these advantages, the incorporation of a CO$_2$ laser into stereotactic methodology provides a mechanism for precise three dimensionally controlled surgical ablation of intracranial intraaxial neoplasms.

We have employed a stereotactic laser technique for the precision resection of CT defined tumor volumes since January 1980[4-8]. Constant refinement of the methodology has continued. The present report will describe the technique as presently practiced and to review our clinical experience to date.

Surgical Instrumentation

A new stereotactic frame was developed which allows rapid and accurate access to multiple intracranial targets (Fig. 1). The frame is based on the arc-quadrant principle: The patient's head moves with three degrees of freedom within a fixed sphere described by an arc and quadrant. The frame consists of a CT compatible head holder, a base plate, and X, Y, and Z mechanical stage and inner and outer arc-quadrants.

The patient's head is secured in a CT compatible head holder by carbon

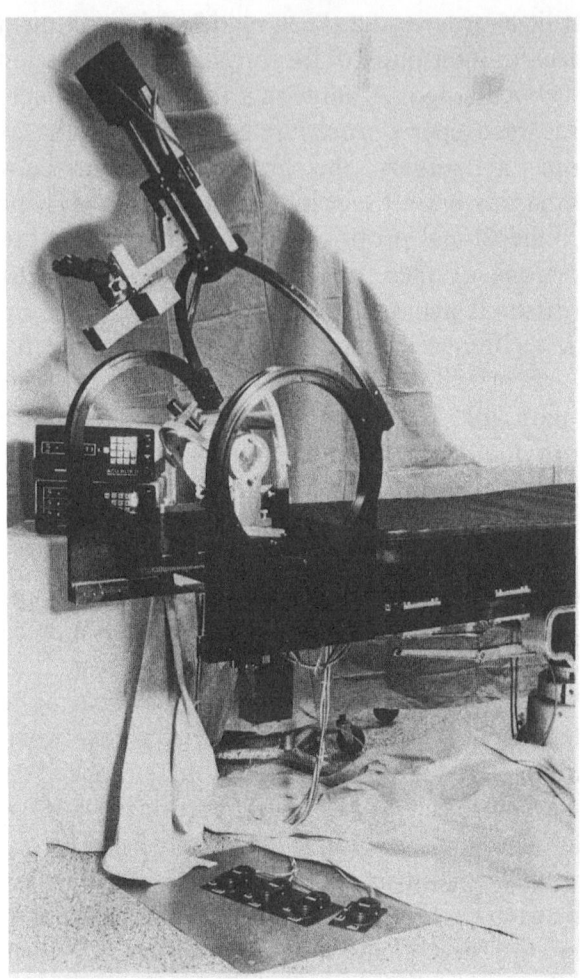

Fig. 1. Arc-quadrant stereotactic system consisting of 400 mm arc quadrant and motorized three dimensional slice system. An operating microscope and CO_2 laser manipulator box run on a carriage perpendicular to the tangent of the arc. The distance of the microscope focus from the focal point of the arc-quadrant and the positions of the patient's head is three dimensional stereotactic space are displayed by the electronic digital read-out system on the left

fiber pins inserted through ⅛ ″ twist drill holes made in the outer table of the skull. The stereotactic head holder fits into the X, Y, and Z mechanical stage.

The mechanical stage is moved by lead screws in three dimensions. Servomotors activated by foot pedals, are used to turn each of the lead screws. Movements of the head in X (right-left), Y (anterior-posterior) and

Z (superior-inferior) are measured by an optical digital readout system*. These digital displays are visible to the surgeon at all times.

An outer arc-quadrant having a radius of 400 mm runs on a slide mechanism at the outer edge of the operating table. It is moved into position whenever stereotactic control is required during any craniotomy. An operating microscope and a CO$_2$ laser manipulator box are attached to a carriage which runs perpendicular to a tangent of the 400 mm arc. The microscope and laser have 400 mm objective focusing lenses respectively.

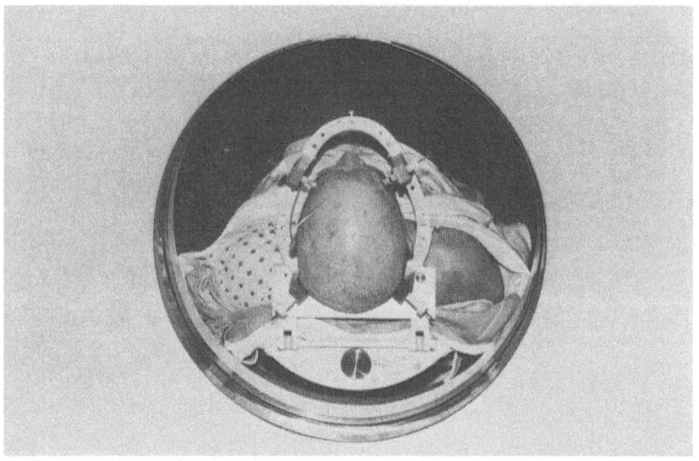

Fig. 2. CT compatible stereotactic headholder which fixed to the patient's skull by carbon fiber pins inserted through the outer table of the skull into the diploe. The head holder fits into the adaptation plate on the GE 8800 scanning table

A Sharplan 743 carbon dioxide laser is utilized. The optical arm connects to the laser micromanipulator box on the stereotactic frame. The aiming beam and carbon dioxide laser beam are manipulated by mirrors on two galvanometers which direct the beams to the focal point of the stereotactic frame. The electrical input to the galvanometers are controlled by a remote joystick which varies the voltage output of a power supply by means of X and Y potentiometers. The joystick, which is controlled by the surgeon, also activates two encoders which input the X, Y position of the laser beam into an operating room computer system**.

----

* Bousch and Lomb, ACCURITE, Analytic Systems Division, Rochester, N.Y.

** Data General Eclipse S 140 mainframe, Data General Corp., Westboro, Massachusetts.

Data Base Acquisition

Patients undergo stereotactic CT scanning on a GE 8800 CT body scanner with their heads fixed in the CT compatible stereotactic head holder (Fig. 2).

A CT compatible localizing system consists of three sets of carbon fiber bars as described previously[3, 4, 8]. Each set consists of three carbon fiber bas attached in an "N" configuration located on either side of the head and

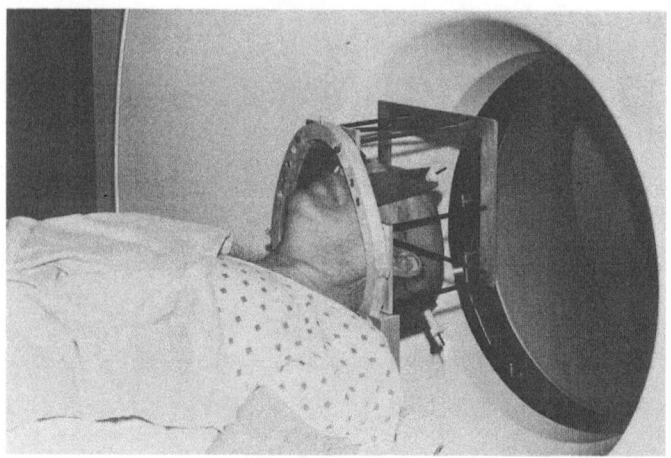

Fig. 3. CT localization system which consist of three sets of three carbon fiber rods arranged in the shape of the letter "N"

anteriorly. The localizing system attaches to the stereotactic head holder (Fig. 3). The localizing device creates a set of nine artifacts on each CT slice (Fig. 4). The height and inclination of each slice is related to the distance between the middle reference mark and the two marks created by the vertical elements on each localizing set.

Following CT scanning, the data tape from the CT scan is read into the operating room computer system. The surgeon views each CT slice on a Ramtek raster display terminal. The reference marks are automatically digitized by the computer by an intensity detection program. The surgeon outlines the margins of the tumor on serial CT slices by utilizing the cursor and trackball (Fig. 5).

The computer records the tumor outlines into a three dimensional matrix. An interpolation program creates intermediate slices at 1 mm intervals. The slices are filled in with 1 mm cubes and then given a thickness of 1 mm. Thus, a three dimensional volume is established in the computer matrix. The surgeon also selects a central point in the tumor and the computer calculates the X, Y, and Z adjustments on the stereotactic frame to bring this point in the tumor into the focal point of the stereotactic arc-quadrant. The tumor volume may be sliced by computer perpendicular to any specified surgical viewline centered at the central point selected by the surgeon.

The surgical viewline describes the angles from horizontal and vertical

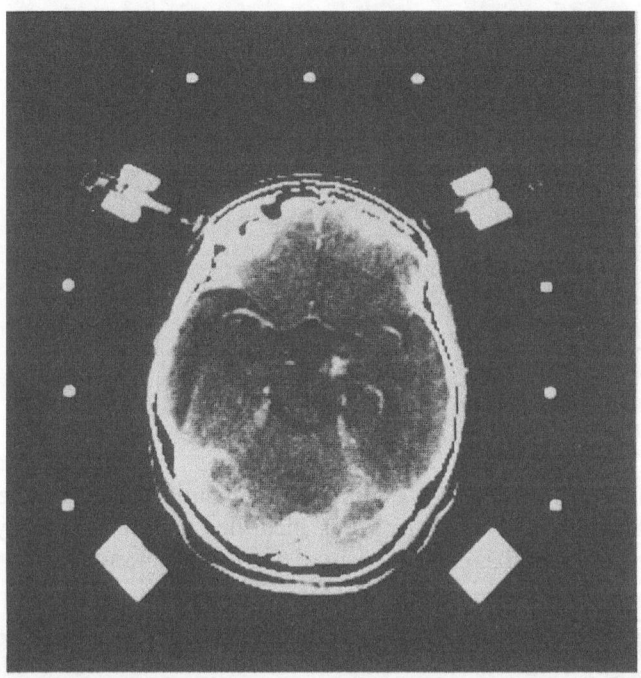

Fig. 4. Stereotactic CT slice showing nine (9) reference marks. The height and inclination of each slice is calculated from the position of the middle reference mark in reference to these resulting from the vertical elements in each localizing set

planes along which the tumor will be approached. In practice, deep-seated tumors are approached through relatively nonessential brain tissue in a direction parallel to major white matter projections. This is specified to the computer as collar and arc angle settings on the stereotactic frame which correspond to angles from horizontal and vertical planes respectively.

Surgical Procedure

The patient is placed under general anesthesia and the stereotactic head holder is fixed into the receiving yoke of the X, Y, and Z mechanical slide. The initial X, Y, and Z settings calculated by computer are made on the stereotactic frame. A linear incision is made in the scalp. A series of stainless steel balls are placed at 5 mm intervals through the tumor along the surgical

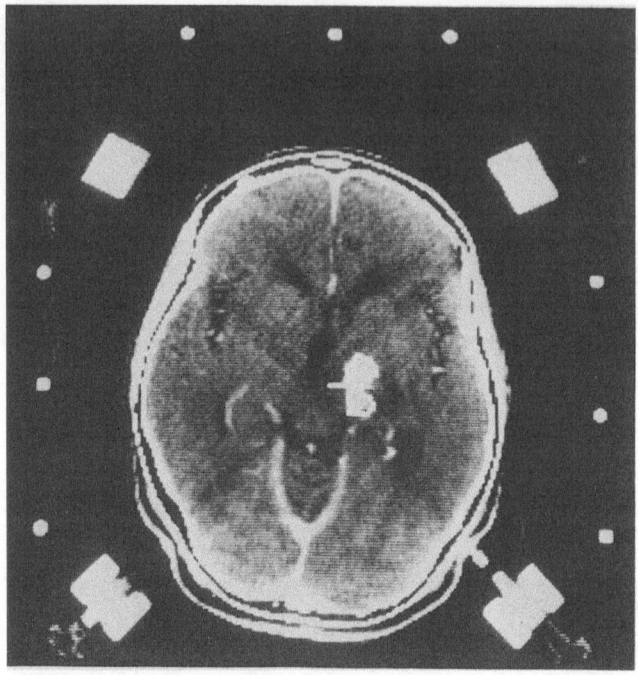

Fig. 5. Digitizing planar contours of tumor on sequential CT slices. The position of the CT localizing reference marks are identified automatically by computer utilizing an intensity detection program

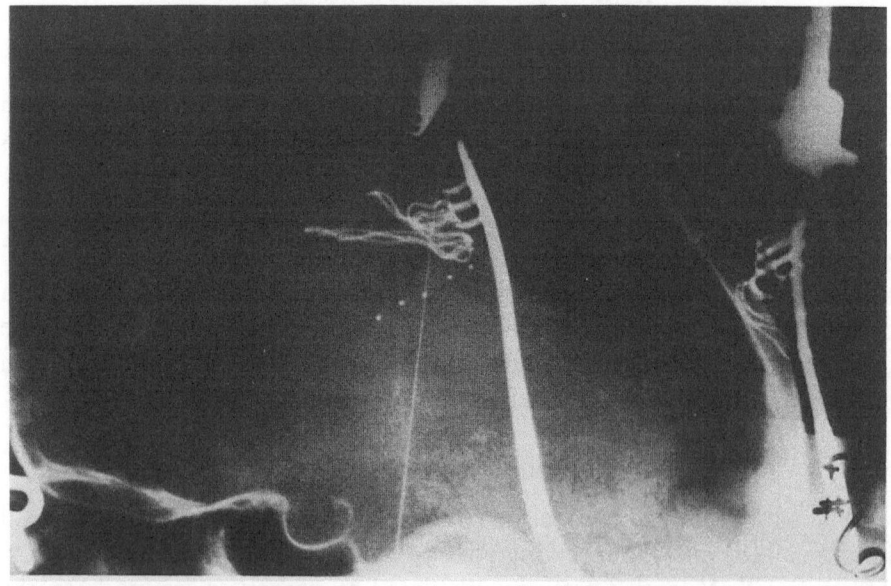

Fig. 6. Stainless steel reference balls are placed at 5 mm intervals through the tumor along the surgical viewline utilizing a stereotactically directed biopsy canula

viewline utilizing an insulated biopsy canula, directed by the inner arc-quadrant, through a ⅛ " twist drill opening of the skull. AP and lateral teleradiographs are obtained in order to document the position of the steel balls (Fig. 6). These serve as a reference for intracranial spatial shifts of the tumor after craniotomy and dural opening. Movement of the tumor within the intracranial space can be detected on subsequent AP and lateral

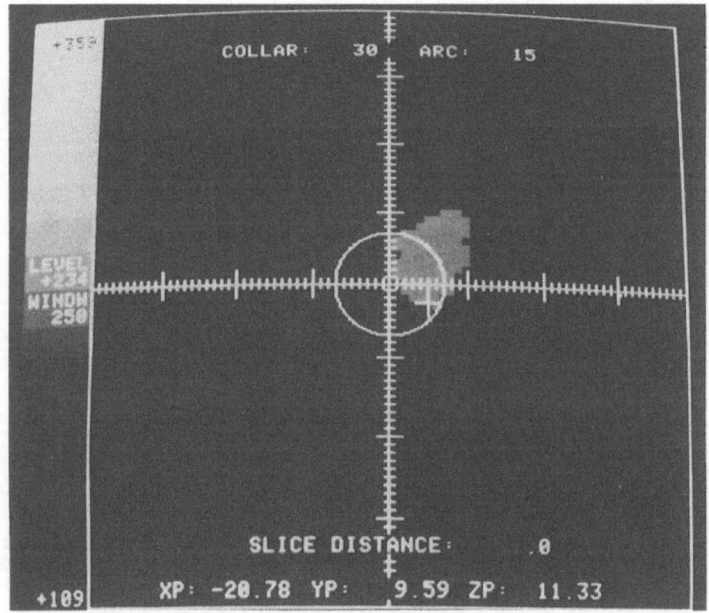

Fig. 7. Computer generated display showing section of tumor sliced along surgical viewline, the outline of the stereotactic retractor and the position of the surgical laser in reference to the tumor represented by a cursor

teleradiographs and the position of the tumor correspondingly shifted within the three dimensional computer matrix.

A trephine craniotomy is done, the dura is opened in a cruciate manner and the 400 mm arc-quadrant is moved into place and secured. Utilizing the carbon dioxide laser at 60 to 80 watts of power, a linear incision is made in cortex and white matter as the microscope and laser are advanced toward the focal point of the stereotactic frame. A stereotactic retractor directs its blades toward the focal point of the frame. At the outer border of the tumor whose margins are indicated by computer, the incision is undercut slightly and the stereotactic retractor opened. This creates a shaft at the bottom of which is the superficial boundary of the tumor. The surgeon monitors the position of the surgical laser displayed as a cursor on the graphics monitor in a calibrated relationship to the outline of the tumor as a surgical plane is developed around the tumor (Fig. 7). The slices displayed are those derived from the CT based tumor volume and represent the level at which the microscope and laser are focused. After cutting around the tumor outline, the retractor is advanced slightly and the surface area of the slice is vaporized. The tumor is vaporized slice by slice progressing from the most

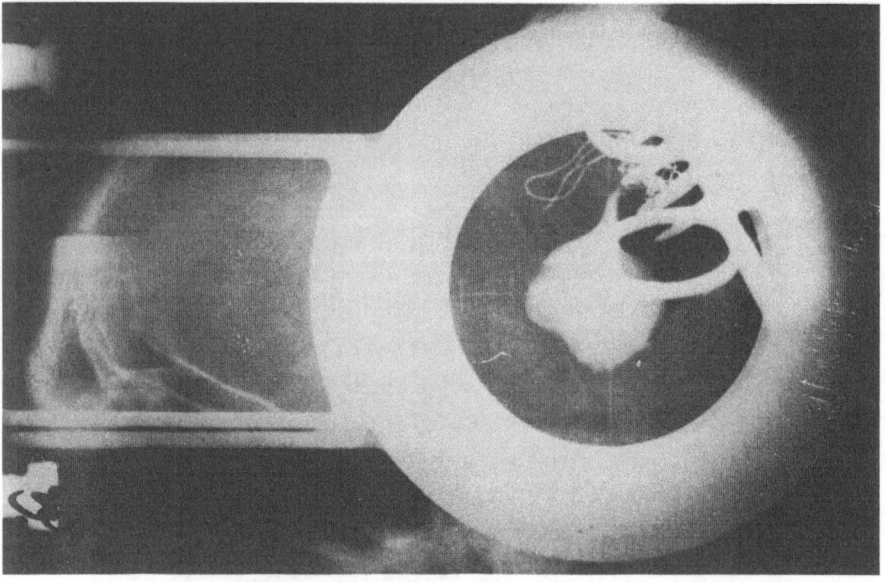

Fig. 8. Cotton balls soaked in Hypaque® to demonstrate cavity produced by stereotactic laser vaporization

superficial level to the deepest. Serial AP and lateral teleradiographs are obtained at various stages in this process. Occasionally, a cotton soaked with Hypaque is inserted to enhance the radiographic appearance of the cavity being produced by laser vaporization (Fig. 8).

Clinical Material

To date, 41 procedures have been performed on 36 patients having tumors in locations indicated by Table 1 and histologies outlined in Table 2. Patients ranged in age from 10 to 73 years. Postoperatively, eighteen patients were improved from their preoperative neurologic level when examined two weeks postoperatively. Sixteen patients had not changed neurologically: Six were neurologically normal, five were hemiplegic before and after the procedure. Six patients were neurologically worse following stereotactic laser craniotomy. Two developed a homonymous hemianopsia

Table 1. *Locations of Tumors in 41 Computer-Assisted Stereotactic Laser Procedures*

Thalamus	
Right	4
Left	6
Basal ganglia	
Right	1
Corpus callosum	3
Central	
Right	10
Left	9
Frontal	
Right	3
Third ventricle	3
Deep temporal	1
Occipital	1
Total	41

Table 2. *Tumor Histology from 41 Stereotactic Laser Procedures*

Glioblastoma	13
Astrocytoma grades II–III	11
Meningioma	3
Metastatic	8
Ganglioglioma	2
Cavernous hemangioma	2
Teratoma	1
Arteriovenous malformation	1
Total	41

following occipital approaches to thalamic neoplasms, three had worsening of hemiparesis noted preoperatively. One additional patient was comatose postoperatively. There have been two infections. One patient's infection responded appropriately to treatment while the other's did not and was the cause of the only postoperative mortality four weeks following surgery.

Thirty-two patients demonstrated no evidence of contrast-enhancing residual of the tumor on the initial postoperative scan after the stereotactic laser microsurgical procedure. Representative cases are demonstrated in

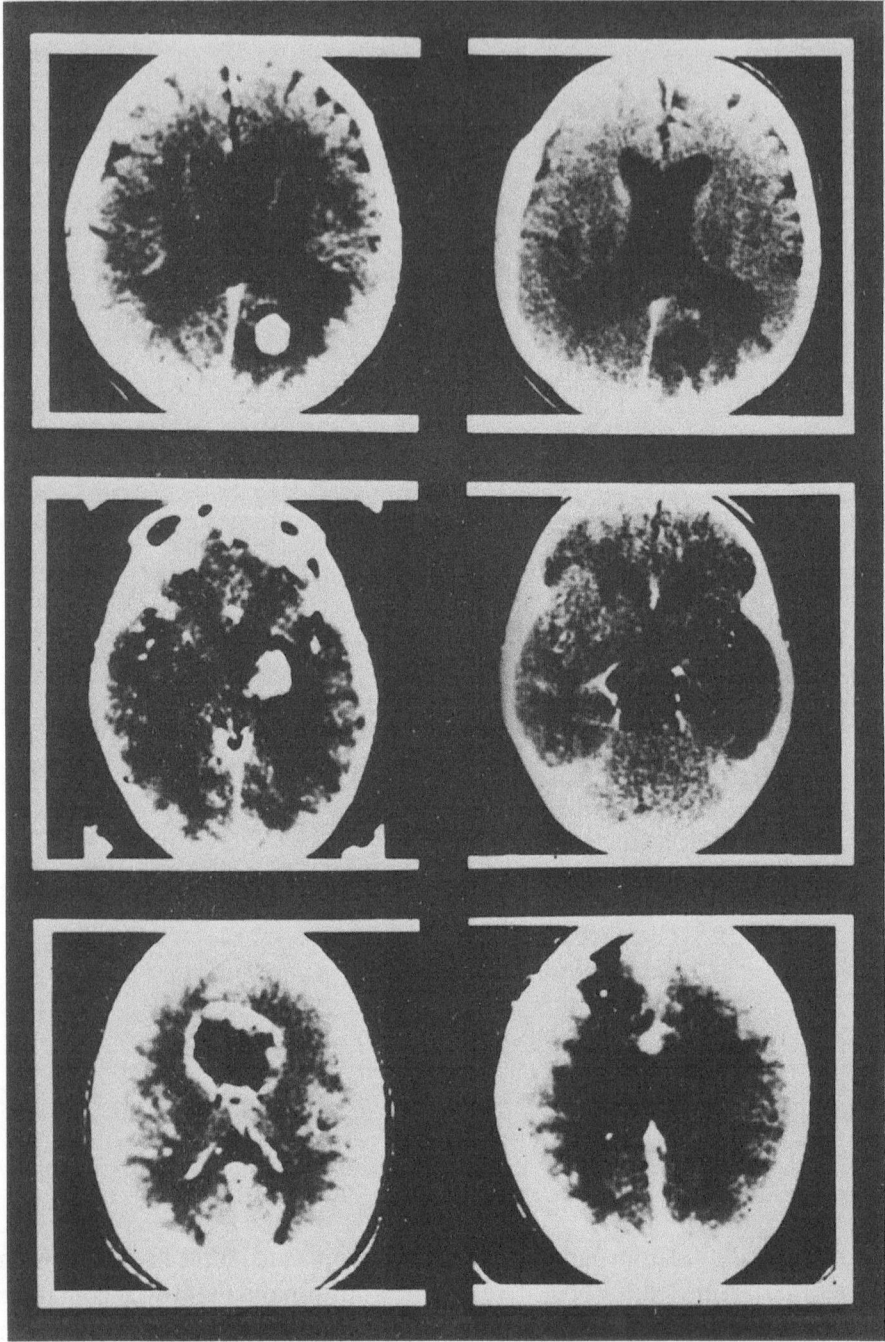

Fig. 9. Representative pre- and postoperative CT scans in (top) metastatic adenocarcinoma (middle) thalamic astrocytoma (bottom) septal glioblastoma

Fig. 9. Nine patients, all with large tumors, demonstrated a small amount of residual tumor on follow-up CT scanning. Four of these patients underwent a second procedure to remove residual tumor. Of thirteen patients with glioblastomas, nine had CT recurrence of their neoplasm within three to eleven months following the stereotactic laser procedure. Two patients with Grade III astrocytomas remain free of clinical or CT evident disease three years and twenty-six months following the procedure.

Discussion

We have developed a technique which provides precise three dimensional control in removing inrraaxial neoplasms by stereotactic laser craniotomy. The technique allows the surgeon to plan the surgical approach through nonessential brain tissue which may not be the shortest route to the tumor. The stereotactic technique significantly reduces the risk of surgical disorientation in locating a deep-seated lesion. The surgical laser in this system is directed with controlled three dimensional precision and its position is monitored on-line by computer. In the future, it will be possible to direct the surgical laser by means of a computer digital-to-analog output.

Our experience demonstrates that some cases treated by computer assisted stereotactic laser surgery do better than others. In general, these are patients with well demarcated primary and metastatic tumors. To date, none of our metastatic tumors have recurred. Less aggressive primary neoplasms have benefitted significantly from this procedure since a significant amount of the tumor may be removed by this method. In most cases, all of the tumor detected by CT scanning can be extirpated.

Our results with glioblastomas have been disappointing. Although neurologic improvement was usually noted in the early postoperative period, these patients usually had tumor recurrence within the same time period as those treated by standard surgical techniques. Tumor recurrence was usually noted in the hypodense area surrounding the contrast enhancing region resected by the surgical procedure. This would indicate that the margins of a malignant glioma may extend beyond the boundaries suggested by CT scanning as also noted by others[1]. Other three dimensional data bases such as Nuclear Magnetic Resonance (NMR) may be incorporated into our technique in order to guide a more thorough removal of tumor tissue. In addition, hematorporphyrin derivative (HPD) photoradiation may be incorporated into our procedure to destroy cells remaining after stereotactic laser extirpation[2, 9]. Here, laser light of the appropriate wavelength would be directed into the cavity produced by stereotactic laser vaporization.

Up to the present, our efforts have been centered on developing a methodology. It is not yet clear where this methodology will be best applied.

Nevertheless, computer assisted stereotactic laser microsurgery has been found to supply a margin of safety to surgery for many intraaxial lesions which becomes more advantageous to deeper a lesion lies below the cortical surface. In addition, the technique lends itself to the future incorporation of other technologies, such as ultrasound and two dimensional imaging matrixes which can be utilized to increase the stereotactic data base prior to or during the surgical procedure.

References

1. Daumas-Dupont, C., Monsaingeon, V., Szenthe, L., Szikla, G., 1982: Serial Biopsies: A double histological code of gliomas according to malignancy and 3-D configuration, and aid to therapeutic decision and assessment of results. Applied Neurophysiol. *45* (4–5), 431–437.
2. Dougherty, T. J., Kaufman, J. E., Goldfarb, A., Weishaupt, K. R., Boyle, D., Mittleman, A., 1978: Photoradiation therapy for the treatment of malignant tumors. Cancer Res. *38*, 2628–2635.
3. Goerss, S., Kelly, P. J., Kall, B., 1982: A simple CT stereotactic adaptation system. Neurosurgery *10*, 375–379.
4. Kelly, P. J., Alker, G. J., Jr., Goerss, S., 1982: Computer assisted stereotactic laser microsurgery for the treatment of intracranial neoplasms. Neurosurgery *10*, 324–331.
5. Kelly, P. J., Alker, G. J., Jr., 1980: A method for stereotactic laser microsurgery in the treatment of deep-seated CNS neoplasms. Applied Neurophysiol. *43*, 210–215.
6. Kelly, P. J., Alker, G. J., Jr., 1981: A stereotactic approach to deep-seated central nervous system neoplasms using the carbon dioxide laser. Surg. Neurol. *15*, 331–334.
7. Kelly, P. J., Alker, G. J., Jr., Zoll, J. G., 1982: A microstereotactic approach to deep-seated arteriovenous malformations. Surg. Neurol. *17*, 260–262.
8. Kelly, P. J., Alker, G. J., Jr., Kall, B., Goerss, S., 1983: Precision resection of intra-axial CNS lesions by CT-based stereotactic craniotomy and computer monitored CO_2 laser. Acta Neurochir. (Wien) *68*, 1–9.
9. Lawes, E. R., Jr., Cortese, D. A., Kinsey, J. H., Eagen, R. T., Anderson, R. E., 1981: Photoradiation therapy in the treatment of malignant brain tumors: A phase I (feasibility) study. Neurosurgery *9*, 672–678.
10. Stellar, S., Polanyi, T. G., Brédemeir, H. C., 1970: Experimental studies with the carbon dioxide laser as a neurosurgical instrument. Med. Biol. Eng. *8*, 549–558.

The Use of Lasers in Nerve Repair

Isabelle L. Richmond

Microsurgical Research Center, Eastern Virginia Medical School,
Norfolk, Virginia (U.S.A.)

Contents

Introduction 175
The Biology of Nerve Coaptation 176
Current Microsurgical Techniques for Nerve Repair 176
Laser Repair of Peripheral Nerves 177
References 182

Introduction

In contrast to current neurosurgical applications of the CO_2 laser which utilize high power densities (12,000–50,000 watts/cm^2) to achieve coagulation or vaporization of tissue, the use of much lower power densities (300–1,200 watts/cm^2) and small focal spot size to achieve tissue welding effects promises to have great potential use in reconstructive microsurgery.

Our study of the use of the CO_2 laser in nerve repair was stimulated by the observations of Neblett and Morris (1983) that microvascular anastomosis could be performed using a highly focused low power beam. A "tissue welding" effect was proposed since a watertight closure with good immediate tensile strength was achieved. In addition, histologic studies of the vessel walls showed excellent reconstitution of the normal layered architecture with a minimum of disruptive scarring. An additional theoretical advantage of the CO_2 laser for microsurgical nerve repair is the expected high absorption by surface moisture and epi- or perineurium which would result in minimal exposure of the internal portion of the fascicle to laser irradiation. In order to understand the specific requirements of a laser technique for nerve repair, the biology of nerve coaptation and current techniques of microsurgical nerve repair will be reviewed briefly.

The Biology of Nerve Coaptation

The peripheral nerves of greatest clinical importance are typically mixed (motor and sensory) nerves with a complex fascicular structure (Sunderland 1968). In primates and man, even lesions in continuity (crush injuries) show poor functional results. Most authors attribute this outcome to two main factors: failure of the regenerating axon sprouts to find the proper distal myelinated "conduit" and the ingrowth of fibrous scar from the epi- or perineural sheath elements. After nerve injury resulting in axontemesis, the distal portion of the axon dies and is phagocytized, leaving an endoneurial tube (Forman *et al.* 1979, Millesi 1982). The proximal axon stumps sprout and grow into the zone of injury. Many of the sprouts fail to reach the distal Schwann tubes resulting in neuromas which further impede the growth of other axon terminals through the injured area (Millesi 1977). Experimental studies of nerve regeneration have investigated the events occurring in the zone of injury. Gutmann *et al.* (1942) noted that regeneration in cut and sutured rabbit nerves was slower and less complete than in crush injuries. There was approximately a two day increase in the time required for the axon sprouts to cross the zone of injury. The same delay was documented in a microsurgical model studied by Forman *et al.* (1979). In addition, the rate of axon elongation after the regenerating axon tips had passed into the distal portion of the nerve was slower in both studies. Speculation about the cause of these phenomena centers around scarring and changes in blood supply at the suture line. It has been conclusively demonstrated in experimental studies that tension at the site of nerve repair results in increased proliferation of connective tissue and in destruction of the regenerating axon sprouts (Millesi 1977, 1982, 1984, Terzis and Strauch 1977).

Current Microsurgical Techniques for Nerve Repair

Application of microsurgical techniques to management of peripheral nerve lacerations has resulted in significant improvement in functional results (Millesi 1982, 1984). Factors responsible for this improvement include use of very fine instruments and microneedles producing less secondary mechanical injury, emphasis on fascicular or grouped fascicular coaptation reducing the amount of connective tissue incorporated into the sutured nerve and in misalignment of nerve fascicles, and the use of ultrafine monofilament suture decreasing the degree of foreign body reaction. However, despite these advances, the clinical results of nerve suture are often disappointing. Fibrous scar can invade the coapted fascicle; suture granulomas further reduce the cross sectional area available for ingrowth of regenerating axon sprouts (Fig. 1). Millesi (1982) emphasizes the importance of careful dissection to obtain fascicles or groups of fascicles containing the minimum amount of connective tissue and the use of a minimum number of sutures (generally one) to achieve coaptation without tension. Although good coaptation of nerve fascicles can be achieved by the use of autologous fibrin clot, the immediate tensile strength of the nerve repair is very low, leading to a significant dehiscence rate unless absolute immobilization is achieved. In fact, Millesi (1982, 1984) describes special

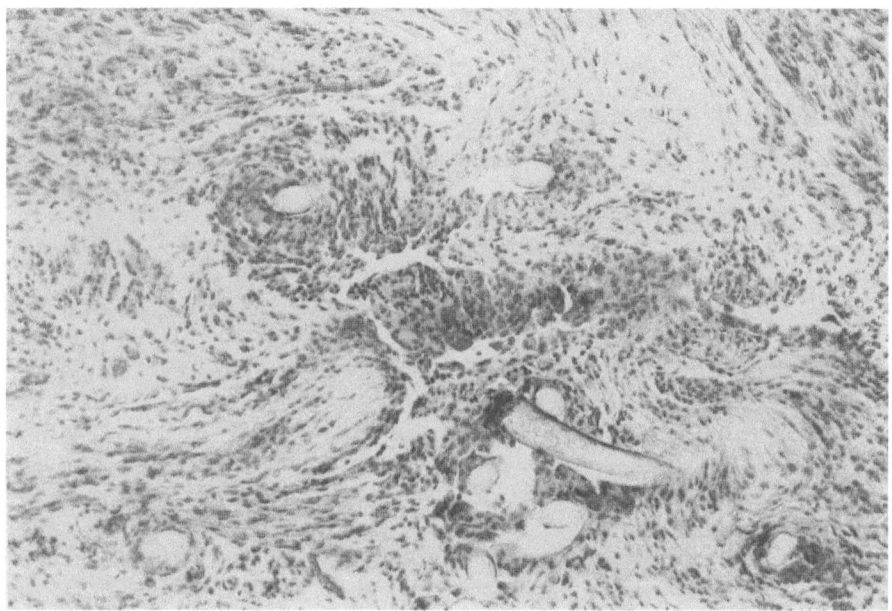

Fig. 1. Suture granulomas, rat sciatic nerve 4 weeks postcoaptation with 10–0 monofilament nylon

precautions necessary to avoid disruption of the coapted fascicles during wound closure, and the "crucial" importance of immobilization during the first two days after repair. Clinically, he recommends application of a plaster cast for 8–10 days postoperatively.

Laser Repair of Peripheral Nerves

The only published report of the use of a laser for nerve coaptation describes the work of Almquist who used an argon laser to coagulate whole blood applied to the apposed fascicles of a rat nerve with results similar to those obtained by suture repair. The author also reported that argon laser irradiation of blood clot applied to primate ulnar nerves which had not been injured had no deleterious effects (Freiherr 1982). The technique described by Almquist offers no significant advantage over the fibrin clot method, and further reports on this technique have not been forthcoming.

The main disadvantage of the fibrin clot technique of nerve coaptation have been poor early tensile strength and the requirement for one or more approximating sutures (Millesi 1977, 1982, 1984). Our experience with the use of the CO_2 milliwatt laser for microvascular anastomosis suggested that this method might provide a nerve coaptation of greater initial tensile strength. In addition, sealing of the epineurium might inhibit outgrowth of

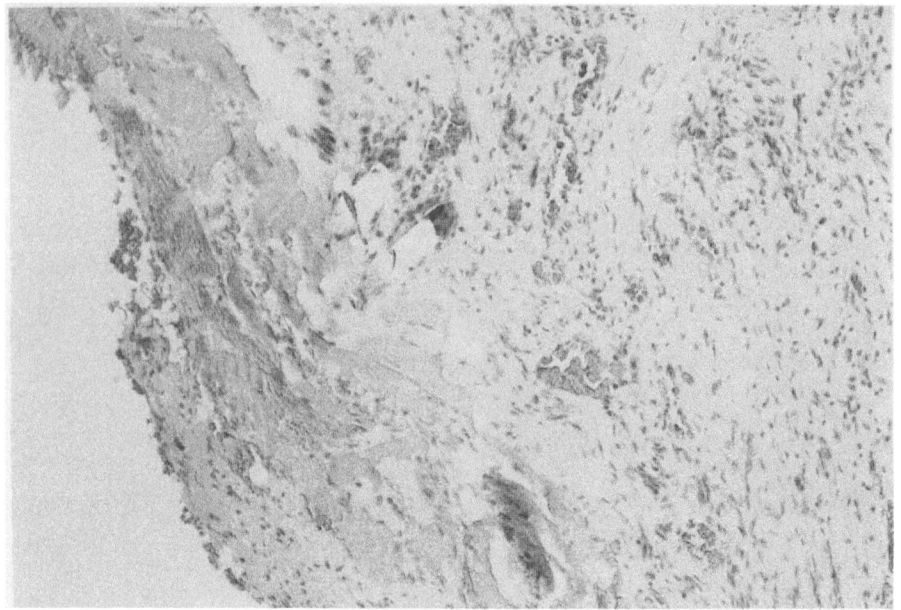

Fig. 2. Neurite outgrowth into muscle near repair site, rat sciatic model 2 weeks postcoaptation

axon sprouts into surrounding muscle, a phenomenon observed frequently in experimental microsuture methods, especially if only one or two approximating sutures are placed (Fig. 2).

Working in collaboration with Dr. Barth Green of the University of Miami, a series of experiments using the rat sciatic model were performed. Both the behavioral and histologic events of nerve regeneration in this system have been described (Forman *et al.* 1979).

The first question we sought to answer was whether CO_2 laser irradiation itself had any harmful effects on the rat sciatic nerve, particularly with respect to fibroblast proliferation. Bilateral sciatic nerve exposure was made and one nerve circumferentially irradiated with the beam at a power setting of 70–80 milliwatts. The contralateral nerve served as the control. A single microsuture was placed in the epineurium to permit identification of the area irradiated. Ten animals were evaluated at intervals of up to 12 weeks.

No behavioral or neurologic deficits were noted. There were no significant histologic differences between control and lased nerves.

A second set of experiments was performed in order to compare laser assisted coaptation with the microsuture method. The sciatic nerves were exposed bilaterally and mobilized in the epineural plane from their emergence from beneath the paraspinous muscles to the bifurcation,

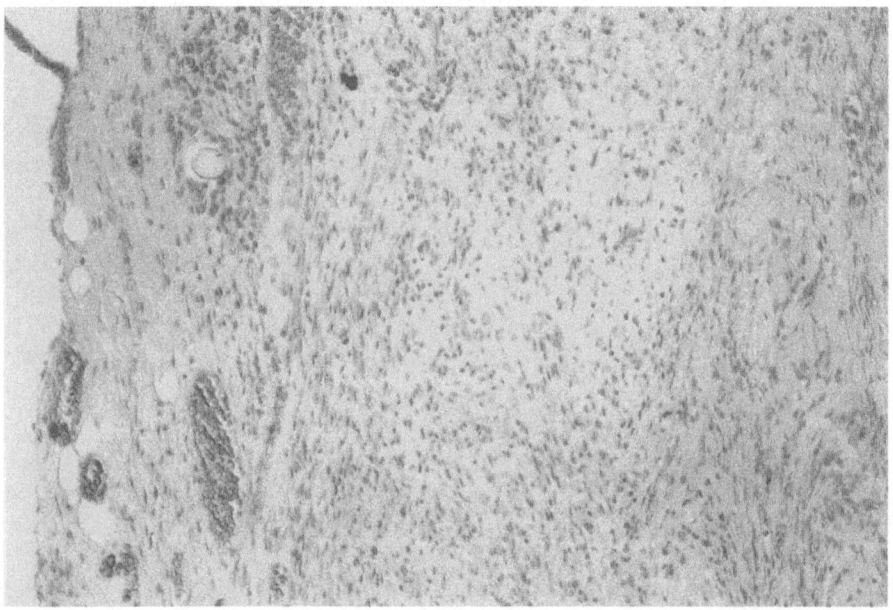

Fig. 3. CO_2 laser assisted coaptation; rat sciatic nerve model, 2 weeks postcoaptation

sharply divided, and the axoplasmic "mushroom" trimmed carefully to allow good epineural coaptation. One nerve was coapted with epineural sutures of 10–0 monofilament nylon. In the other, three stay sutures were placed to bring the epineurium into apposition and then "welded" together using the CO_2 laser beam. Two of the three stay sutures were then removed. One suture was left in place to permit precise localization of the repair site histologically. Animals were allowed to recover from anesthesia and were then reexplored, and the sciatic nerves removed and examined histologically at intervals up to twelve weeks after repair. Parallel experiments were conducted: one at the University of Miami by Dr. Green and his trainees (H. Landy and A. Lang) using the Bioquantum laser (model 7600) and one at the Uniformed Services University of the Health Sciences by the author and her trainee (L. Spetka) using a modification of the Cooper Lasersonics model 350. In both series, a disappointingly high early dehiscence rate

(40–60%) was observed, despite the use of three power ranges: 75–100 mw, 100–150 mw, and 200–250 mw (Landy *et al.* 1985). However, healing in the nondisrupted nerves looked quite favorable histologically, especially in comparison with the marked suture granulomas seen in the conventionally repaired nerves (Fig. 3). Clearly, the early tensile strength of the laser coaptation was not adequate.

Rather than attempt external immobilization of our experimental animals, we searched for an alternate method of avoiding early dehiscence.

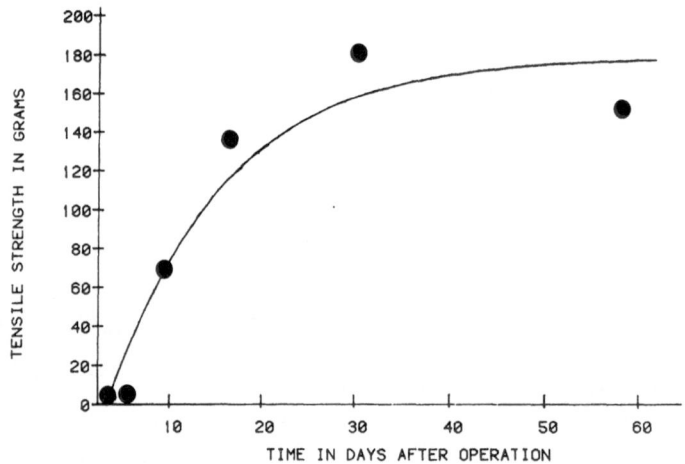

Fig. 4. Relationship between tensile strength and time after operation for sutureless CO_2 laser coaptation using rat sciatic interposition graft model

Discussions with Drs. Millesi and Terzis, who have used the fibrin clot method of nerve coaptation extensively, led to the recommendation that interposition nerve grafts be used in the sciatic model. It is well known that after sharp division of a peripheral nerve, the cut ends retract, producing a gap. Performance of a suture repair even with nerve mobilization by epineural dissection requires tension across the site of coaptation. In the rat sciatic model, sharp transection of the nerve one cm proximal to the bifurcation results in a gap of approximately 1.3 cm. While this gap can easily be bridged using microsutures, fibrin clot coaptation without multiple stay sutures cannot be reliably attained. Therefore, an interposition graft was taken from the contralateral sciatic nerve of the animal (allografts are not tolerated in the Wistar strain, see Zalewski *et al.* 1980, 1982), and cut to just fill the retraction gap left after nerve trimming. Initial coaptation using the fibrin clot method could then be reliably achieved, permitting gentle manipulation of the nerve during epineural lasing without the secondary damage produced by stay sutures. Thus coaptation could be accomplished without tension, since the tensile strength of a fibrin clot rat sciatic coaptation is less than 1 g.

A series of 28 sutureless laser coaptations using 100–125 mw was performed with a 3.6% dehiscence rate in unrestrained animals. (It should be noted that rats with bilateral sciatic nerve palsies are quite cage mobile.) Tensile strength of laser coapted nerves, although initially quite low (8 g),

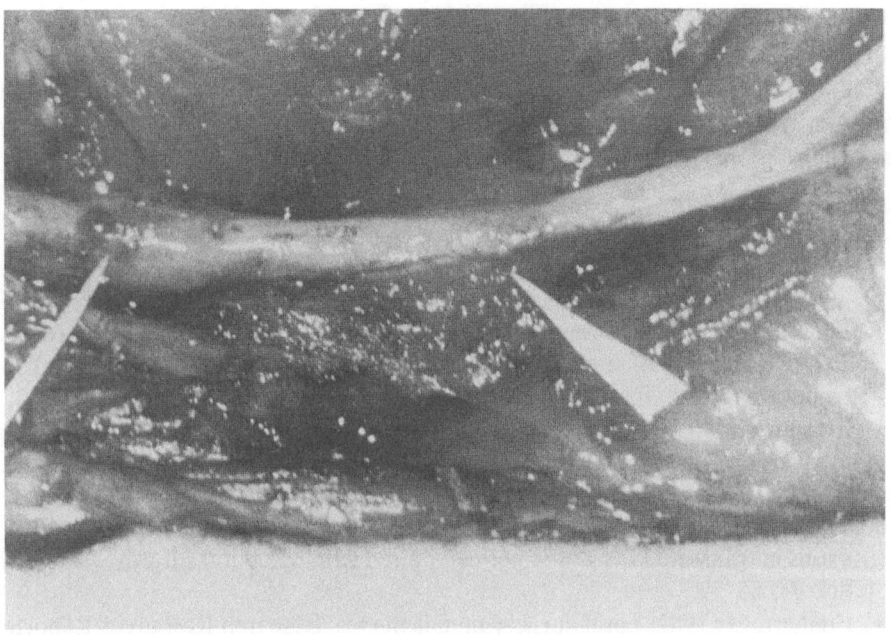

Fig. 5. Gross appearance of interposition graft 8 weeks after sutureless CO_2 laser coaptation (thin marker proximal, wide marker distal)

rapidly rose to levels similar to that for sutured nerves (180 g) at two weeks (Fig. 4).

Functional results were assessed with the pinch test (Behrenberg *et al.* 1977) and with the inclined plane test (Rivlin and Tator 1977). Animals with sciatic transection treated by interposition grafts coapted with either the laser technique or with microsuture showed no significant differences in functional improvement. Since it is well known that nerve regneration is generally very good in this model system, these results are not surprising.

Although histological studies are not yet completed, the gross appearance of the nerves coapted with the laser has been very gratifying. Smooth healing of the epineurium occurred without neuroma formation (Fig. 5). In addition, the laser technique of coaptation was more rapid, requiring a mean time of 11 ± 6 minutes as compared with 21 ± 9 minutes required for the suture technique. This feature could result in significant reduction of operating time in more complex procedures such as brachial plexus reconstruction, requiring multiple cable grafts.

In summary, a sutureless technique for microsurgical nerve repair has been developed using milliwatt CO_2 lasers with a small spot size. An acceptable dehiscence rate has been achieved in the rat sciatic model by the use of an interposition cable graft as commonly employed in nerve reconstruction procedures. The risks of mechanical damage and scar formation are reduced, and the quality of early regeneration appears to be at least as good as that achieved with optimal microsuture methods. The rapidity with which coaptation can be performed offers advantages in complex reconstructive procedures.

References

1. Behrenberg, R. A., Forman, D. S., Wood, D. K., DeSilva, A., Demaree, J., 1977: Recovery of peripheral nerve function after axotomy: Effect of triiodothyronine. Exp. Neurol. *57*, 349–363.
2. Erasmus, M. D., Richmond, I. L., Terzis, J. K., 1985: Nerve repair using interposition grafts and a sutureless laser technique. Abstract presented at Annual Meeting of LANSI, March 1985.
3. Forman, D. S., Wood, D. K., DeSilva, S., 1979: Rate of regeneration of sensory axons in transected rat sciatic nerve repaired with epineural sutures. J. Neurol. Sci. *44*, 55–59.
4. Freiherr, G., 1982: Laser surgery mends nerves. Research Resources Reporter *6*, 1–5.
5. Gutmann, E., Gutmann, L., Medawar, P. B., Young, J. Z., 1942: The rate of regeneration of nerve. J. exp. Biol. *19*, 14–44.
6. Lang, A., Landy, H., Green, B., Richmond, I., Spetka, L., Thomas, J., Reyes, F., Kato, S., 1985: Preliminary results of an ongoing project using micro-laser technique for sciatic nerve anastomosis: A controlled study. Abstract presented at the First Annual Meeting of the Joint Section of Spinal Diseases AANS/CNS, Feb. 1985.
7. Millesi, H., 1977: Fascicular nerve repair and interfascicular nerve grafting. In: Reconstructive Microsurgery (Daniel, R. K., Terzis, J. K., eds.), pp. 430–442. Boston: Little, Brown and Co.
8. Millesi, H., 1982: Peripheral nerve injuries. Scand. J. Plast. Reconstr. Surg. (Suppl. *19*), 25–37.
9. Millesi, H., 1984: Nerve grafting. Clinics in Plastic Surgery *11*, 105–112.
10. Neblett, C., Morris, J., 1983: A study of CO_2 laser assisted microsurgical anastomoses of small vessels. Plastic Surgery Educational Foundation.
11. Rivlin, A. S., Tator, C. H., 1977: Objective clinical assessment of motor function after experimental spinal cord injury in the rat. J. Neurosurg. *47*, 577–581.
12. Sunderland, S., 1968: Nerves and Nerve Injuries. Edinburgh: Livingstone.

13. Terzis, J. K., Strauch, B., 1978: Microsurgery of the peripheral nerve. Clin. Orthop. Rel. Res. *133*, 39–48.
14. Zalewski, A. A., Gulati, A. K., 1982: Evaluation of histo-compatibility as a factor in the repair of nerve with a frozen nerve allograft. J. Neurosurg. *56*, 550–554.
15. Zalewski, A. A., Silvers, W. K., 1980: An evaluation of nerve repair with nerve allografts in normal and immunologically tolerant rats. J. Neurosurg. *52*, 557–563.

Laser Vascular Application:
Reconstructive and Reparative

Charles R. Neblett

Baylor College of Medicine, Houston, Texas (U.S.A.)

Contents

I. Introduction.. 184
II. The Bonding Mechanism 185
III. The M-CO$_2$ Laser.. 186
IV. The Research Animal Model 186
V. Arterial Anastomosis.. 187
VI. Venous Anastomosis 190
VII. Spot-Welding.. 191
VIII. The Growing Anastomosis.. 191
IX. The Reparative Process 192
X. The PP Requirement 193
XI. Conclusion.. 193

I. Introduction

The reconstruction and the repair of vascular structures has been an important goal in neurosurgery for many decades. Advancements have been forthcoming through new instruments, improved suture materials and better visualization. The development of the CO$_2$ laser as a surgical instrument for ablation is well accepted. A microsurgically adapted CO$_2$ laser can provide reconstructive and reparative capabilities. This chapter will highlight the application of an M-CO$_2$ laser system made specifically for these purposes, providing application in the $micro$-mode, with $micron$ spot-size and with $milliwatt$ power exposure.

Arteries and veins can be anastomosed, end-to-end or end-to-side. Arteries, veins and vascular sinuses can be spot-welded. Because of the nature of this bonding mechanism these vessels have the capacity to continue to grow as that tissue grows, thus minimizing the risk of future constrictions. Also the reparative process allows vascular anomalies to be diminished or obliterated through their exposure to a carefully controlled M-CO_2 thermal force close to its reconstructive levels and significantly below its destructive levels.

II. The Bonding Mechanism

The reapproximation of organic tissue is usually achieved through the use of sutures. This time-tested mechanism has proven to be satisfactory. However, it does have limitations. The mechanics of suture placement and the tethering of tissues result in imperfect healing. Additional trauma, hemorrhage, necrosis and the presence of a foreign body excites increasing scar tissue formation. The laser provides a way of enhancing the healing properties through a more natural process.

First, the thermal effect must be considered. If organic tissue is exposed to a temperature of 100 °C, or greater, that tissue is vaporized. Therefore, the temperature must be controlled well below that level. Fifty to 75 °C appears to be the appropriate laser thermal level to affect bonding of tissue. The architecture of the cells is altered but not destroyed. This is accomplished with a power setting ranging from 50 to 150 milliwatts. The spot-size is quite small, varying from 80 to 250 microns. Larger spot-sizes result in a zone of thermally induced cellular damage beyond that required for the anastomosis.

Although the biochemical responses are not completely understood, there do appear to be certain characteristics present. Protein chemistry is altered when heat is applied. The thermal effect of the M-CO_2 laser at 50 to 75 °C momentarily alters protein molecules with some destruction to the skeletal architecture of cells. A denaturation-renaturation process occurs. The hydroxyl and disulfide bonds holding the protein in a tertiary position appear to be altered resulting in an opening, then rejoining of the molecules in a bonding fashion. The beta-helical protein molecules, and those with particularly hydrophobic peripheral amino acids are the most amenable to this bonding process. In essence, an "organic protein glue" is formed.

Through the use of transmission electron microscopy the collagen molecules have been studied. Dr. Peter Clara[1] has shown that the usually randomly positioned collagen molecules appear to be polarized after this laser exposure and become linearly placed across the bonded site. Improved structural integrity results.

---

[1] Peter Clara, M.D., "Lasers in Neurosurgery": Presentation to Texas Association of Neurological Surgeons, May 21, 1983, Houston, Texas.

Intense biochemical studies are still required to further delineate the mechanism of M-CO_2 laser bonding. Certainly, this is one of the most exciting areas for continued research.

III. The M-CO_2 Laser

In order to deliver a precise thermal energy dose to the tissue being bonded, a specific instrument is required. Mr. James Morris[2] has pioneered the research work which has resulted in achieving this process. He, through Bio-Quantum Technologies, Inc., has developed a CO_2 laser designed precisely for this purpose. Although the Bio-Quantum Laser can function exceptionally well as a tool for cutting and vaporizing tissue, it is the reconstructive-reparative capabilities on which this chapter concentrates. All of the studies described herein were performed with this laser.

Because a definite force must be provided by the M-CO_2 laser, it must possess certain specific properties. Precision is essential. The wattage utilized is milliwatts ranging from 50 to 150. This is applied in conjunction with a spot-size varying from 80 to 250 microns. These variables are dependent upon the tissue characteristics including composition and density of the tissue. Specifically, the work in vascular reconstruction of small arteries and veins required a lesser power density obtainable with about 100 milliwatts and 150 microns. However, this is very dependent on the chemistry of the tissue. Once these tissue parameters are established then more exact laser energy doses can be applied.

Spot sizes also requir rather stringent control. The parameters described for milliwatts applies here also, and only small variations are reasonable. The more delicate the tissue, the fewer microns the reconstructive process demands. Eighty to 250 microns is the usual requirement. Should the spot-size be larger than one-tenth the vessel diameter, undue changes take place in the surrounding cells and result in undesirable tissue damage, as our current experience indicates.

Microscopic delivery is required for the accurate control of the M-CO_2 laser and for the immediate visual appreciation of tissue changes indicative of fusion.

IV. The Research Animal Model

The Sprague-Dolly 250–300 gram rat was the basic animal model. Anesthesia was obtained with intraperitoneal Ketamine (200 mg/kg of body weight). A routine inguinal incision was made and the femoral artery exposed. The profundus femoral artery was sacrificed by sealing (200 milliwatts) and then cutting (500 milliwatts) with the laser. Microvascular

---

[2] Mr. James Morris, Bio-Quantum Technologies, Inc., 8275 El Rio, no. 180, Houston, TX 77054.

clamps were placed on the artery. It was divided with microscissors. The artery was freed of all blood using normal saline. Blood should not remain within the lumen or at the anastomotic site. The diameter of the rat femoral artery ranges from 0.5 to 1.0 mm. Three 10/0 vascular sutures were put into place approximately 180° apart and the sutures were left long to allow their use for traction. The adventitia was not removed.

The operation was performed with microsurgical technique. Attached directly to the microscope was the Bio-Quantum 7600 Microsurgical CO_2 Laser System. The focal distance was 300 mm. The spot-size was 150 microns, and the wattage was 80 to 100 milliwatts. Tension was placed on two of the three stay sutures and the interface between the arteries' edges was sealed with the laser, either with continuous or with interrupted exposures. Bonding could be determined by the change in the tissue's appearance. This process was repeated two additional times between the other stay stitches. The distal clamp was then removed and the anastomotic site observed for any evidence of blood leakage. If any leakage was noted, the clamp was reapplied and the area of incomplete bonding was reexposed to the laser after the blood had been lavaged from the lumen. The proximal clamp was then removed and a distal patency test performed. A closure of the incisional site was performed utilizing standard technique.

V. Arterial Anastomosis

The rat's femoral and carotid arteries, as well as the pig's and dog's femoral artery and aorta were used. The vessel to be anastomosed was prepared as previously described. The femoral artery of the rat has served as the most frequently used animal model. Hundreds of these operations have been performed. To tabulate the results, 200 consecutive procedures were recorded. Patency was achieved in 91% of the arteries. All 200 were initially patent, but six arteries were found to be not-patent during the follow-up period.

The patency rate should be very high. With increasing experience the long-term patency should be above 95%. In five percent minor constrictions were present, none sufficient to produce any significant hemodynamic alterations. The histological studies which followed confirmed what had been recorded at the time of surgery—that additional laser exposure had been required. If a bleeding site was present, the bonding process was repeated and the arterial wall was occasionally overexposed. As a result, that portion of the vessel wall had scar tissue formation and thus a regional stricture.

The reverse may also be seen at an anastomotic site. Should bleeding occur in the process of attempting to reweld the tissue, blood may remain in the interface between arterial walls and the resultant bond is weakened. A pseudoaneurysm may form. This did occur in three of the 200 anastomes, and it has been reported in other femoral artery anastomosis studies.

Two important points should be emphasized. First, the technique must be perfected to minimize this possibility. This can be accomplished through experience and meticulous operative technique. Second, if and when an aneurysm develops, the histologic characteristics will be somewhat different than true aneurysms. Aneurysms which form in conventional anastomoses

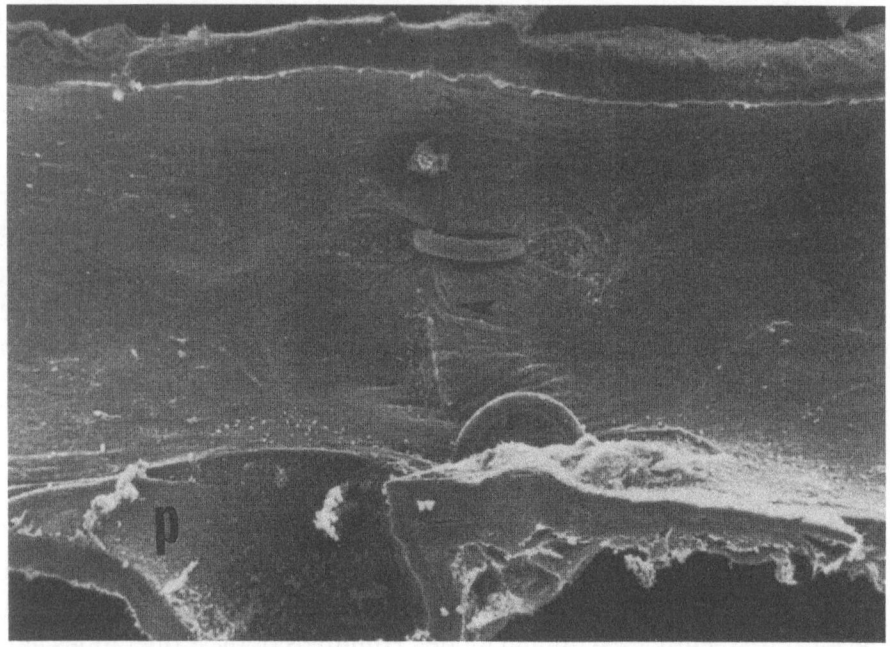

Fig. 1

possess less connective tissue about the weakened area and appear to be more friable. The connective tissue surrounding the pseudoaneurysm in the laser anastomoses is denser and appears structurally stronger. They are also less frequently seen in the laser anastomoses than with conventional suturing technique.

A similar experience has been noted with other arteries in the rat, dog and pig. The larger arteries require a moderate increase in the wattage and spot-size. Also two or four stay stitches may be used instead of the standard three.

An end-to-side artery-to-artery laser assisted anastomosis can be performed. Four stay stitches are used, one at either end of the anastomosis and one on either side. The histologic appearance and patency rate are essentially the same.

The histology was performed by Dr. Sharon Thomsen[3]. Immediately postoperatively the amount of endothelial damage was much less in the lasered area compared to the standard suture anastomosis, in part due to fewer stitches being required. However, it began to be deposited on the denuded areas (Fig. 1).

By the first postoperative day, and using scanning electron microscopy,

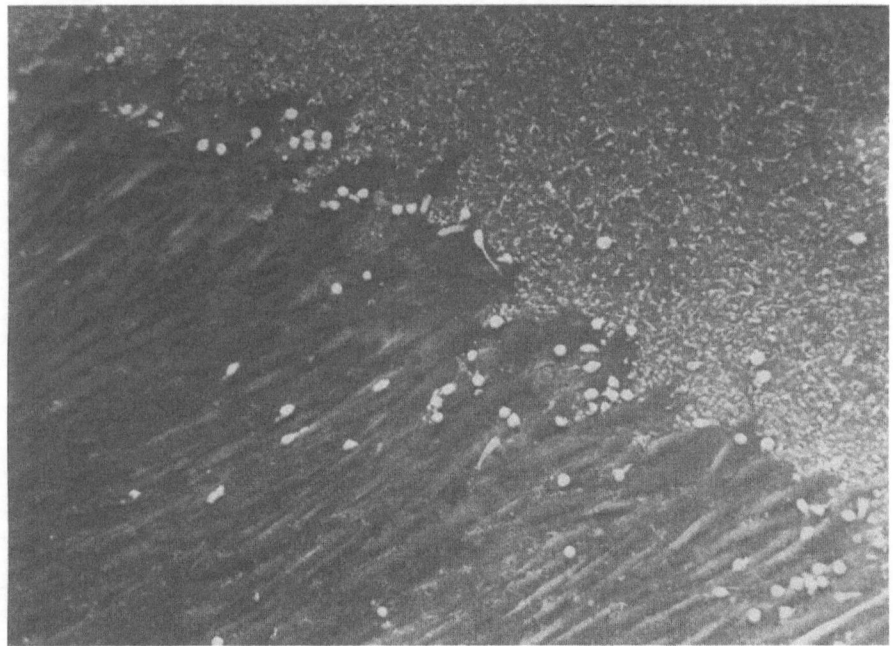

Fig. 2

most of the damaged endothelium had sloughed. The fibrin deposition was becoming more organized. Platelets as well as a few red and white blood cells were adherent to the exposed internal elastic lamina with the greatest density at the anastomotic site.

Endothelial cell proliferation begins by the seventh postoperative day, but only at the border of the intact endothelium and at the islands of intact endothelium closer to the anastomotic site. At the boundary of the proliferating endothelial cells and the exposed fibrin covering the internal elastic lamina are an increasing number of white blood cells. They appear to be cleaning necrotic debris or organizing the fibrin prior to the endothelial advancement (Fig. 2).

Reendothelialization continued and by the third postoperative week the

[3] Sharon Thomsen, M.D., Associate Professor, Department of Pathology, University of Miami, Miami, Florida.

anastomotic site was completely covered by continuous, intact endothelial cells. It was noted that the long axis of the endotheal cells was parallel to the longitudinal axis of the artery.

By the sixth week reendothelialization was complete (Fig. 3).

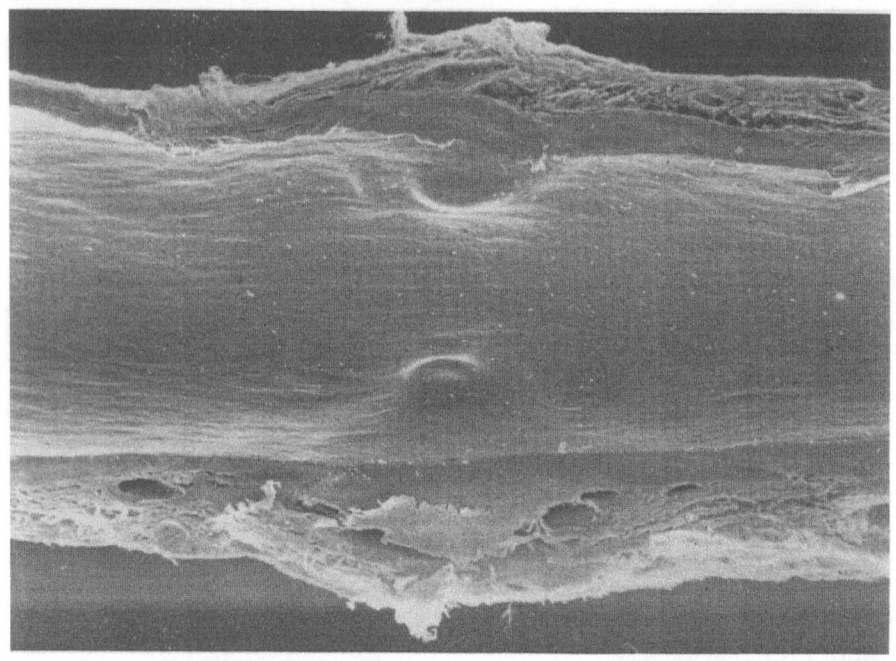

Fig. 3

VI. Venous Anastomosis

Venous anastomoses have been performed in all of these animal models. A similar surgical technique was utilized. Dr. Renee Hartz[4], Associate Professor of Cardiovascular Surgery at Northwestern University, uses a mattress stitch to evert the edges of the vein. She believes this facilitates the bonding process. We have not found this to be necessary. It is Dr. Hartz' opinion that this technique will have significant application in human general and cardiovascular surgery. Also the histology and patency is similar to that observed in arterial anastomoses.

Artery-to-vein anastomoses can be achieved, either end-to-end or end-to-side. The variances in the vessel wall thickness have proven not to be of significance.

---

[4] Renee Hartz, M.D.: Personal communication.

VII. Spot-Welding

Hemostasis is an essential feature of any surgical procedure. Should a bleeding diathesis develop in a vascular structure (artery, vein or vascular sinus) it must be secured. As well, preservation of that vascular structure is desired. Suturing the opening may be technically difficult and/or impossible. Obliteration of that vascular structure may be required to obtain hemostasis.

Spot-welding can help achieve this goal. First, hemostasis must be obtained. A suitable tissue to cover the opening must then be provided. The vessel's own adventitia is ideal. Adventitia-connective tissue from adjacent structures may be used. This material, high in collagen, is then placed to cover the diathesis. It should be thin. Good apposition between that material's edge and the involved vessel's edge is essential. The laser welding process occurs at this interface. Third, specially made liquid collagen may be directly applied and laser affixed.

Several technical features should be observed. The tissue used needs to be high in collagen. Most adventitia fulfills this criteria. Prepare a thin "patch". Thick patches tend to pull away from the parent vessel resulting in nonbonding. If bonding is not accomplished initially, repeated laser exposures may be required and the vessel may constrict. The constriction can be temporary due to vessel wall spasm or permanent due to tissue damage and excessive scar tissue formation. Keep the tissue moist. The initial laser force should be of about 150 microns and 50 milliwatts. After the edges first appear to adhere, increase the power to 100 milliwatts to enhance the initial bond.

An opening as large as 25 percent of the diameter of the vessel can be closed with this technique. The histological appearance of the spot-welded area reveals a limited amount of scar proliferation. The area is strong and not prone to future rupture or aneurysmal dilatation.

It should be noted that the spot-welding technique may be used in other settings. The surgeon can reinforce an anastomotic area or add to an area of aneurysmal or AVM weakness or diathesis.

In summary, this procedure may be of benefit when the surgeon is confronted with any of several unexpected, potentially serious problems. Therefore, it is recommended that the Bio-Quantum Laser be placed on the microscope for all surgical procedures, just as you would place a movie camera. It will then be available for use in certain emergencies.

VIII. The Growing Anastomosis

Preservation of normal growth pattern potentials is very desirable. For example, in pediatric vascular surgery, an anastomotic site becomes a future coarctation. With progressive flow compromise the stricture must be removed and another anastomosis provided. Thus the question: does the laser anastomosis have the capability of "growing" as that tissue expands? Dr. Denton Cooley[5] and Dr. O. Howard Frazier[6] assisted in the study of this problem.

Nine miniswine at two months of age underwent a femoral artery anastomosis with M-CO_2 laser technique. These animals were chosen because of their vascular similarity to humans and because of their rapid growth. The artery preparation and opening were both as previously described. After approximation of the edges with 10/0 vascular stitches the anastomosis was provided with the laser at 150 microns and 125 milliwatts.

By the thirteenth postoperative week the pig was sacrificed. The average weight had increased 350 percent. One hundred percent patency was demonstrated by angiography and histology. The external diameter had increased 80 percent and there was no evidence of stenosis. Minimal fibrosis and scar tissue reaction was elicited.

It was concluded that the laser assisted anastomotic site does indeed possess the capacity to continue with its normal growth pattern.

IX. The Reparative Process

With the proper control provided by the M-CO_2 laser many goals can be accomplished. It is applied routinely in a destructive mode. This chapter stresses the other end of the spectrum, reconstruction. Let us focus for a moment on its controlled use just beyond the classic reconstructive area, the reparative mode.

The reparative process allows the surgeon to selectively alter the cellular characteristics and arrangements of the organic tissue through exposure to the thermal effect of the M-CO_2 laser. Changes in the reconstructive mode have been discussed, and those in the destructive mode have been repeatedly chronicled. Thermal forces just greater than those at the reconstructive level are reparative.

The realignment of collagen cells in linear fashion is one important component in the process. Clinical applicability has already been demonstrated in the treatment of vascular anomalies. The argon and neodymium YAG lasers as well as the bipolar coagulation forceps have been used for this purpose.

The M-CO_2 laser provides the control to shrink and firm up the tissues. For example, an aneurysmal dilatation can be diminished in size using the laser at 250 microns and 100 to 150 milliwatts. The same process applies to

---

[5] Denton A. Cooley, M.D., Sergeant-in-Chief, Cardiovascular Surgery, St. Luke's Episcopal Hospital, Houston, Texas.

[6] O. Howard Frazier, M.D., Cardiovascular Surgeon, St. Luke's Episcopal Hospital, Houston, Texas.

AVMs. A variation in this theme can be appreciated when normal venous plexuses are sealed in the process of removing a disc herniation or, for that matter, when performing any spinal surgery.

The reparative process is an important capability provided by the laser. However, you should remember these two considerations. First, it is the precise control of the M-CO_2 laser which allows you to achieve this goal. Do not attempt this process without precise microscopic, micron and milliwatt control. Second, appreciate that this is another application mode in an ever increasing spectrum of laser surgery.

X. The PP Requirement

In order to achieve hemostasis, the historic principles required "*Pressure* and *Patience*". I term this the "PP Requirement". As neurosurgery was modernized we were provided with improved instruments, sutures, machines and visualization. The technical advancements of the M-CO_2 laser add another quantum leap. There are at least seven "P's" which have application.

Prompt: The tissue bonding process is instantaneous. The time expenditure in the technical part can be minimized.

Precise: The byword is, "the more delicate the surgery, the more precise the process". Precision is measured in microns and milliwatts. The delivery system is through a microscope with a bias manipulator. The tolerance variation is limited to only a few percentile.

Patent: Patency is desirable, frequently essential. The patency rate with the M-CO_2 laser assisted anastomosis is in the very high 90 percentile range.

Powerful: The anastomosis site is strong. An adequate tensile strength is provided.

Pure: Arguably, the most important "P" is the purity of the process. With little or no foreign body to excite tissue reactions, the repair proceeds unincumbered.

Process—the Spectrum: Conceptualize the laser application as the light itself, a spectrum of varying colors. It is not simply divided into two extremes, the destructive mode on one extreme, the reconstructive mode on the other. For example, adjoining the reconstructive area is the reparative arena. Many more subdivisions will follow.

XI. Conclusion

New technologies in neurosurgery provide genuine excitement. This chapter highlights the application of the M-CO_2 laser technique in a very well-controlled microscopic-micron-milliwatt mode. Adherence to strict parameters is critical. The result of this application is the organic fusion of vascular structures.

Arterial and venous anastomoses can be achieved with particular emphasis on otherwise extremely difficult small vessel (< 1 mm) anastomoses. The process can be achieved with more rapidity (prompt), with greater precision, with good tensile strength (powerful), with high rates of patency and with an enhanced healing process (pure).

The net result is a better, simpler operative procedure which can supplement current techniques. Controlled increases in the thermal force of the M-CO_2 laser allow for the vascular reparative process. Reconstructive-reparative laser vascular surgery is rapidly progressing from the laboratory to the clinical arena.

Application of Laser for Vaporization of Atherosclerotic Disease

GARRETT LEE, MING C. CHAN, RICHARD M. IKEDA, and DEAN T. MASON

The Western Heart Institute, St. Mary's Hospital and Medical Center,
San Francisco, California (U.S.A.)

Contents

General Considerations 196
The Atherosclerotic Plaque Obstruction 197
Immediate Laser Effects on Atherosclerotic Obstruction 198
Laser Delivery System 202
Long-Term Laser Effects on Atherosclerotic Obstruction 203
Laser Effects on Thrombotic Obstruction.. 204
Risks of Laser Treatment 204
Clinical Laser Recanalization 206
Catheter to Target Plaque for Laser Vaporization 206
Conclusions.. 208
Acknowledgments... 208
References... 208

Atherosclerotic disease accounts for significant morbidity, disability and mortality in man. As the disease progressively narrows the arterial lumen, blood flow is decreased to vital organs and structures such as the brain, heart, kidneys and leg muscles. The disease may also predispose afflicted vessels to thrombosis and embolism. Hence, cerebrovascular accidents, myocardial infarction, renal infarction, ischemia and gangrene of the lower extremities are all conditions that are frequently a consequence of atherosclerosis. Each year in the United States alone, an estimated 500,000 individuals are victims of stroke and 164,000 die; and approximately 1,500,000 develop myocardial infarction and 559,000 die[1].

Current methods of treatment in atherosclerotic patients to increase blood supply to vital organs include 1. bypass graft surgery, 2. surgical endarterectomy, 3. transluminal balloon angioplasty to fracture the atherosclerotic vascular wall by intravascular compression of the plaque and thus dilating the vessel lumen, and 4. use of thrombolytic agents such as streptokinase or urokinase to dissolve freshly organized vascular thrombus. Recently, enthusiasm has been generated by a new mode of therapy with future potential—laser recanalization of atherosclerotic disease. Since our early experiments using balloon angioplasty in human cadaver coronary arteries in the late 1970s[2], we conceived the applicability of laser technology to penetrate through an intravascular atherosclerotic obstruction which would create a channel large enough for adequate blood flow and would also allow passage of a balloon catheter for further expansion by transluminal angioplasty. The basic experimental and clinical progress of this new developing technology are reviewed herein.

General Considerations

Fundamentally, the interaction between a laser beam and biologic tissue involves the absorption of light energy by the tissue and the conversion of this energy into heat which results in the tissue vaporization effect. Further, the interaction depends on the physical properties of the beam and the biologic tissue. The three commonly used lasers in medicine are the argon (wavelength between 488–514 nm), neodymium-yttrium-aluminum-garnet (Nd : YAG) (1,069 nm) and carbon dioxide (CO_2) (10,600 nm). The narrow wavelengths produced by each specific laser medium will be preferentially absorbed by components of target tissue with matching absorbing peaks at those wavelengths. Since the hemoglobin in blood demonstrates major spectrophotometric absorption peaks between wavelengths of 400 and 600 nm, argon laser energies would be expected to be largely absorbed by blood. Thus argon lasers can be applied for photocoagulation of bleeding ulcers. On the other hand, since most biologic tissue contains water, the CO_2 laser, highly absorbed by water, can remove very thin tissue layers and make precise depth control possible by varying the power density.

The concept of power density is important in predicting the response of biologic tissue to laser radiation. Power density may be defined as the available instantaneous power (usually expressed in watts) per unit area; in practical terms, power density is calculated as the measured output of the laser divided by the cross-section of the area of the beam. Higher power densities coupled with shorter delivery times generally results in smaller degrees of thermal damage caused by dissipation of heat from target tissue into adjacent non-target tissue.

Power density differs from cumulative power or energy density (usually expressed in joules per unit area), which is a product of instantaneous power in watts and time in seconds. It is possible to achieve the same cumulative power in the same target area with two differing laser applications; for example, one of 12 watts at 0.5 seconds and another of 3 watts at 2 seconds both result in an energy of 6 joules. Thus, the four-fold increase in time coupled with a similar decrease in instantaneous power results in greater destructive accumulation of heat. The higher power density of 12 watts is almost instantly dissipated by vaporization of target tissue, whereas the lower power density of 3 watts is only sufficient to liquefy or char the target tissue. In the latter case, this heated material continues to absorb heat for 2 seconds without any dissipating mechanism other than transfer of thermal energy by continued contact with underlying tissue.

The Atherosclerotic Plaque Obstruction

Since the target tissue properties determine, in part, the degree of laser energy absorption, it is important to understand the physical characteristics of the atherosclerotic plaque. The atherosclerotic plaque is a raised, pearly gray to yellowish gray lesion, that bulges the intima into the vascular lumen. It is principally composed of mixtures of lipoid, fibrous and calcified materials. The ingredients in plaque are so heterogeneous that no two plaques are identical[3]. Spectrophotometric absorption studies to characterize the plaque are difficult to obtain. The ratio of fat to fibrous components tends to be higher in early developing plaque and lower in older plaques. Calcification, when present, tends to occur in aged plaques and in late fibrotic lesions in which the collagen has become hyalinized[3, 4]. Thus, newly formed plaques, in general, tend to have substances of lower density and older plaques tend to be composed of high density material. Plaques may ulcerate or rupture and may give rise to thrombo-embolic complications or lead to intimal hemorrhage.

Myointimal cells, myofibroblasts and lipid-filled macrophages comprise the plaque's main cellular components while the dense connective tissue is composed mostly of collagen fibers with infiltrations of macrophages and other white blood cells. Deep within the plaque's thickened intima are necrotic debris and varying amounts of lipid material. Biochemical analysis of plaque reveals heterogeneous mixtures of cholesterol, cholesterol esters, lipoproteins, proteoglycans, phospholipids, glycerol esters, and calcium salts.

Certain vascular sites are more prone to develop atherosclerotic lesions than others[4]. Frequent sites of occurrence include the carotid arteries, circle of Willis, coronary arteries, abdominal aorta, and arteries of the lower extremities. Infrequent sites include the mammary arteries and arteries of the upper extremities. Large and medium sized arteries are more often affected than smaller arteries[3, 4]. Lesions are more prone to develop near the orifices of branch vessels or at the bifurcation. Fortunately, from the operative viewpoint, in most patients with symptomatic coronary disease (*i.e.,* unstable angina), the distal half of the coronary arteries generally have less atherosclerotic narrowing than the proximal half[5].

Immediate Laser Effects on Atherosclerotic Obstruction

The acute effects of laser radiation on human cadaver atherosclerotic coronary disease have been documented by several studies[6-9]. When diseased vessels are exposed to argon, Nd-YAG or CO_2 laser energies,

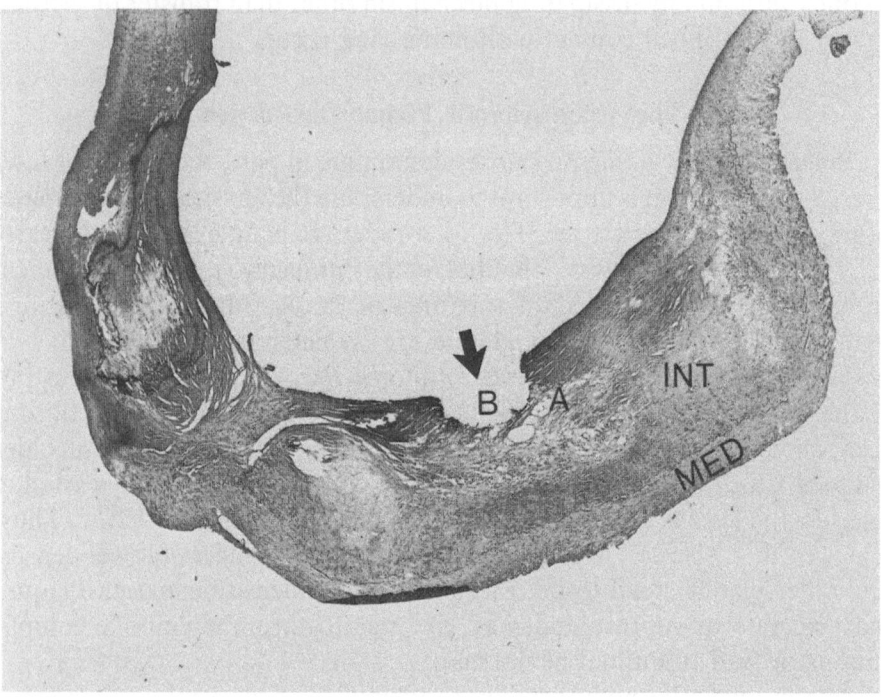

Fig. 1. Longitudinally opened human epicardial coronary artery exposing the inner luminal lining of the atherosclerotic plaque. An argon laser beam (7 watts, 0.4 seconds) directed perpendicular (arrow) to the hyalinized fibrous and lipid intimal area (*A*) of the plaque created a punched-out crater (*B*). *INT* intima, *MED* media. (Reproduced with permission from Lee, G., *et al.,* Am. Heart J. *105*, 886, 1983, Fig. 1)

thermal injury takes place producing a vaporized area or crater (Fig. 1). On microscopic cross-sectional examination of severely obstructed human atherosclerotic coronary artery, laser radiation adjacent to the existent narrowed channel can significantly widen luminal diameter (Fig. 2) or create a new channel for blood to flow (Fig. 3). Around the vaporized area is a charred lining (Figs. 2, 3, and 4). The charring is greater the longer the duration of laser exposure. Adjacent and beyond the charred lining may be an area of acoustic injury where there may be disruption and boiling of cellular and noncellular material (Fig. 4).

During the lasing process, solid or liquid matter is converted into gas. Analysis of the gaseous products of irradiated plaque reveals water vapor, carbon dioxide, nitrogen, hydrogen and light hydrocarbon fragments[10]. The rate of laser vaporization varies with tissue density. Rapid vaporization

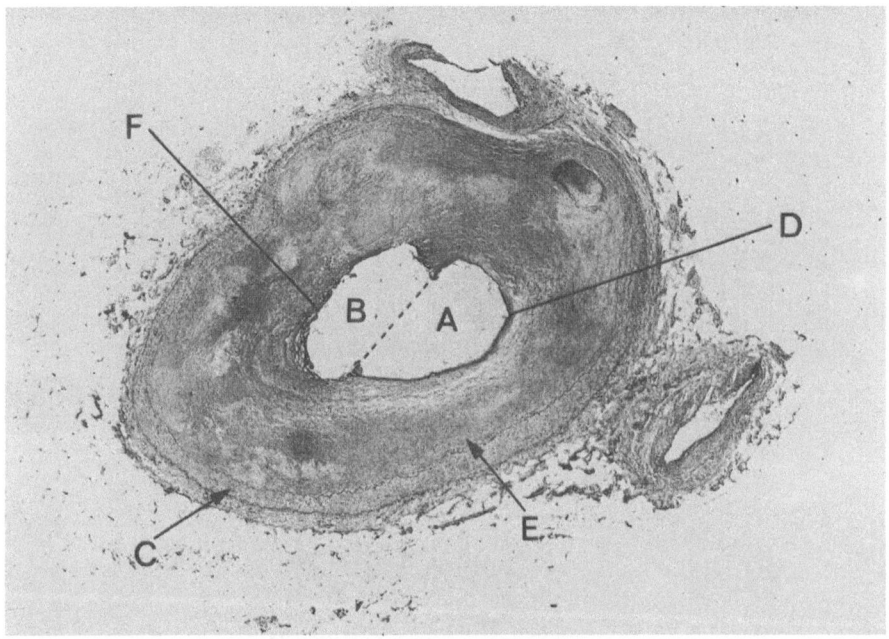

Fig. 2. Cross-section of obstructed human epicardial coronary artery. Following laser vaporization of hyalinized fibrous obstructing plaque (*B*), there was relief of stenotic lumen (*A*) with consequent two-fold widening of vessel patency. *C* coronary artery smooth muscle wall; *D* endothelial stenotic lining; *E* circumferential atherosclerotic hyaline plaque; *F* remnants of fibrous collagen charred by laser radiation. (Reproduced with permission from Lee, G., *et al.,* Am. Heart J. *102*, 1074, 1981, Fig. 1)

can be achieved with plaque containing materials of lower densities such as lipid-laden deposits. Laser penetration is retarded by high density deposits such as heavily calcified plaque. Moreover, greater extent of charred remnants may be found in the laser-induced channel of calcified plaque (Fig. 5) than in hyalinized plaque obstruction[6]. In lipid-laden plaque occluded coronary artery, no charred debris is found in its laser-treated passageway.

The ability of laser to penetrate plaque depends not only upon the absorptive characteristics of plaque material, but also on the physical and thermal properties of the laser beam. Thus, the higher the power intensity, the longer the laser exposure, and the more focused the beam, the greater is

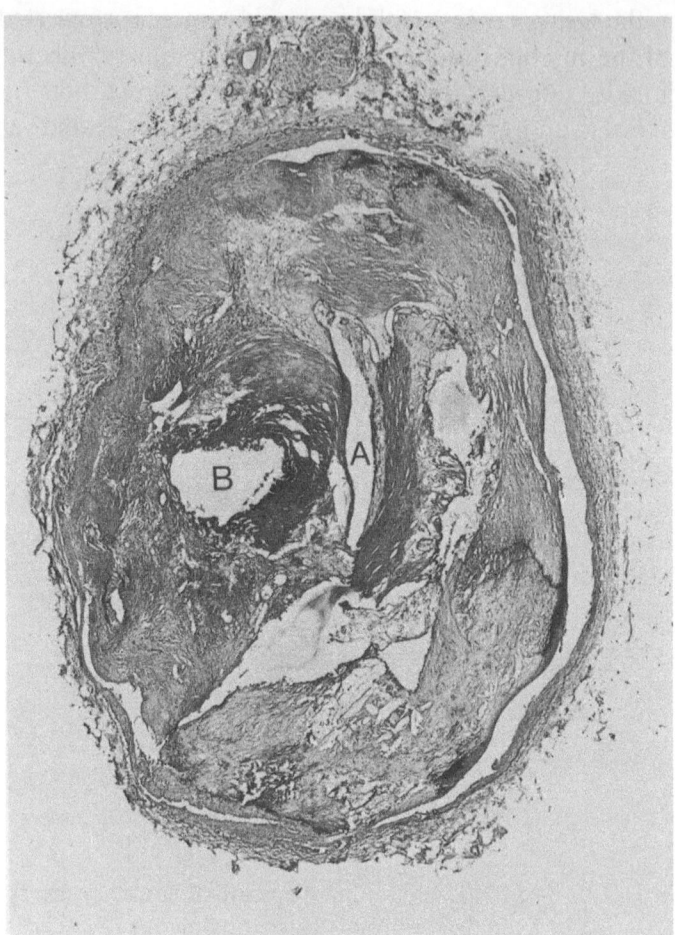

Fig. 3. Cross-section of a severely obstructed human atherosclerotic coronary artery with its slit-like lumen (*A*). Exposure from a CO_2 laser (40 watts, 0.4 seconds) vaporized a hyalinized fibrous area creating a new channel (*B*) near the original lumen (*A*). There is now a two-fold widening of vessel patency with the newly created channel. Note the dark rim and the tiny fragments in the channel. (Reproduced with permission from Lee, G., *et al.*, Am. Heart J. *105*, 888, 1983, Fig. 4)

the depth of plaque penetration. In one report in air, using a CO_2 laser with a 0.2 mm focal spot, plaque dissolution occurred at 1 to 2 joules; plaque and media were penetrated at 2.5 to 5 joules, and perforation of the vessel wall took place at greater than 7.5 joules[7]. Furthermore, deeper penetration of laser energy occurred under dry than wet conditions. In studies using CO_2 laser, injury to plaque occurred with a minimum total energy of 2.5 joules. Under saline solution, similar degree of plaque damage required a total

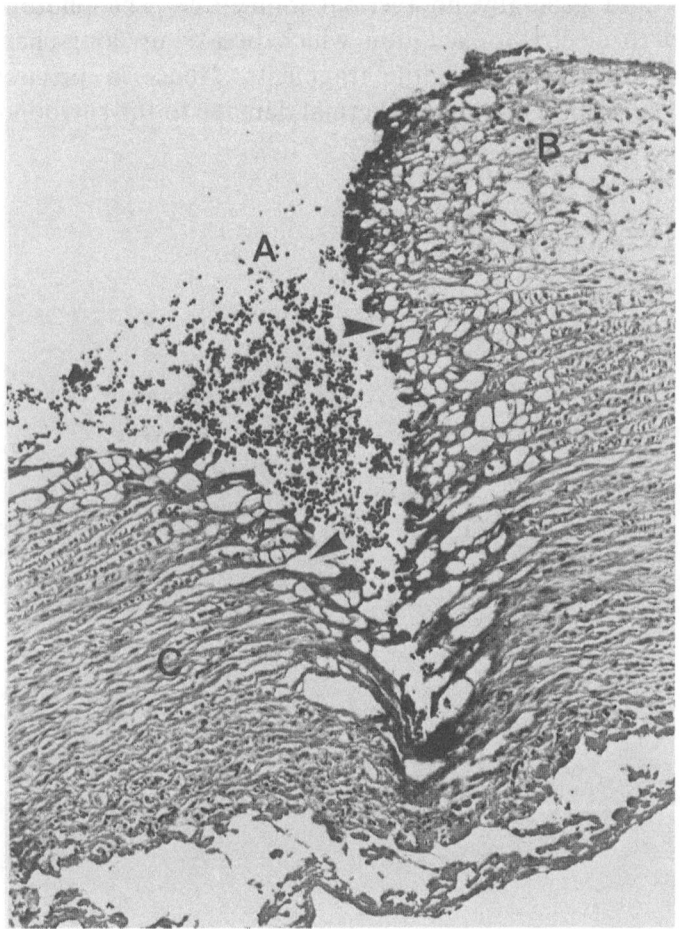

Fig. 4. Rabbit atherosclerotic aorta subjected to argon laser exposure produced a vaporized crater (*A*) with deep penetration through the atherosclerotic plaque (*B*) and the medial layer (*C*) of the vessel. Note the red blood cells filling the crater covered by a charred lining. Note also lacunae formation (arrows) in the zone adjacent to the charred lining. (Reproduced with permission from Lee, G., *et al.,* Am. J. Cardiol. *53,* 291, 1984, Fig. 2)

energy of greater than 5 joules. In addition, there are selective dyes that can be used to enhance or attenuate laser absorption on atherosclerotic plaque or the vascular wall[11].

The absorption of ultraviolet light (193, 248, 308, 351 nm) upon atherosclerotic disease from an excimer laser results in a different ablative outcome than with absorption of visible (argon) or infrared (Nd:YAG, CO_2) radiation. Ultraviolet light causes photochemical ablation of the atheroma and generally no thermal injury[12, 13]. The photon energy is converted to electrical excitation which breaks up long-chain polymer molecules into smaller volatile fragments. Hence, a precisely defined incision can result without any thermal damage to the surrounding tissue.

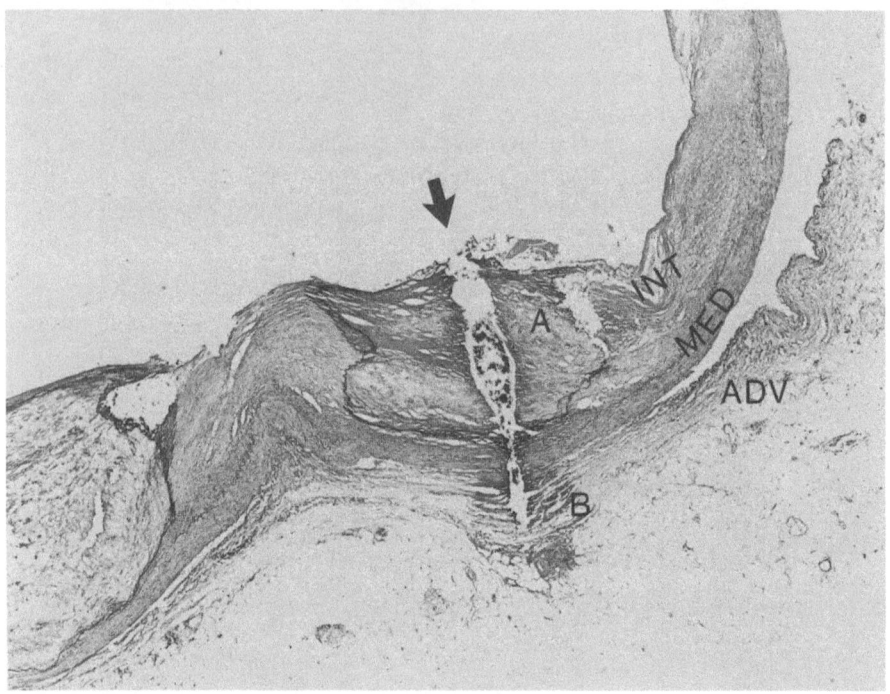

Fig. 5. Longitudinal section of human atherosclerotic coronary artery. An argon laser created a channel through a calcified atherosclerotic plaque (*A*) with extension through the entire vascular wall from the intima (*INT*) to the adventitial layer (*ADV*) and surrounding fat (*B*). Note the charred remnants within the channel adjacent to calcified and hyalinized areas in the intima and media (*MED*) but not fragments adjacent to the lipid area (*B*) of the adventitia. (Reproduced with permission from Lee, G., *et al.,* Am. Heart J. *105,* 886, 1983)

The depth of penetration varies directly with the cumulative number of ultraviolet pulses emitted while the width of the radiated channel remains unchanged. While application of ultraviolet light using excimer laser has certain advantages, the mutagenic or toxic effect of ultraviolet laser energies is still unknown.

Laser Delivery System

The development of flexible optical fibers has made it possible to propagate light internally into body cavities and, coincidentally, to transmit images formed by optical fiber bundles within internal organs back to the viewer without open surgical exposure. A laser light beam is confined internally in the optical fiber owing to refractive properties of the fiber, and incident energy can be conducted to its target with very little energy loss. The light is directed coaxially as close as possible along the central axis of the blood vessel, dissolving plaque adjacent to the stenotic lumen and thereby extending the diameter of the stenotic channel.

Both argon and Nd:YAG laser energies can be transmitted through flexible optical fibers made of silica quartz. However, optical fibers used to deliver the long wavelength CO_2 energies or the ultrashort wavelength excimer light (*i.e.*, 193 nm) are not yet readily available, since the materials that transmit the beam may not be technologically feasible at the present time or may be toxic under physiologic conditions.

The use of a fiberoptic laser heated metal cap can also instantaneously vaporize atherosclerotic plaque upon contact[14]. The concept was based on our findings, using an electrically heated metal cap device to dissolve fatty-fibrous plaque in the late 1970s. The quantity of plaque removal was largely dependent on the contact time and the physical characteristics of the plaque. The laser cautery cap was also effective in melting human thrombus.

Long-Term Laser Effects on Atherosclerotic Obstruction

The chronic effects of laser radiation on atherosclerotic disease were demonstrated by inducing aortic atherosclerosis in swine fed a hyperlipidemic diet[15]. The aorta was surgically opened and the diseased intima was exposed to CO_2 laser beam with a spot diameter of 0.9 mm utilizing energies of less than 10 joules. The vaporized craters measured approximately 2 mm in diameter and 1 mm in depth. Two days following laser treatment, the crater was covered with platelet-fibrin thrombi. By 2 weeks, the crater was still depressed but the surface had rapidly endothelialized, with some fibrin and platelets remaining. By 8 weeks, the lased site was still visible as a re-endotheliazed crater. Moreover, thrombogenic complications did not occur under these experimental conditions. Thus this study demonstrated that the vaporized crater had a lasting effect.

The long-term laser effects on the underlying normal vascular wall were studied in canine carotid and femoral arteries[16]. The endothelial surface of the artery was subjected to laser radiation and lased site was biopsied from 2 to 30 days after treatment. Within 4 days following therapy, the laser-induced crater area in the vascular wall had fibrin clot deposition. Between 4 to 7 days, there was mild inflammation and collagen had infiltrated the crater. By 9 days, the endothelial lining had healed. As in the swine experiments, the laser-induced vascular injury stimulated reendothelialization and clot deposition without causing thrombotic occlusion in the artery.

Long-term studies in atherosclerotic arteries of Rhesus monkeys fed an atherogenic diet have also been performed to determine whether the effects of laser radiation can accelerate the atherosclerotic process[17]. Following several argon laser exposures (1.5 to 2.5 joules) upon the femoral arteries and aorta, light and electron microscopic examination after 2 to 60 days showed that the vaporized crater had significantly less atherosclerosis than the unlased plaque border. Thus, there was no evidence of increased atherosclerotic development following laser therapy.

Laser Effects on Thrombotic Obstruction

Since vascular thrombosis often accompanies atherosclerotic disease, the effect of laser radiation on human thrombus has been studied[18]. Blood was obtained from normal human volunteers and allowed to clot. The clotted samples were cut to fixed lengths of 3 to 11 mm. The argon laser energy required to penetrate greater depths of thrombus increased in a linear dose fashion. The longer the red blood clot, the higher is the energy necessary to penetrate through that clot.

The spectrophotometric scan of freshly formed thrombus demonstrated a typical absorption curve for hemoglobin pigments, and hence, argon energies are easily absorbed by the red blood clot. Clots devoid of red blood cells or hemoglobin pigment are not absorbed by argon radiation and thus lacked recanalizing effect[19]. Since argon energies are poorly absorbed in water, freshly formed thrombus might better be dissolved with a thrombolytic agent, such as streptokinase, urokinase, or tissue plasminogen activator.

Risks of Laser Treatment

One of the major complications of laser recanalization is vessel perforation (Fig. 6). A slightly misdirected beam from an optical fiber can deliver a thermal burn through an atherosclerotic plaque and beyond the arterial wall. Thus far, a laser-beam wavelength that is absorbed by plaque but spares the normal vascular wall has not been found. In in-vivo dog experiments to determine the feasibility of laser catheter intervention into the coronary artery, a coronary guiding catheter was inserted into the right carotid artery, and the distal tip of the catheter was positioned at the left coronary orifice under fluoroscopic guidance. A flexible 400 μm central core quartz fiber was advanced through the coronary catheter into the proximal left coronary artery without untoward effects. Laser energies approximating those used to vaporize plaque were transmitted into the coronary lumen from an argon laser source. The resulting laser burns perforated the coronary artery which led to cardiac tamponade, causing hemodynamic and electrical instability. On postmortem examination, there was evidence of coronary perforation and perivascular hemorrhage. When thermal injury extended beyond the coronary artery into the cardiac muscle, there was also myocardial necrosis and hemorrhages[20]. Further, in addition to thermal trauma, mechanical perforation during the passage of the optical fiber can occur. This injury is more likely in arteries that are small and tortuous and particularly at branching sites.

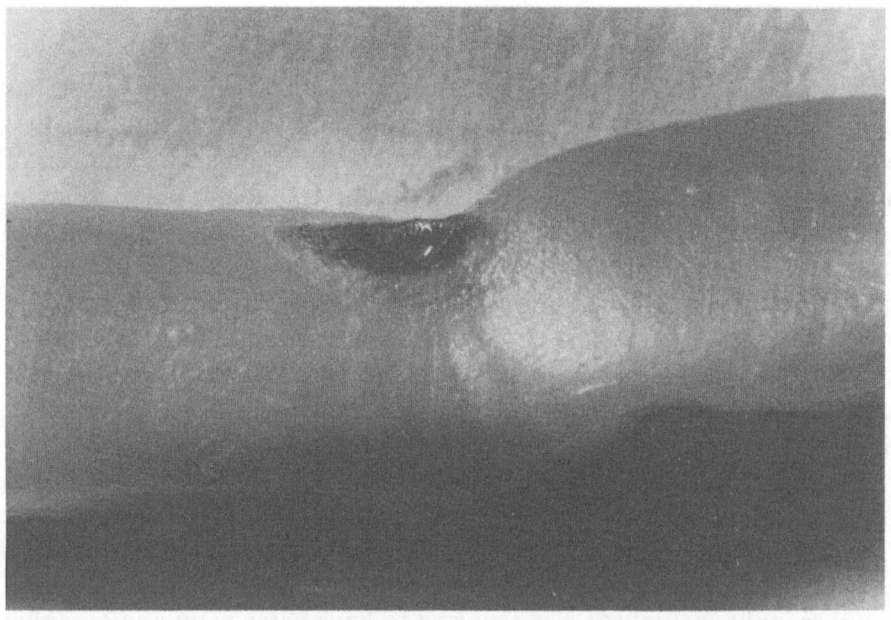

Fig. 6. Dog carotid artery perforation produced by argon laser energies delivered by 400 μm diameter core flexible quartz fiber (5 watts, 3 seconds) inserted into the vessel from the right side of the photo. Note the charred exit site of the laser beam

Another risk of laser phototherapy was observed in rabbits that were fed an atherogenic diet and allowed to develop atherosclerotic lesions[21]. Low-level laser energies from an argon laser were applied via flexible 400 μm diameter core quartz fiber to vaporize the plaque lesions. In animals examined immediately after laser treatment, a vaporized crater was produced within the atherosclerotic plaque at the endothelial surface; in others, the medial layer was also injured. Importantly, in half of the animals that were followed one to 14 days following the procedure, aortic aneurysms with muscular wall damage had resulted. These problems may be avoidable by applying catheter laser angioplasty while visualizing specific plaque target sites and/or using safe dose increments of laser energies.

Further, the delivery of argon laser energies into blood exposes human red blood cells to intense heat. As a result, there was lysis of erythrocytes as demonstrated by a drop in hematocrit and an increase in plasma hemoglobin[22]. Although thrombogenic complication did not develop in one study[15], there exists the potential of a break in the intimal lining following laser therapy with exposure of the subintimal layers initiating platelet aggregation and vascular thrombosis. Moreover, prolonged lasing in an intravascular blood medium can predispose the flexible quartz fiber tip to thrombus formation, as seen by echocardiography[23], and when a thrombus has developed, the risk of thrombo-embolic phenomenon is also present.

Clinical Laser Recanalization

The use of laser energies to reopen obstructed atherosclerotic vessels has been tried in humans with coronary or peripheral vascular disease. The first report was in a patient who had left leg claudication and a 95% stenosis of the deep femoral artery[24]. Under fluoroscopic guidance, a peripheral balloon angioplasty catheter was passed into the orifice of the left profunda femoral artery and situated near the stenotic lesion. A 200 μm silica fiber was inserted through the balloon catheter and into the stenotic obstruction. Power intensity of approximately 4.1 watts from an argon source for a total duration of 26 seconds was applied. Although no postoperative angiogram was performed, the report indicated that the patient had improvement in clinical symptoms and in distal blood flow using a Doppler flowmeter.

In another report, 5 patients with coronary disease had their stenosed native vessel (left anterior descending or right coronary artery) treated by laser recanalization during bypass graft surgery[25]. An 85 μm quartz fiber was utilized transmitting total argon energies between 60–1,231 joules. However, only one patient was reported to have patency on angiographic restudy 25 days after the procedure. A review of this "successful" case showed different angiographic techniques to compare the pre-laser and post-laser treatments; contrast dye was injected down the stenotic native coronary artery before treatment and through the saphenous bypass graft, filling the lesion in a retrograde manner, after laser angioplasty.

In a third study, percutaneous transluminal laser recanalization was performed in patients with obstructed femoral or popliteal arteries[26]. An optical fiber (200 μm diameter) coupled to a Nd : YAG laser was inserted into a balloon catheter placed against the atheromatous plaque. Power intensity of 12 watts and a total duration of exposure between 90 to 150 seconds were applied to penetrate and enlarge the arterial stenotic lumen. During the procedure, cooling was done using a dilute blood perfusate. No adverse effects were reported by this technique.

Catheter to Target Plaque for Laser Vaporization

A fiberoptic laser catheter was conceived by us in the late 1970s to target plaques for laser vaporization[27-29]. It incorporated features of balloon

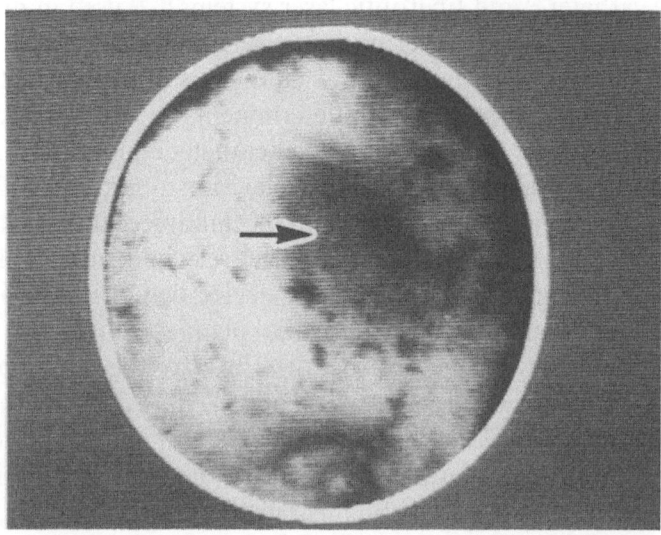

Fig. 7a. Atherosclerotic plaque obstruction (arrow) observed from the viewing channel of the fiberoptic laser catheter. The implanted plaque is surrounded by the normal smooth vascular wall lining

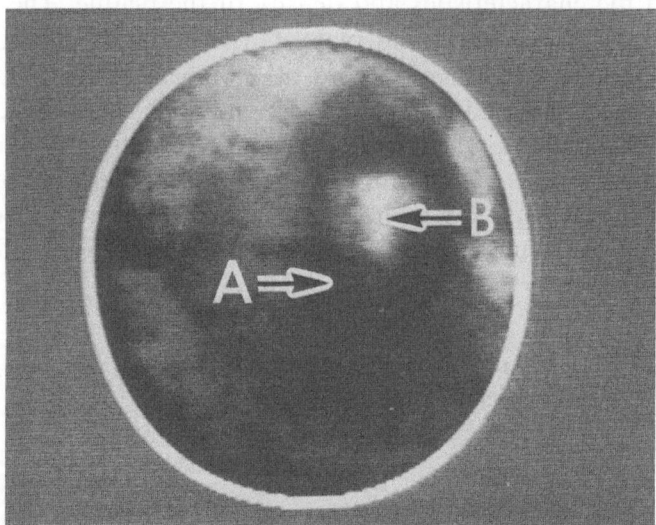

Fig. 7b. Atherosclerotic plaque (*A*) with vaporized hole (*B*) within the center of the plaque following argon laser radiation. (Reproduced with permission from Lee, G., *et al., Cath. Cardiovasc. Diagn. 10*, 14, 1984, Fig. 2)

angioplasty catheter[30] and fiberoptic laser systems[31, 32] used in medicine at that time. Designed for use in peripheral vessels, the prototype catheter was tested in living arteries of animals and in animals implanted with human atherosclerotic vascular segments to determine its feasibility. The catheter assembly consists of a 3 mm outer diameter catheter connected to a viewing handpiece, which could be connected to a television monitor. The device has three hollow passageways extending from the handpiece to the catheter tip. These include channels for viewing, laser delivery and suction/flushing[29].

Early experimental studies using this device demonstrated its ability to visualize and vaporize atherosclerotic plaques implanted in living animals[28, 29]. By observing the obstruction (Fig. 7a), the laser energies can be directed to the diseased target area for controlled thermal treatment (Fig. 7b), avoiding the normal vessel wall and thereby minimizing the risks of perforation and aneurysm formation. Furthermore, the visualization of the obstructed area can also help distinguish plaque from thrombus, which is important since different energies may be required for laser absorption.

Conclusions

Laser energies can be delivered by tiny flexible optical silica fiber to effectively vaporize atherosclerotic plaque as well as thrombotic obstruction. The depth of plaque penetration varies with the applied laser energy and the characteristics and density of the plaque. The vaporized crater is covered with fibrin and platelets but is rapidly endothelialized. There was no increased atherosclerotic development at the treated area as compared to the unlased atherosclerotic site. The major risks of laser therapy are vascular perforation, aneurysm formation, and thrombo-embolic complications. A handful of patients with atherosclerotic disease have received intravascular laser recanalization, but more research and technical improvements are needed to render the procedure safe.

Acknowledgments

We thank the San Francisco Laser Center for their support and Ms. Leslie Silvernail for her secretarial assistance.

References

1. American Heart Association: Heart Facts. American Heart Association, Dallas, 1984.
2. Lee, G., Ikeda, R. M., Joye, J. A., Bogren, H., DeMaria, A. N., Mason, D. T., 1980: Evaluation of transluminal angioplasty of chronic artery stenosis. Value and limitations assessed in fresh human cadaver hearts. Circulation *61*, 77–83.
3. Roberts, W. C., Buja, L. M., 1972: The frequency and significance of coronary arterial thrombi and other observations in fatal myocardial infarction. A study of 107 necropsy patients. Am. J. Med. *52*, 425–443.

 4. Crawford, T., 1977: Blood and lymphatic vessels. In: Pathology, 7th edition (Anderson, W. A. D., Kissane, J. M., eds.), pp. 879–927. St. Louis: C. V. Mosby Company.

 5. Roberts, W. C., Virmani, R., 1979: Quantification of coronary arterial narrowing in clinically-isolated unstable angina pectoris. An analysis of 22 necropsy patients. Am. J. Med. *67*, 792–799.

 6. Lee, G., Ikeda, R. M., Kozina, J., Mason, D. T., 1981: Laser dissolution of coronary atherosclerotic obstruction. Am. Heart J. *102*, 1074–1075.

 7. Abela, G. S., Normann, S., Cohen, D., Feldman, R. L., Geiser, E. A., Conti, C. R., 1982: Effects of carbon dioxide, Nd-YAG and argon laser radiation on coronary atheromatous plaques. Am. J. Cardiol. *50*, 1199–1205.

 8. Choy, D. S. J., Stertzer, S., Rotterdam, H. Z., Bruno, M. S., 1982: Laser coronary angioplasty: Experience with 9 cadaver hearts. Am. J. Cardiol. *50*, 1209–1211.

 9. Lee, G., Ikeda, R., Herman, I., Dwyer, R. M., Bass, M., Hussein, H., Kozina, J., Mason, D. T., 1983: The qualitative effects of laser irradiation on human arteriosclerotic disease. Am. Heart J. *105*, 885–889.

10. Clarke, R. H., Donaldson, R. F., Isner, J. M., 1984: Identification of photoproducts liberated by in vitro laser irradiation of atherosclerotic plaque, calcified valves and myocardium. (Abstract) Lasers Surg. Med. *3*, 358).

11. Chan, M. C., Lee, G., Seckinger, D. L., Reis, R. L., Lee, M., Rink, J., Mason, D. T., 1984: Pretreatment with vital dyes to enhance or attenuate argon laser energy absorption in blood vessels. (Abstract) Circulation *70* (Suppl. II) 298 .

12. Grundfest, W., Litvack, F., Forrester, J., Fishbein, M., Morgenstern, L., McDermid, S., Pacala, T., Rider, D., Laudenslager, J., 1984: Pulsed ultraviolet lasers provide precise control of atheroma ablation. (Abstract) Circulation *70* (Suppl. II), 35.

13. Isner, J. M., Clarke, R. H., Donaldson, R. F., Muller, D. F., Foxall, T. L., Laliberte, S. M., Libby, R., Alroy, J., Ucci, A. A., 1984: The excimer laser: Gross, light microscopic, and ultrastructural analysis of potential advantages for use in laser therapy of cardiovascular disease. (Abstract) Circulation *70* (Suppl. II), 35.

14. Lee, G., Ikeda, R. M., Chan, M. C., Dukich, J., Lee, M. H., Theis, J. H., Bommer, W. J., Reis, R. L., Hanna, E. S., Mason, D. T., 1984: Dissolution of human atherosclerotic disease by fiberoptic laser-heated metal cautery cap. Am. Heart J. *107*, 777–778.

15. Gerrity, R. G., Loop, F. D., Golding, L. A. R., Erhart, L. A., Argentyl, Z. B., 1983: Arterial response to laser operation for removal of atherosclerotic plaques. J. Thorac. Cardiovasc. Surg. *85*, 409–421.

16. Abela, G. S., Conti, C. R., 1983: Laser revascularization: What are its prospects? J. Cardiovasc. Med. *8*, 977–984.

17. Abela, G., Franzini, D., Crea, F., Pepine, C. J., Conti, C. R., 1984: No evidence of accelerated atherosclerosis following laser radiation. (Abstract) Circulation *70* (Suppl. II), 323.

18. Lee, G., Ikeda, R. M., Stobbe, D., Ogata, C., Chan, M. C., Seckinger, D. L., Vazquez, A., Theis, J., Reis, R. L., Mason, D. T., 1983: Effect of laser radiation

on human thrombus: Demonstration of a linear dissolution dose relationship between clot length and energy density. Am. J. Cardiol. *52*, 876–877.

19. Lee, G., Seckinger, D. L., Vazquez, A., Stobbe, D., Rosenthal, P., Chan, M. C., Ikeda, R. M., Reis, R. L., Mason, D. T., 1984: Laser irradiation of human thrombus: Selective absorption of radiation for red blood clots but not white clots. (Abstract) J. Am. Coll. Cardiol. *3*, 489.

20. Lee, G., Seckinger, D., Chan, M. C., Embi, A., Stobbe, D., Thomson, R. V., Sanchez, N. A., Ikeda, R. M., Reis, R. L., Mason, D. T., 1984: Potential complications of coronary laser angioplasty. Am. Heart J. *106*, 1577–1579.

21. Lee, G., Ikeda, R. M., Theis, J. H., Chan, M. C., Stobbe, D., Ogata, C., Kumagai, A., Mason, D. T., 1984: Acute and chronic complications of laser angioplasty. Vascular wall damage and formation of aneurysms in the atherosclerotic rabbit. Am. J. Cardiol. *53*, 290–293.

22. Theis, J. H., Lee, G., Ikeda, R. M., Stobbe, D., Ogata, C., Lui, H., Mason, D. T., 1983: Effects on laser irradiation on human erythrocytes: Considerations concerning clinical laser angioplasty. Clin. Cardiol. *6*, 396–398.

23. Bommer, W. J., Lee, G., Rebeck, K., Stobbe, D., Ogata, C., Ikeda, R., Mendizabal, R., Reis, R. L., Mason, D. T., 1983: Two-dimensional echocardiography of argon-laser vapor trails: Monitoring of catheter position and prevention of potential complications. (Abstract) Circulation *68*, 259.

24. Ginsburg, R., Kim, D. S., Guthaner, D., Toth, J., Mitchell, R. S., 1984: Salvage of an ischemic limb by laser angioplasty: Description of a new technique. Clin. Cardiol. *7*, 54–58.

25. Choy, D. S. J., Stertzer, S. H., Myler, R. K., Marco, J., Fournial, G., 1984: Human coronary laser recanalization. Clin. Cardiol. *7*, 377–381.

26. Geschwind, H., Boussignac, G., Teisseire, B., Vieilledent, C., Gaston, A., Becquemin, J. P., Mayiolini, P., 1984: Percutaneous transluminal laser angioplasty in man (Letters to the Editor). Lancet *I*, 844.

27. Lee, G., Ikeda, R. M., Dwyer, R. M., Hussein, H., Dietrich, P., Mason, D. T., 1982: Feasibility of intravascular laser irradiation for in vivo visualization and therapy of cardiocirculatory diseases. Am. Heart J. *103*, 1076–1077.

28. Lee, G., Ikeda, R. M., Stobbe, D., Ogata, C., Theis, J., Hussein, H., Mason, D. T., 1983: Laser irradiation of human atherosclerotic obstructive disease: Simultaneous visualization and vaporization achieved by a dual fiberoptic catheter. Am. Heart J. *105*, 163–164.

29. Lee, G., Ikeda, R. M., Stobbe, D., Ogata, C., Embi, A., Chan, M. C., Reis, R. L., Mason, D. T., 1984: Intraoperative use of dual fiberoptic catheter for simultaneous in vivo visualization and laser vaporization of peripheral atherosclerotic obstructive disease. Cathet. Cardiovasc. Diagn. *10*, 11–16.

30. Gruntzig, A. R., Myler, R. K., Hanna, E. S., Turina, M. I., 1977: Coronary transluminal angioplasty. (Abstract) Circulation *56*, 84.

31. Dwyer, R., Haverback, B. J., Bass, M., Cherlow, J., 1975: Laser induced hemostasis in the canine stomach: Use of fiberoptic delivery system. J.A.M.A. *231*, 486–489.

32. Dwyer, R. M., Yellin, A. E., Craig, J., Cherlow, J., Bass, M., 1976: Gastric hemostasis by laser phototherapy in man. J.A.M.A. *236*, 1383–1384.

Photoradiation Therapy with Hematoporphyrin Derivative in the Management of Brain Tumors

ROBERT E. WHAREN, JR., ROBERT E. ANDERSON, EDWARD R. LAWS, JR.

Department of Neurologic Surgery, Mayo Clinic, Mayo Medical School, Rochester, Minnesota (U.S.A.)

Contents

Clinical Studies 219
Limitations and Future of Photoradiation Therapy 222
Acknowledgement... 223
References 223

Hematoporphyrin is a naturally occurring compound similar to the heme of hemoglobin without the iron ligand (Fig. 1). Since the observation by Lipson[44-46] in 1960 that a derivative of hematoporphyrin (HpD) had superior tumor localizing characteristics when compared to hematoporphyrin, all subsequent clinical studies have used HpD.

Despite the use of HpD for the detection of malignancy, the use of photosensitization for the treatment of tumors received scant attention until the 1970s. In 1972 Diamond et al.[17] and in 1975 Granelli et al.[34] reported the capability of hematoporphyrin to kill glioma cells both in vitro and in vivo upon exposure to white light. Systemically injected HpD caused extensive tumor necrosis in rats with subcutaneously implanted gliomas when exposed to light, while neither light alone nor porphyrin alone had any effect. Dougherty in 1975[23] described instances of complete eradication of experimental tumors using HpD and red light. Red light delivered twenty-four hours after drug administration prevented recurrences for at least 90 days in nearly half of a group of mice with subcutaneous mammary tumors. The use of red light at 630 nm provided much better tissue penetration when compared to violet light, and resulted in a useful degree of tumor destruction.

The first reports of HpD photoradiation therapy of human tumors appeared in 1978[25] and 1979[26] when Dougherty found that cutaneous metastases of breast cancer and malignant melanoma could be selectively ablated by photoradiation therapy with HpD and red light. Since these

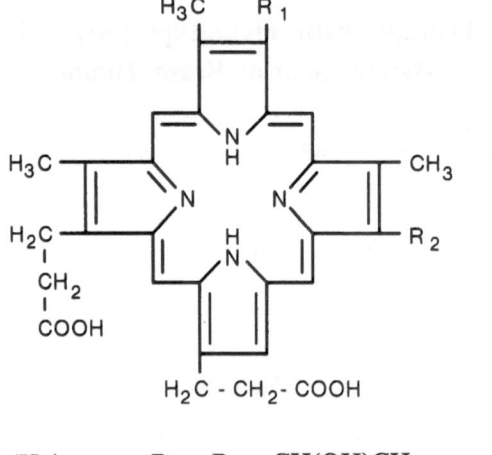

1. Hematoporphyrin (Hp) $R_1 = R_2 = CH(OH)CH_3$
2. Hematoporphyrin (HOAC) $R_1 = CH(OH)CH_3$ $R_1 = CH(OAC)CH_3$
   monoacetate $R_2 = CH(OAC)CH_3$ or $R_2 = CH(OH)CH_3$

3. Hematoporphyrin (HOAC²) $R_1 = R_2 = CH(OAC)CH_3$
   diacetate

4. Hydroxyethylvinyl (Hvd) $R_1 = CH(OH)CH_3$ $R_1 = CH = CH_2$
   deuteroporphyrin $R_2 = CH = CH_2$ or $R_2 = CH(OH)CH_3$

5. Acetoxyethylvinyl (Avd) $R_1 = CH(OAC)CH_3$ $R_1 = CH = CH_2$
                                        $R_2 = CH = CH_2$ or $R_2 = CH(OAC)CH_3$

6. Protoporphyrin (Pp) $R_1 = R_2 = CH = CH_2$

Fig. 1. Structure of hematoporphyrin and some of the components of HpD

initial reports, the concepts of HpD photoradiation therapy have been applied to the treatment of a. number of malignancies including lung cancer[15, 21, 35], bladder cancer[2, 36, 40], head and neck tumors[10, 16, 64, 65], ocular tumors[54], and brain tumors[31, 43, 48, 55, 56, 63] with some success. The report by Hayata[35] of the primary treatment of bronchial carcinoma with complete removal of small early lesions and a three-year tumor-free survival are very encouraging and have been confirmed by Doiron[21].

The application of photoradiation therapy in neurosurgery was initially very encouraging. A number of investigators have reported the capability of HpD to selectively kill glioma cells both in vitro[17, 34] and in vivo[17, 31, 34, 43, 48, 55,

[56, 63]. More recent reports have described initial attempts in the use of photoradiation therapy for the treatment of malignant brain tumors[31, 43, 48, 55, 56, 63], and although the results are equivocal, it is evident that despite major differences in the protocols by various investigators HpD phototherapy is capable of tumor cell destruction in man. Rounds[59] and Bonnet[7] both warned, however, that hematoporphyrin is not entirely contained within neoplastic tissue and that some HpD accumulates in brain tissue. This small amount of HpD within normal brain tissue can produce significant morbidity and mortality in experimental animals upon application of a sufficient dose of light.

HpD is usually administered clinically (following sterile preparation) as a piggyback infusion at a dose of 3–5 mg/kg[43] over 5 to 10 minutes into a freely running intravenous line of D 5.02% saline. Thus far there has been no toxicity associated with the administration of HpD in this manner. There has been some attempt to standardize the preparation of HpD, and indeed the product has recently been marketed as Photofrin I and subsequently Photofrin II (PHOTOFRIN Medical Inc., Cheektowaga, N.Y.).

Although hematoporphyrin (Hp) has been clearly established as a photosensitizer in cell-free systems[8, 39, 62], further studies have demonstrated that simple hematoporphyrin is ineffective as a photosensitizer when tested in cellular systems either in vitro[22, 42, 49] or in vivo[3, 22, 27, 41]. Actual intracellular[18] or intraorganelle uptake of porphyrin appears necessary for photosensitization in both intact cells and liposomes[60]. Kessel[41] has suggested that hematoporphyrin may be too hydrophilic to cross the cell membrane and, thus, is an ineffective photosensitizer for intact cells. Although some[47] have suggested that hematoporphyrin is an effective photosensitizer of experimental tumors, Dougherty[22] has shown that pure hematoporphyrin is ineffective and that certain preparations of Hp contain "impurities" which are entirely responsible for the photosensitizing ability of Hp in cellular systems.

Despite the well established property of HpD to localize within tumors, the mechanisms of its uptake and retention in malignant tissue have not yet been clearly established. Initial reports suggesting the preferential uptake of porphyrin by tumor cells[11, 52] have been substantially refuted[12]. Dougherty[25, 26] suggested that a more rapid clearance of HpD from normal tissue than from malignant tissue provided the basis for the preferential localization of HpD. This differential clearance of HpD was considered a property of the microenvironment of a tumor where increased vascular permeability and inadequate lymphatic drainage resulted in trapping of protein-bound HpD[51, 53, 61] in the interstitial fluid for longer periods than in normal tissues[21, 32, 57].

Because tumors appear to accumulate mainly porphyrin aggregates, Moan[50] thought that the preferential accumulation of HpD in tumors was not a property of the tumor cells but rather was related to other factors in the tumors such as vascular permeability and lymphatic drainage as proposed previously by Dougherty[28]. In addition, the high concentration of HpD noted in stromal and reticuloendothial areas of tumors, notably in macrophages[21], suggested that phagocytosis may participate in the accumulation of porphyrin aggregates[6, 50]. Dougherty has proposed that the aggregates are retained in tumors and serve as a reservoir for monomeric porphyrins subsequently diffusing into cells.

Table 1. *Concentration of HpD in Human Gliomas Determined by Fluorescence Assay*

Case	Histology	Injected HpD concentration, mg/kg	Time after injection, hours	HpD concentration determined by fluorescence, µg/ml
1	grade III oligoden-droglioma	5	48	0.1
5	grade III mixed astro-oligoden-droglioma	5	24	2.5
3	grade II–III mixed astro-oligoden-droglioma	5	24	1.7

Christensen et al.[13] have also observed that in tissue cultures, the photodynamic effects of HpD varied depending upon the stage of the cell cycle with cells in interphase being the most susceptible while cells in the early G_1 phase were the least susceptible.

Thus, although the active components of HpD have been studied and even isolated[29] the mechanism of the localization of HpD in neoplastic tissue remains obscure. Indeed, some of the difficulty has been the complex and variable nature of the HpD mixture of porphyrins. Many authors have suggested the advantages of working with a pure substance rather than a mixture, but thus far few have pursued this possibility. El-Far and Pimstone[30] have recently reported the efficacy of uroporphyrin-I as a selective tumor localizer. This is a pure compound which when compared to HpD had a 7–20-fold greater tumor localizing ability with exceedingly small amounts accumulating in normal tissues. Further work with this and similar compounds needs to be pursued. The actual concentration of HpD achieved in human tumors has been quantitated by Wharen et al.[63] using a microfluorescence assay (Table 1). HpD concentrations of 1.7–2.5 µg/ml were obtained in two cases of malignant gliomas 24 hours following the IV administration of 5 mg/kg of HpD, while simultaneous biopsies of surrounding normal brain tissue yielded values of 0.1–0.4 µg/ml and HpD tumor/brain ratios of 6–17. Clearly, it appears that a small amount of HpD does cross the BBB into normal tissue[66]. The distribution of HpD in normal brain or tumor and its location within the cell have not yet been determined. Whether this small amount of HpD can be damaging to normal cells during photoradiation therapy has recently been investigated[59]. Under the appropriate experimental conditions in mice, significant morbidity and mortality was produced upon application of light to the brain following HpD administration. This phototoxicity was considered a result of oxygen deprivation in brain tissue resulting from mitochondrial damage, as HpD is reported to concentrate in mitochondria[4]—the first organelle to show damage from light exposure[14]. The extrapolation of this observation to the human brain is difficult but does reveal that the use of HpD in its present form may not be free from potential toxicity and further studies are certainly needed.

The optimum time to administer photoradiation therapy following drug administration would be when the HpD concentration in tumor versus normal brain is maximum, privided that the absolute amount in normal brain is low enough to be nontoxic. Although Wharen et al.[63] noted a ratio approximately two-fold higher at 4 hours compared to 24 hours after drug administration, Boggan et al.[5] found maximal ratios at 24 hours. This ratio will also be dependent upon the HpD preparation, and further development is necessary before the timing of photoradiation therapy after drug administration can be optimized.

The toxicity of HpD in clinical applications has thus far been limited primarily to skin sensitization. Patients must remain out of bright sunlight for approximately 4 weeks following drug administration[43, 48]. McCulloch et al.[48] have also reported one patient who developed cerebral edema following the administration of 150 joules/cm² of red light 48 hours after the injection of 5 mg/kg of HpD. As suggested by El-Far et al.[30] and Dougherty[29] the use of a more pure preparation of HpD or a different porphyrin such as uroporphyrin-I may limit or eventually eliminate at least the skin toxicity.

Anderson et al.[1] investigated the effect of optical spectrum, power density, HpD concentration, and HpD preparation on the HpD tumor cell killing efficiency of MEWO cells in culture. Using a trypan blue exclusion assay, cell survival curves were obtained following irradiation with violet (405 nm), red (630 nm), and white light (340–680 nm) at energies of 0–320 joules and at power densities of 20–160 mw/cm² for cells exposed for six

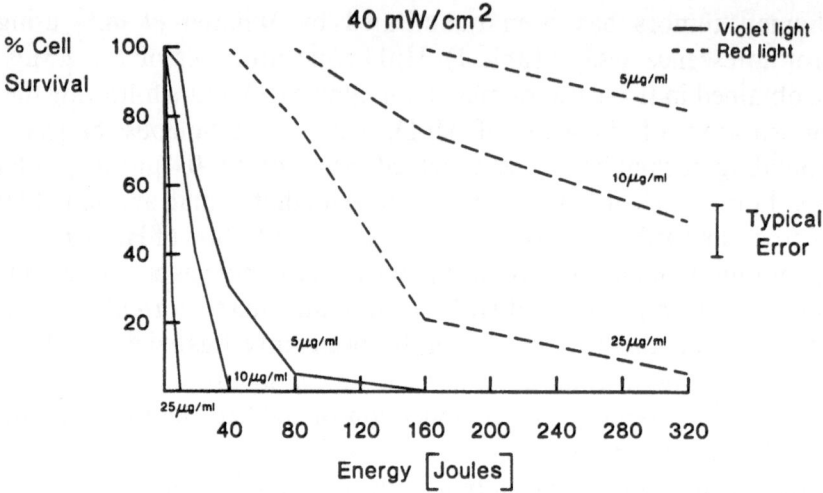

Fig. 2. HpD tumor cell killing efficiency-red vs. violet light

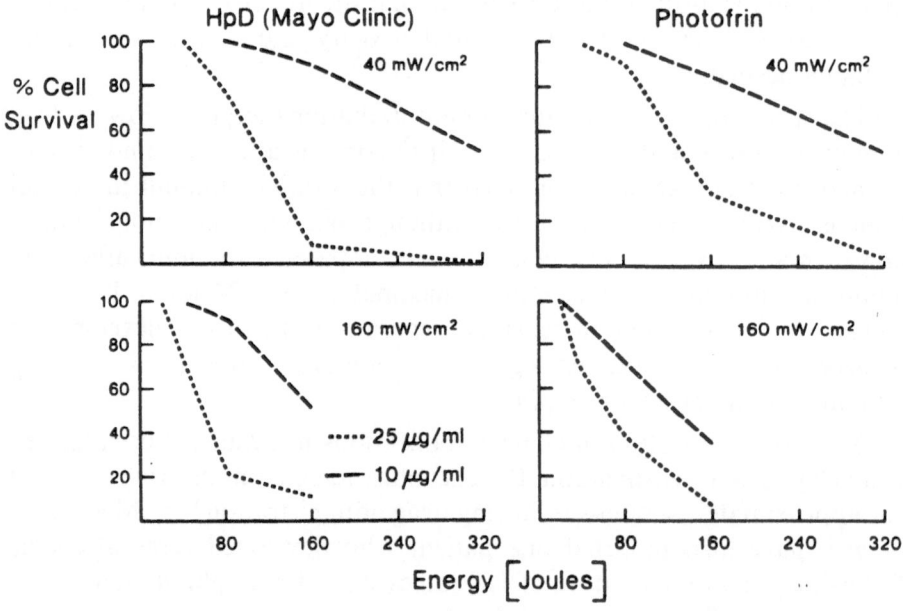

Fig. 3. Tumor cell killing efficiency-red light irradiation

hours to HpD concentrations of 0–25 µg/ml. All studies were performed for both Photofrin I and for Mayo Clinic preparations of HpD.

The survival curves (Fig. 2) demonstrated a consistant pattern with an increasing slope and decreasing shoulder to the curve at increasing concentrations of HpD. Identical curves were obtained for both Mayo Clinic HpD and Photofrin I. The ratio of the killing efficiency of violet light to red light was approximately 20:1. For red light (Fig. 3), a twofold

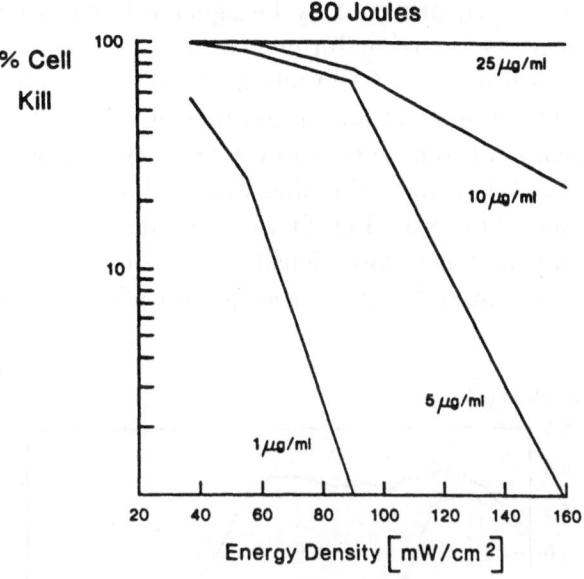

Fig. 4. Violet light irradiation

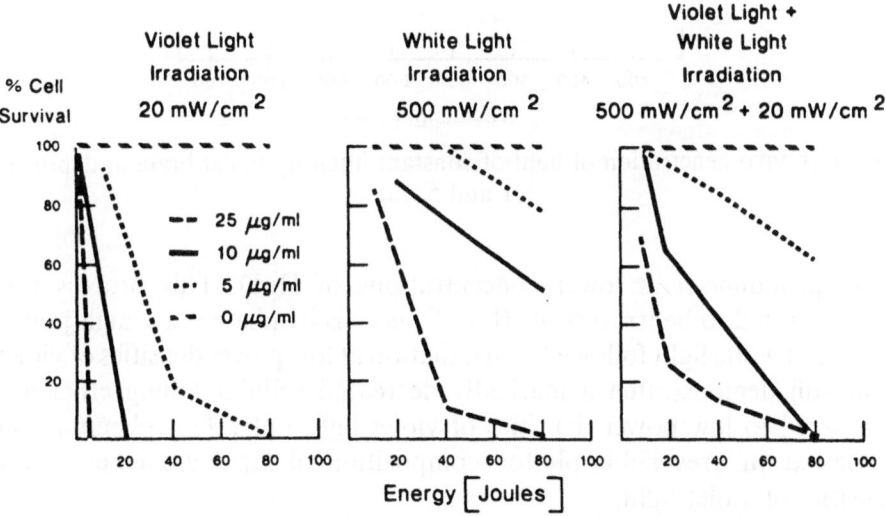

Fig. 5. Effect of high energy density white light on HpD cell killing efficiency

increase in cellular killing efficiency was observed at higher power densities of 160 mw/cm² compared to a lower power density of 40 mw/cm². One hundred and ten joules of red light at a power density of 40 mw/cm² produced a 50% cell kill compared to only 55 joules required at a power density of 160 mw/cm², at an HpD concentration of 25 µg/ml. This phenomenon of an decreased killing efficiency of red light at lower power densities has also been observed by Dougherty[24] who attributed it to a partial repair process occurring during exposure. Gomer *et al.*[33], however, found that the cytotoxicity of CHO cells in cultures was independent of the dose rate of red light at lower power densities of 0.5 to 60 mw/cm². Using 2.5 nm increments of red light from 620–640 nm, the most efficient wavelengths of red light for cell killing were 627.5 to 632.5 nm.

For violet light, however, (Fig. 4) a marked decrease in cellular killing efficiency is found at higher power densities. This decrease in cellular killing efficiency at higher power densities varied greatly with concentration, being

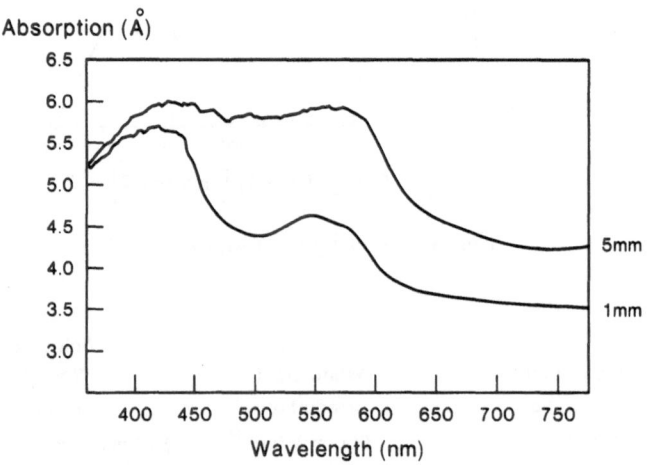

Fig. 6. In vivo penetration of light of constant intensity in cat brain at depths of 1 and 5 mm

more pronounced at lower concentrations of HpD. This process was demonstrated to be irreversible (Fig. 5) as cells irradiated at a high power density of white light followed by irradiation at low power densities of violet light still demonstrated a markedly decreased cellular killing efficiency compared to low power densities of violet light only. This phenomenon suggested an irreversible photodecomposition of HpD at higher power densities of violet light.

After all the drug and light parameters have been maximized in HpD photoradiation therapy, the limiting factor in its clinical application may remain the penetration of light through brain and tumor tissue[19]. Light penetration into tissue is determined by the optical characteristics of the tissue, the wavelength of the light, and the concentration of the photosensitizer that has been used. Photons are either absorbed or scattered and the ultimate penetration of light is both wavelength and tissue dependent in an exponential manner[20].

Fig. 6 demonstrates the relative penetration of light through in vivo cat brain as a function of wavelength and demonstrates the significantly greater depth of penetration of red light (630 nm) compared to violet light (405 nm). Dougherty[28], however, has recently stated that the useful penetration of visible light in adult brain at 630 nm is on the order of 1–1.5 mm. If that is the case, then the depth of penetration of light at 630 nm represents a significant limiting factor for the use of photoradiation therapy in brain and brain tumors. It is known, however, that the penetration of light through tissue continues to improve by several orders of magnitude as the wavelength increases from approximately 600 nm–1.1 m[58]. Thus, the possibility exists that photoradiation therapy at these wavelengths might provide a more effective depth of tissue penetration.

Clinical Studies

HpD photoradiation therapy (HpD-PRT) has been used clinically in neurosurgery for approximately 5 years in the treatment of malignant brain tumors. The photoradiation therapy has been applied by two techniques. Initial attempts involved the stereotactic insertion of fiberoptic probes into the tumor delivering red light (630 nm) produced by an argon-pumped dye laser. More recently, HpD-PRT has been applied by irradiating the tumor bed following resection of the tumor both for recurrent tumors and at the time of the initial resection.

The technique of inserting quartz fiberoptic probes stereotactically into the tumor for the administration of PRT has been described by Laws et al.[43]. Five patients with recurrent malignant gliomas were administered photoradiation therapy 48–72 hours following the IV piggyback infusion of 5 mg/kg HpD over 30 minutes. PRT was applied by the insertion of a single 400 μm diameter quartz fiber probe into the center of the tumor through an 18 gauge thin wall needle. The fiberoptic probe was coupled to an argon-pumped dye laser producing 300–400 mw of red light at 630 nm at the tip of the fiberoptic probe. The light was applied for 45 minutes. Pre- and postoperative CT scans demonstrated a slight decrease in the size of the tumor in all five patients but it did not appear to have a significant effect on patient survival. This study does demonstrate, however, both the feasibility of the technique and the fact that the technique is capable of tumor cell destruction.

Forbes et al.[31] using a similar technique for the treatment of gliomas in two patients have also reported that although it is not yet possible to assess the efficacy of photoradiation therapy, the technique does produce significant tumor cell destruction. More recently, Jacques[38] has discussed the possibility of applying HpD-PRT by fiberoptic probes inserted through the Shelden/Jacques stereotactic system following the stereotactic resection of a tumor with the use of a CO_2 laser. The combining of these two technologies of HpD-PRT and stereotaxis for the treatment of malignant brain tumors is an intriguing possibility which is currently being investigated.

Recently, photoradiation therapy has been administered by the irradiation of the tumor bed following resection of the tumor. Initially, the HpD was given approximately 24 hours prior to surgery. However, since the observation[63] that the concentration of HpD in the tumor was greater at 4 hours compared to 24 hours after HpD administration, with a greater

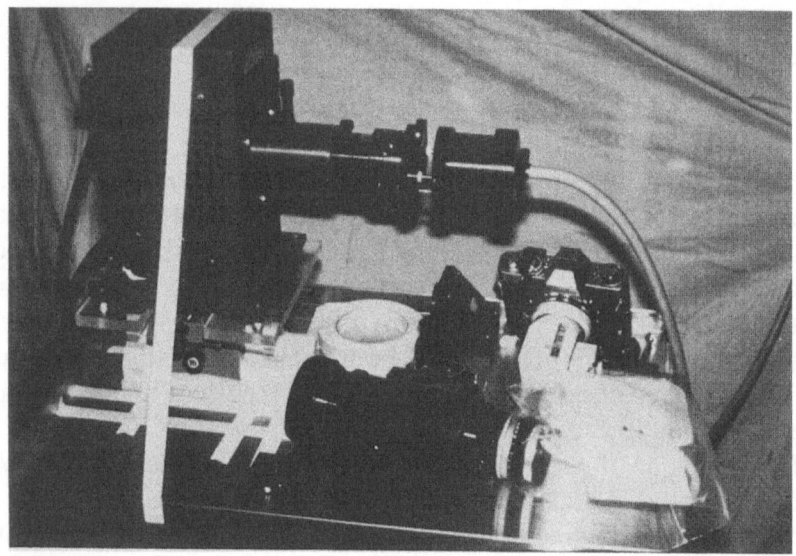

Fig. 7. Clinical photoradiation arrangement with xenon arc lamp and fiberoptic cable

tumor to brain ratio at 4 hours as well, patients now receive the drug approximately 4 hours prior to surgery. The light source used is a filtered xenon arc lamp producing red light (630 nm) which is directed through a 1 cm fiberoptic cable for irradiation (Fig. 7) having an output of approximately 300 mw at the fiber tip. Fig. 8 demonstrates how the light and fiberoptic probe are positioned for irradiation of the tumor bed. Before irradiation with red light is applied, the tumor bed is first illuminated with violet light (405 nm) from the filtered xenon arc lamp and the area is observed for red fluorescence both with the naked eye and also through a Starlight scope (Nitec, Standard Equipment Co., Milwaukee, Wisconsin) low light image detector (Fig. 9). The tumor bed is then irradiated for one hour with red light. In addition, in an effort to achieve more uniform and thorough irradiation, a light diffusing medium is first applied which fills the cavity of the tumor bed and the light is then evenly dispersed by directing the

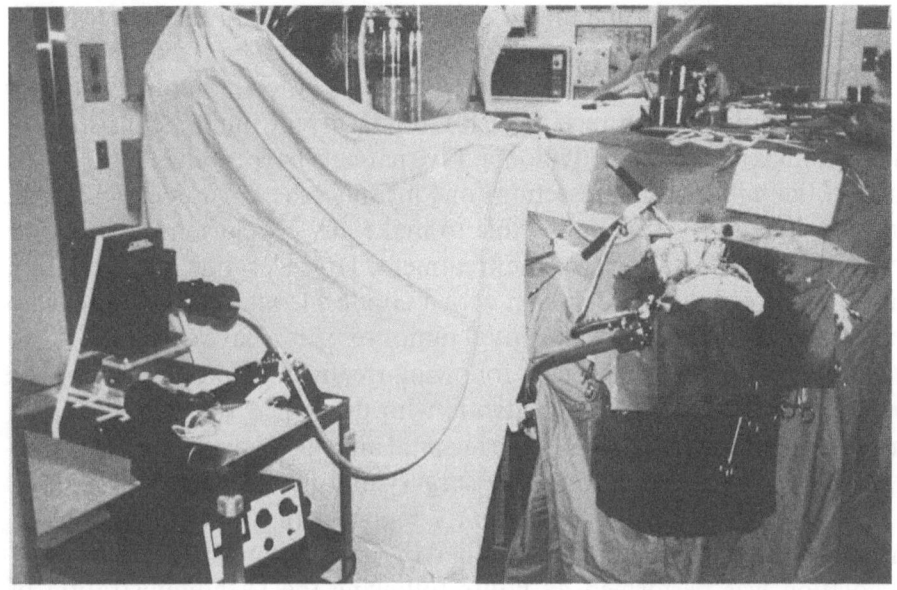

Fig. 8. Photoradiation in the operating room. Tumor bed is illuminated by fiberoptic probe

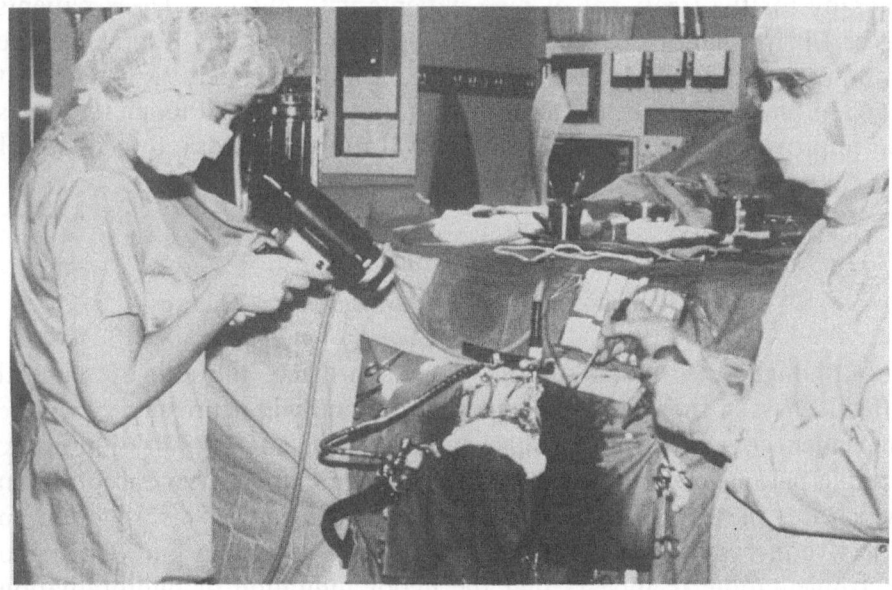

Fig. 9. Tumor fluorescence can be detected by a low light photomultiplier scope

tip of the fiberoptic probe into the diffusion medium in the center of the tumor bed.

Fourteen patients have now been treated by photoirradiating the tumor bed. Nine patients have received PRT for recurrent tumors consisting of eight gliomas and one ependymoma. Five patients have received PRT at the time of the initial tumor resection (one medulloblastoma, one metastasis, and three gliomas). It is impossible to make any conclusions at this time regarding the effectiveness of the treatment. However, one patient with a medulloblastoma and one patient with a Grade 4 frontal astrocytoma who received PRT at the time of the initial tumor resection have continued to do well now greater than two years following treatment. Complications have been few and consist of two patients who developed second degree sun burns following discharge from the hospital and one patient who developed transient cerebral edema following surgery and PRT.

Mc Cullough *et al.*[48] have recently reported the use of HpD-photo-radiation therapy in a similar manner by irradiation of the tumor bed. Irradiation was performed 48 hours following the IV administration of 5 mg/kg HpD using 100–200 J/cm^2 at 630 nm obtained from a filtered 1,000 w incandescent lamp[37]. Using this technique metastatic tumors were effectively prevented from recurrence, and two patients with glioblastoma probably received some benefit[48].

Perria[55, 56] has also reported the application of HpD photoradiation therapy for the treatment of nine patients with gliomas. These patients received irradiation of the tumor bed 24–96 hours following the administration of 2.5–5 mg/kg of HpD using approximately 9 J/cm^2 of light at 632.8 nm obtained from a 25 mw helium-neon laser. Although there was no improvement in the length of survival, tumor necrosis to a depth of 1.5 cm was observed.

Limitations and Future of Photoradiation Therapy

Although these initial reports are encouraging, the ultimate clinical effectiveness of the use of photoradiation therapy in neurosurgery will be dependent upon a more thorough understanding and optimization of the various parameters involved in the photodynamic effect. The concepts upon which this therapy is based are sound, and with further investigation an effective therapy may be forthcoming. Given our current knowledge and instrumentation, it appears that the major limitation of photoradiation therapy in neurosurgery is the limited penetration of light through brain tissue. The future of photoradiation therapy may well involve more effective drug-light combinations operating at longer wavelengths which have a much greater penetration through normal and neoplastic tissue.

Acknowledgement

The authors are grateful to Mrs. Mary Beth Wharen, Ms. Bernita Bruns and Mrs. Constance Hoeft for their assistance in the preparation of the manuscript. Portions of this manuscipt and its accompanying Tables and Illustrations have been published elsewhere[1, 43, 63].

References

1. Anderson, R. E., Wharen, R. E., Jones, C. A., et al., 1984: HpD tumor cell killing efficiency as a function of power density, optical spectrum, concentration, and HpD preparation—decomposition of HpD at high power densities. The Clayton Foundation Symposium on Porphyrin Localization and Treatment of Tumors. Santa Barbara, CA, April 24–28, 1983 (Doiron, D., ed.), pp. 483–500. New York: Allan R. Liss.

2. Benson, R. C., Farrow, G. M., Kinsey, J. H., 1982: Detection and localization of in situ carcinoma of the bladder with hematoporphyrin derivative. Mayo Clinic Pro. 57, 548–555.

3. Berenhaum, M., Bonnett, R., Scourides, P. A., 1982: In vivo biological activity of the components of hematoporphyrin derivative. Br. J. Cancer 45, 571–581.

4. Berns, N. W., Dahlman, A., Johnson, F. M., et al., 1982: In vitro cellular effects of hematoporphyrin derivative. Cancer Research 42, 2325–2329.

5. Boggan, J. E., Berns, M., Edwards, M., 1984: Uptake, distribution, and retention of hematoporphyrin derivative in metastatic and intrinsic rat tumor models. The Clayton Foundation Symposium on Porphyrin Localization and Treatment of Tumors, Santa Barbara, CA, April 24–28, 1983 (Doiron, D., ed.). New York: Allan R. Liss.

6. Bonnett, R., Berenbaum, M. C., 1983: HpD—A study of its components and their properties. In: Porphyrin Photosensitization (Kessel, D., Dougherty, T. J., eds.), pp. 241–260. New York: Plenum Publishing Corp.

7. Bonnett, R., Berenbaum, M. C., Kaur, H., 1983: Chemical and biological studies on hematoporphyrin derivative. Presentation at the International Symposium on Porphyrins in Tumor Phototherapy, Milan, Italy, May, 1983.

8. Brun, A., Hording, G., Romelo, I., 1981: Protoporphyrin-induced photohemolysis—differences related to the subcellular distribution of protoporphyrin in erythropoietic protoporphyria and when added to normal red cells. Int. J. Biochem. 13, 225–228.

9. Bugelski, P. J., Porter, C. W., Dougherty, T. J., 1982: Autoradiographic distribution of hematoporphyrin derivative in normal and tumor tissue of the mouse. Cancer Res. 41, 4606–4612.

10. Carpenter, R. J., III, Neel, H. B. III, Ryan, R. J., et al., 1977: Tumor fluorescence with hematoporphyrin derivative. Ann. Otol. Rhinol. Laryngol. 86, 661–666.

11. Carrano, C. J., Tsatsui, M., McConnell, S., 1975: Tumor localizing agents: The transport of meso-tetra (P-sulfurphenyl) porphine by Vero and HEp-2 cells in vitro. Chem. Biol. Interact. 21, 233–248.

12. Chang, C., Dougherty, T. J., 1978: Photoradiation therapy: Kinetics and thermodynamics of porphyrin uptake and loss in normal and malignant cells in culture. Abstr. Rad. Res. Soc. 74, 498.

13. Christensen, T., Moan, J., et al., 1979: Photodynamic effect of haematoporphyrin throughout the cell cycle of the human cell line NHIK 3025 cultivated in vitro. Br. J. Cancer 34, 64.

14. Coppola, A., Viggiani, E., Salzarulo, L., et al., 1980: Ultrastructural changes in lymphoma cells treated with hematoporphyrin and light. Am. J. Pathol. 99, 175–181.

15. Cortese, D. A., Kinsey, J. H., 1982: Hematoporphyrin-derivative phototherapy for local treatment of cancer of the tracheobronchial tree. Ann. Otol. Rhinol. Laryngol. 91, 652–655.

16. Dahlman, A., Wile, A. G., Burns, R. G., et al., 1983: Laser photoradiation therapy of cancer. Cancer Res. 43, 430–434.

17. Diamond, I., Granelli, S., McDonagh, A. F., et al., 1972: Photodynamic therapy of malignant tumors. Lancet 2, 1175–1177.

18. Dixit, R., Mulchtar, H., Bickers, D. R., 1983: Destruction of microsomal cytochrome P-450 by reactive oxygen species generated during photosensitization of hematoporphyrin derivative. Photochem. Photobiol. 37, 173–176.

19. Doiron, D. R., Svaasand, L. O., Profio, A. E., 1981: Light dosimetry in tissue: application to photoradiation therapy. Adv. Exp. Med. Biol. 160, 63–76.

20. Doiron, D. R., 1984: Photophysics and instrumentation. The Clayton Foundation Symposium on Porphyrin Localization and Treatment of Tumors. Santa Barbara, CA, April 24–28, 1983 (Doiron, D., ed.), pp. 41–73. New York: Allan R. Liss.

21. Doiron, D. R. (ed.), 1984: The Clayton Foundation Symposium on porphyrin localization and treatment of tumors. Santa Barbara, CA, April 24–28, 1983. New York: Allan R. Liss.

22. Dougherty, T. J., 1983: Hematoporphyrin as a photosensitizer of tumors. Photochem. Photobiol. 38, 377–379.

23. Dougherty, T. J., Drindey, G. B., Fiel, R., et al., 1975: Photoradiation therapy II. Cure of animal tumors with hematoporphyrin and light. J. Nat. Cancer Inst. 55, 115–119.

24. Dougherty, T. J., Gomer, C. J., Weishaupt, K. R., 1976: Energetics and efficiency of photoinactivation of murine tumor cells containing hematoporphyrin. Cancer Res. 36, 2330–2333.

25. Dougherty, T. J., Kaufman, J. E., Goldfarb, A., et al., 1978: Photoradiation therapy for the treatment of malignant tumors. Cancer Res. 38, 2628–2635.

26. Dougherty, T. J., Lawrence, G., Kaufman, J. E., et al., 1979: Photoradiation in the treatment of recurrent breast carcinoma. J. Nat. Cancer Inst. 62, 231–237.

27. Dougherty, T. J., Boyle, D. G., Weishaupt, B. W., et al., 1983: Photoradiation therapy-clinical and drug advances. In: Porphyrin Photosensitization (Kessel, D., Dougherty, T. J., eds.), pp. 3–15. New York: Plenum Publishing Corp.

28. Dougherty, T. J., 1984: Recent advances in photoradiation therapy (PRT). The Clayton Foundation Symposium on porphyrin localization and treatment of tumors. Santa Barbara, CA, April 24–28, 1983 (Doiron, D., ed.). New York: Allan R. Liss.

29. Dougherty, T. J., Potter, W. R., 1984: Structure and properties of HpD active component. The Clayton Foundation Symposium on porphyrin localization

and treatment of tumors. Santa Barbara, CA, April 24–28 (Doiron, D., ed.). New York: Allan R. Liss.

30. El-Far, M. A., Dimstone, N. R.,1984: Superiority of uroporphyrin I over other porphyrins in selective tumor localization. The Clayton Foundation Symposium on Porphyrin Localization and Treatment of Tumors. Santa Barbara, CA, April 24–28 (Doiron, D., ed.). New York: Allan R. Liss.

31. Forbes, I. J., Cowled, P. A., Leong, A. S., et al., 1980: Phototherapy of human tumors using hematoporphyrin derivative. Med. J. Aust. 2, 489–493.

32. Goldacre, R. J., Sylven, B., 1962: On the access of blood-borne dyes to various tumor regions. Br. J. Cancer 16, 306–322.

33. Gomer, C. J., Doiron, Dr., Dunn, S., et al., 1984: Examination of action spectrum, dose rate, and mutagenic properties of hematoporphyrin derivative photoradiation therapy. The Clayton Foundation Symposium on Porphyrin Localization and Treatment of Tumors. Santa Barbara, CA, April 24–28, 1983 (Doiron, D., ed.). New York: Allan R. Liss.

34. Granelli, S. G., Diamond, I., McDonagh, A. F., et al., 1975: Photo-chemotherapy of glioma cells by visible light and hematoporphyrin. Cancer Res. 35, 2567–2570.

35. Hayata, Y., Kato, H., Konaka, C., 1982: Hematoporphyrin derivative and laser photoradiation in the treatment of lung cancer. Chest 81, 269–277.

36. Hisazumi, H., Misaki, T., Miyoshi, N., 1983: Photoradiation therapy of bladder tumors. J. Urology 130, 685–687.

37. Jacka, F., Blake, A. J., 1983: A lamp for cancer phototherapy. Aust. J. Physics 36, 221–226.

38. Jacques, S., 1984: Photoradiation and lasers in the treatment of central nervous system neoplasms: Adaptation to the Sheldon-Jacques CT based computerized stereotactic system. Clayton Foundation Symposium on Porphyrin Localization and Treatment of Tumors (Doiron, D., ed.). Santa Barbara, CA, April 24–28, 1983. New York: Allan R. Liss.

39. Jori, G., Reddi, E., Rossi, E., et al., 1980: Porphyrin-sensitized photoreactions and their use in cancer therapy. Med. Biol. Environ. 8, 140–154.

40. Kelly, J., Snell, M. E., Berenbaum, M. C., 1975: Photodynamic destruction of human bladder carcinoma. Brit. J. Cancer 31, 237.

41. Kessel, D., 1982: Components of hematoporphyrin derivatives and their tumor-localizing capacity. Cancer Res. 42, 1703–1706.

42. Kessel, D., Chou, T. H., 1983: Tumor-localizing components of the porphyrin preparation hematoporphyrin derivative. Cancer Res. 43, 1994–1999.

43. Laws, E. R., Cortese, D. A., Kinsey, J. H., et al., 1981: Photoradiation therapy in the treatment of malignant brain tumors: A phase I (feasibility) study. Neurosurgery 9, 672–678.

44. Lipson, R. L., Baldes, E. J., The photodynamic properties of a particular hematoporphyrin derivative. Arch. Derm. 82, 517–520.

45. Lipson, R. L., Baldes, E. J., 1960: Photosensitivity and heat. Arch. Derm. 82, 517–520.

46. Lipson, R. L., Baldes, E. J., Olsen, A. M., 1961: The use of a derivative of hematoporphyrin in tumor detection. J. Nat. Cancer Inst. 26, 1–8.

47. Malik, Z., Djaldetti, M., 1980: Destruction of erythroleukemia, myelocytic leukemia, and Burkett lymphoma cells by photoactivated protoporphyrin. Int. J. Cancer 26, 495–500.

48. McCulloch, G. A., Forbes, I. J., LeeSee, K., et al., 1984: Phototherapy in malignant brain tumors. The Clayton Foundation Symposium on Porphyrin Localization and Treatment of Tumors, Santa Barbara, CA, April 24–28, 1983 (Doiron, D., ed.), pp. 709–718. New York: Allan R. Liss.

49. Moan, J., Christensen, T., Sommer, S., 1982: The main photosensitizing components of hematoporphyrin derivative. Cancer Lett. 15, 161–166.

50. Moan, J., Sommer, S., 1983: Uptake of the components of hematoporphyrin derivative by cells and tumors. Cancer Lett. 21, 167–174.

51. Morgan, W. T., Muller-Eberhard, U., 1972: Interactions of porphyrins with rabbit hemopexin. J. Biol. Chem. 247, 7181–7182.

52. Mossman, B. T., Gray, M. J., Silberman, L., 1974: Identification of neoplastic versus normall cells in human cervical cell culture. Obstet. Gynec. 43, 635–639.

53. Muller-Eberhard, U., Morgan, W. T., 1975: Porphyrin-binding proteins in serum. Ann. NY Acad. Sci. 244, 624–650.

54. Murphree, A. L., Doiron, D. R., Gomer, C. J., et al., 1984: Hematoporphyrin derivative photoradiation treatment of ophthalmic tumors. The Clayton Foundation Symposium on Porphyrin Localization and Treatment of Tumors, Santa Barbara, CA, April 24–28, 1983 (Doiron, D., ed.). New York: Allan R. Liss.

55. Perria, C., Capuzzo, T., Cavagnaro, G., 1980: First attempts at the photodynamic treatment of human gliomas. J. Neurosurg. Sci. 24, 119–129.

56. Perria, C., 1981: Photodynamic therapy of human gliomas by hematoporphyrin and He-Ne laser. IRCS Med. Sci. (Cancer) 9, 57–58.

57. Peterson, H. I., Applegren, K. L., 1973: Experimental studies in the uptake and retention of labelled proteins in a rat tumor. Eur. J. Cancer 9, 543–547.

58. Preuss, L. E., Bolin, F. P., Cain, B. W., 1982: Tissue as a medium for laser light transport-implications for photoradiation therapy. In: Lasers in Medicine and Surgery (Leon Goldman, ed.). Proc SPIE 357, 77–84.

59. Rounds, D. E., Jacques, S., Shelden, C. H., et al., 1982: Development of a protocol for photoradiation therapy of malignant brain tumors: Part I. Photosensitization of normal brain tissue with hematoporphyrin derivative. Neurosurgery 11, 500–505.

60. Suwa, K., Kimura, T., Schaap, A. P., 1977: Activity of singlet molecular oxygen with cholesterol in a phospholipid matrix. A model for oxidative damage of membranes. Biochem. Biophys. Res. Comm. 73, 785–791.

61. Tipping, E., Ketterer, B., Koskelo, P., 1978: The binding of porphyrins by ligandin. Biochem. J. 169, 509–516.

62. Tomio, L., Reddi, E., Jori, G., et al., 1980: Hematoporphyrin as a sensitizer in tumor phototherapy: effect of medium polarity on the photosensitizing efficiency and role of the administration pathway on the distribution in normal and tumor-bearing rats. Springer Ser. Opt. Sci. 22, 76–82.

63. Wharen, R. E., Anderson, R. E., Laws, E. R., 1983: Quantitation of hematoporphyrin derivative in human gliomas, experimental central nervous system tumors, and normal tissues. Neurosurgery 12, 446–450.

64. Wile, A. G., Dahlman, A., Berns, M. W., 1983: Laser photoradiation therapy of recurrent human breast cancer and cancer of the head and neck. In: Porphyrin Photosensitization (Kessel, D., Dougherty, T. J., eds.), pp. 47–52. New York: Plenum Press.
65. Wile, A. G., Novotny, J., Mason, G. R., et al., 1984: Photoradiation therapy of head and neck cancer. Am. J. Clin. Oncol. (CCT) 6, 39–43.
66. Wise, B. L., Taxdal, D. R., 1967: Studies of the blood brain barrier utilizing hematoporphyrin: Short communication. Brain Res. 4, 387–389.

Anesthesiological Techniques in Laser Neurosurgery

R. Urciuoli

Institute of Neurosurgery, University of Turin (Italy)

The introduction of laser use in neurosurgery has modified operative techniques and improved the quality of surgical management, as well as influencing general anesthesia. Surgical and anesthesiological procedures in neurosurgery, more than in the other surgical fields, are strictly complementary. Surgery may be facilitated and its consequences better controlled but anesthesiological procedures may also cause serious damage indirectly to healthy tissue surrounding a lesion. However selective and less traumatic surgical maneuvers can facilitate anesthesia and limit the negative effects of drugs and anesthetic techniques by allowing less prolonged administration and lower doses of drugs, and by requiring less complicated and dangerous techniques or reducing at least the time of their use. The direct relationship of anesthesia to cerebral physiology and intracranial dynamics in surgical procedures suggests on the operative field some anesthesiological considerations for those operations in which laser sources (CO_2-Nd-YAG and argon) are routinely employed.

From a general point of view, the operative advantages of laser use have extended surgical treatment to deeper and larger lesions or near vessels, nerves or critical brain areas such as brain stem; this obliges the anesthesiologist to face more serious clinical problems. On the other hand, some of the surgical advantages, such as a more radical and selective surgery with fewer side effects, an easier hemostasis with considerable reduction of blood loss and shortening of surgical time[4-6], reduce anesthesiological problems in terms of patient management. This allows a quick and very good healing, improving postoperatory course[1, 3, 9].

Parameters generally accepted for evaluation of patient's surgical risk are in this way changed.

From a strictly anesthesiological point of view, some considerations are referred to laser advantages which directly interact with the anesthesiological procedures, some others are referred to a selection of proper anesthetic agents and techniques to make laser use safer.

The main advantage of laser is represented by the fact there is no interference with routine intraoperative monitoring systems such as ECG, arterial and venous pressure, EEG, evoked potentials, avoiding the display interruption of records of vital function parameters in the more critical moments of the operation.

Laser used intermittently provides greater surgical precision during manipulation and retraction in the area of the midbrain and removal of

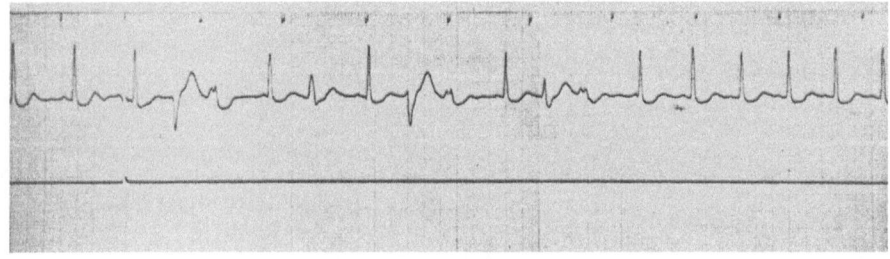

Fig. 1. ECG recording during posterior fossa surgery (tumor around the brain stem). Mechanical dissection produces cardiac disritmias which disappear with the use of the laser

tumors near the brain stem, and does not cause cardiovascular and respiratory changes as frequently can be noticed using traditional surgical techniques (Fig. 1). Besides the thermic effect a direct laser influence on the functional activity of the nervous tissue has been indicated. The very low extension of laser effect on the tissue is shown by EcoG recordings during surgical treatment of cerebral tumors[12]. Bioelectrical activity of the surrounding cerebral tissue irradiated with laser is not compromised (Fig. 2).

The brain stem auditory evoked potentials (BAEP) also, registered during neurosurgical procedures in posterior fossa tumors, are not altered by the effects of laser[9, 10, 13]. The Vth wave generally accepted as indicative of brain stem activity appears unchanged in amplitude and latence time (Fig. 3). Technical aspects of general anesthesia during laser use as a surgical instrument must follow the basic principles for anesthesia in neurosurgical patients.

More careful anesthesiological procedures are required in controlling the harmful effects of laser beam on the eyes of the patient. The possibility of perforation or burning of the endotracheal tube and inappropriate or inadvertent movements of the patient during operation may destroy normal adjacent tissues.

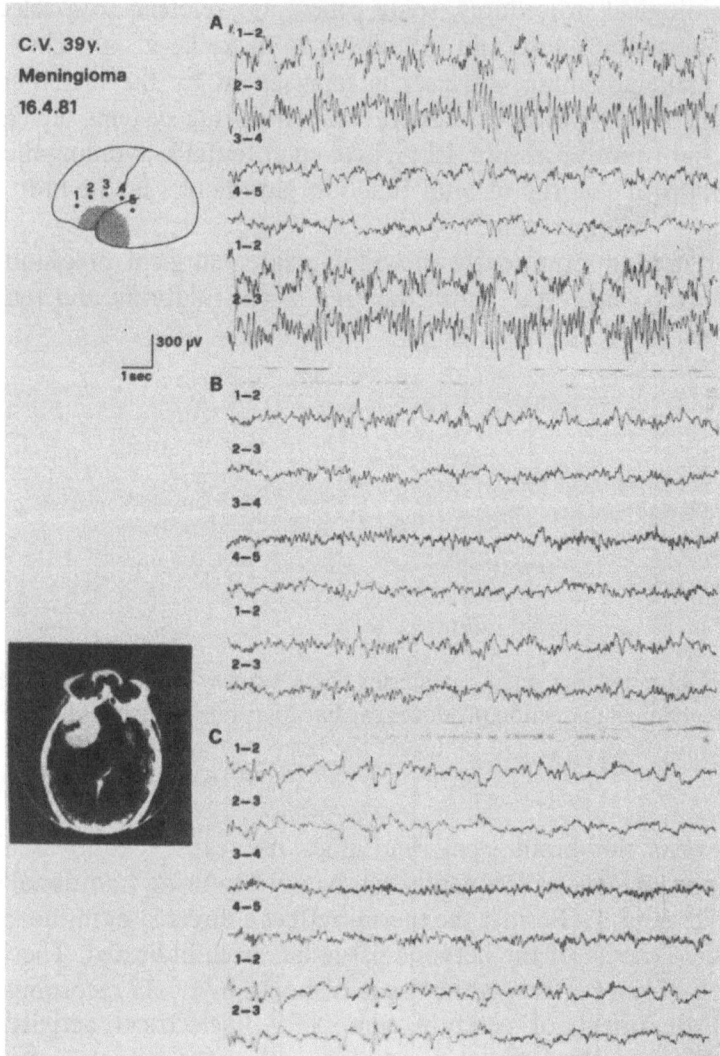

Fig. 2. EcoG recordings in a case of temporal left meningioma, before (*A*), during CO_2 and Nd : YAG laser irradiation (*B*), after complete removal of the tumor (*C*). A reduction of the EcoG voltage and a disappearance of the delta waves are observed during laser irradiation

The eyes have to be protected always by wave length specific protective lenses for the different laser sources.

Endotracheal tube and anesthesia apparatus have to be protected by sponges or foil wrap to absorb CO_2 laser energy or reflect argon and Nd-YAG laser beam; the latter is preferable because of the potential damage caused by a reflected beam. This is the major concern in transphenoidal and skull base surgery[3, 13].

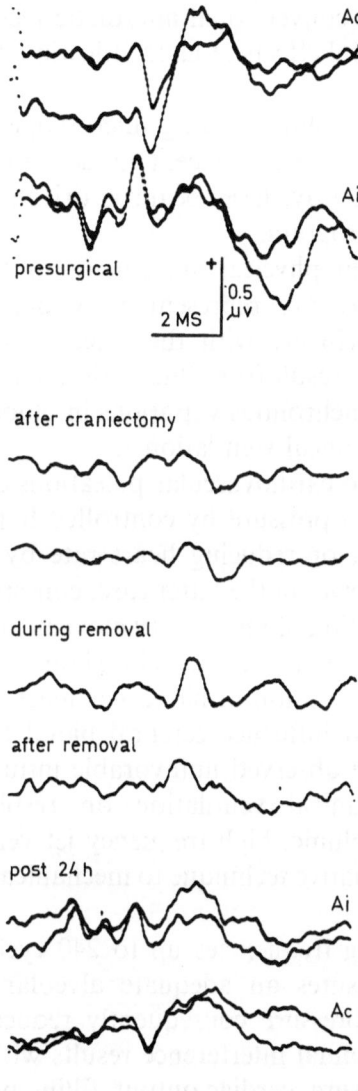

SL f 64 y R.c.p.a. meningioma left BAEP

Fig. 3. BAEP recorded before, during and after removal of a cerebello- pontine angle meningioma. The record shows a reduction in the amplitude of the waveform components during surgical procedure. The latency and amplitude of the Vth wave is preserved

An adequate deep general anesthesia is the obvious solution to the control of the inadvertent or inappropriate patient's movements. These movements, even if limited, can modify surgical field position in respect of the previously fixed focal spot of the laser, and this will result in a larger area of tissue contact with laser beam or in a reduction of laser power density because of altered focus on spot size at target.

Finally, some of the conventional anesthetic techniques also must be modified to avoid harmful effects of laser following physical movement of the exposed brain surface.

These movements, amplified during microscope use, may switch the laser beam to the undamaged adjacent tissue and become particularly dangerous when, as recently, laser beam is driven by computer with a previously fixed work program.

It is well known that physical movements of the exposed brain in neurosurgical procedures are represented by phasic pulsation of the cerebral surface in synchrony with the arterial pulse waves and with respiration. They mainly result from fluctuation in cerebral blood volume related to respiratory synchronous variations in blood pressure that occur during traditional mechanical ventilation[11].

Movements related to cardiovascular pulsations can be reduced either depressing blood arterial pressure by controlled hypotension during the short time of laser use, or reducing heart rate by beta blocker drugs. Pulsations, which are slower in the latter case, consent a better immobility for a longer time. Reduction of respiratory movements is hotly debated for the close link between ventilation and cerebral homeostasis. A modification in ventilation causes a variation in blood gas tension (PaO_2-$PaCO_2$) and respiratory pressure that influence cerebral blood flow and intracranial pressure. Because of the observed unfavorable influence of conventional positive-pressure mechanical ventilation on respiratory synchronous fluctuations in blood volume, high frequency jet ventilation (HFJV) has been applied as an alternative technique to mechanically slower and deeper respiration.

This system, allowing frequencies up to 240 cycles/minute with very small tidal volume, ensures an adequate alveolar ventilation and by reducing peak airway pressure consequently reduces hemodynamic influence. In this way minimal interference results with circulatory parameters such as blood pressure, cardiac output, filling pressure, heart rate.

Mean intracranial pressure and the peak of intracranial pressure, observed during a single respiratory cycle, are also significantly reduced, and a very stable cerebral surface is produced[2, 11].

High frequencies and low volumes, associated with ventilatory oscillations at rates up to 40 Hz, reduce even small fluctuations in the brain occurring simultaneously with inspiration at the time of the peak airway or arterial pressure and depending on direct transmission of intrathoracic pressure. The ventilatory system employed in our experience was a Soxil-Jet Ventilator. Its main advantage lies in the adoption of a new mechanical rotating valve as a flow chapper, in place of the conventional electrovalve, which gives good clean-shaped pulses at much higher frequencies and a life expectancy of years (Fig. 4).

After induction of anesthesia with thiopentone and endotracheal intubation, anesthesia can be maintained as neurolept-analgesia. Ventilation must then be changed to high frequency jet ventilation, after the dura is opened, at frequencies of 260 cycles/minute at 12–10 ml/kg volumes, with ventilatory oscillation at rates up to 40 Hz, and continued till end of laser use. Using this method, additional humidification to the anesthesia circuit must be supplied to avoid drying of the mucous membranes of the tracheo-

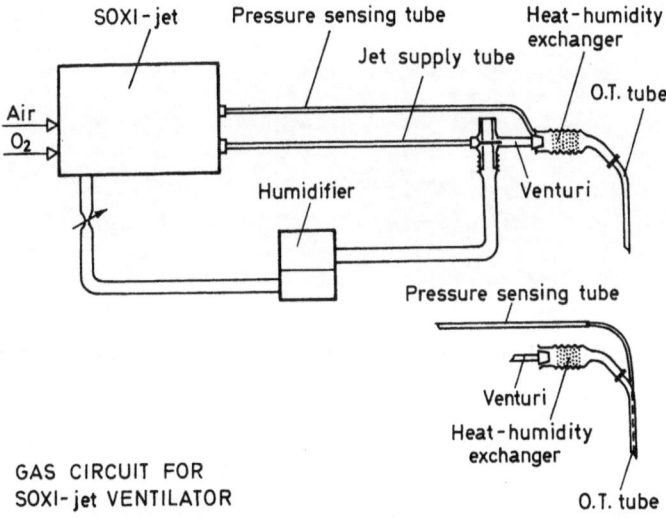

Fig. 4. Soxi-jet ventilator system (SOXIL S.p.A., Milano)

bronchial tree. While no problem occurs in maintaining normal levels of arterial CO_2 tension, arterial O_2 tension appears to be strictly dependent on the percent of oxygen and ventilatory oscillation rate. In order to overcome this problem, a controlled increase of the percent of oxygen or a variation of ventilatory oscillation rate are required.

To accomplish this goal a continuous monitoring of blood gas tension is required. Because this is very difficult using blood gas analysis, it is useful to use a transcutaneous gas monitor which is a noninvasive method and is widely used. Recent experience shows that a transconjunctival oxygen tension monitor can be used, with the advantage of monitoring the oxygen tension in a tissue bed vascularized by the internal carotid artery and therefore reflecting intracranial oxygenation[7, 8] (Figs. 5 and 6).

The ever increasing use of laser will certainly bring other anesthesiological problems, which have to be evaluated case by case and requiring new procedures according to the different surgical and clinical needs.

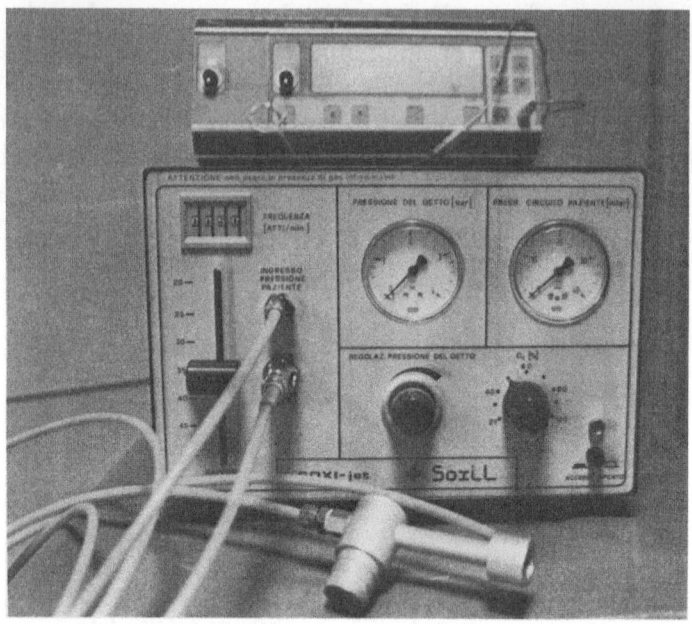

Fig. 5. Soxi-jet ventilator with transconjunctival oxygen monitoring system

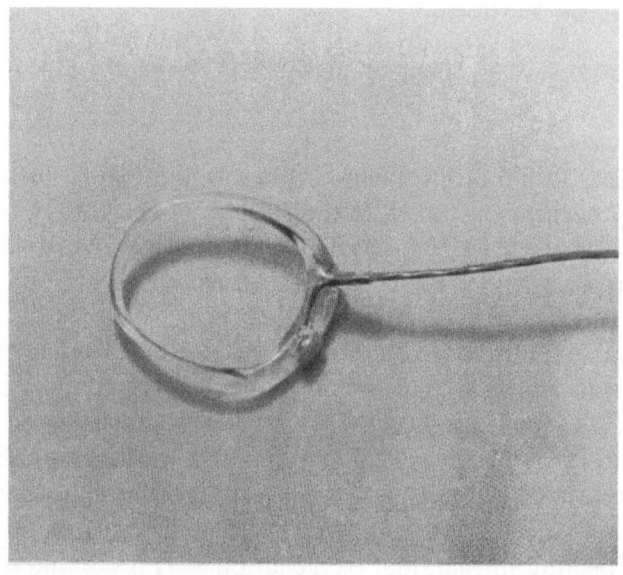

Fig. 6. Transconjunctival electrode for oxygen continuous monitoring (ORANGE 1®)
(Orange Medical Instruments, Costa Mesa, California)

References

1. Alexander, A., Birch, M. D., 1973: Anaesthetic considerations during laser surgery. Anesth. Analg. (Cleve) *52*, 53–58.
2. Carlon, G. C., Ray, C., Jr., Pierri, M. K., Groeger, J., Howland, W. S., 1982: High-frequency jet ventilation. Theoretical considerations and clinical observations. Chest *81*, 350–353.
3. Cerullo, L. J., Koht, A., 1983: Anesthesiologic considerations in laser neurosurgery. Laser in Surgery and Medicine *3*, 35–38.
4. Fasano, V. A., Urciuoli, R., Ponzio, R. M., 1982: Photocoagulation of cerebral arteriovenous malformations and arterial aneurysms with the neodymium: yttrium aluminum garret or argon laser: preliminary results in twelve patients. Neurosurgery *11*, 754–760.
5. Fasano, V. A., 1984: Experiences on the use of various laser sources (CO_2-argon-Nd-YAG) in neurosurgery. In: Proceedings of the American Congress on Laser Neurosurgery II, pp. 32–38. Chicago.
6. Fasano, V. A., Lombard, G. F., Urciuoli, R., Benech, F., Ponzio, R. M., Menzio, D., 1984: The influence of the advanced technologies on the traditional surgical techniques. In: Proceedings of the American Congress on Laser Neurosurgery II, pp. 52–58. Chicago.
7. Fatt, I., Deutsch, T. A., 1983: The relation of conjunctival PO_2 to capillary bed PO_2. Critical Care Med. *11*, 445–448.
8. Isemberg, S. J., Shoemaker, W. C., 1983: The transconjunctival oxygen monitor. Amer. J. Ophthalmol. *95*, 803–806.
9. Koht, A., 1981: Anesthesiological considerations in laser microneurosurgery. In: Proceedings of the First American Congress on Laser Neurosurgery, pp. 67–69. Chicago.
10. Koht, A., Slodan, T. B., 1984: The use of evoked potential and cortical mapping during laser neurosurgery. In: Proceedings of the First Congress of L.A.N.S.I., p. 11. Salzburg.
11. Todd, M. M., Tautant, S. M., Shapiro, H. M., 1981: The effects of high-frequency positive pressure ventilation on intracranial pressure and brain surface movement in cats. Anesthesiology *54*, 496–504.
12. Urciuoli, R., Bergamasco, B., Benna, P., Lo Russo, G., 1981: EcoG changes during cerebral tumor laser surgery. In: Laser Tokyo 81 (Atsumi, K., Nimsakul, N., eds.), pp. 16–19. Internat. Society for Laser Surgery.
13. Urciuoli, R., 1982: Laser use in neurosurgery and anaesthetic considerations. In: Proceedings of American Congress of Soc. Neurosurgical Anesthesia and Neurologic Supportive Care, pp. 33–38. Las Vegas.
14. Urciuoli, R., 1984: High frequency jet ventilation in neurosurgical procedures by laser use. In: Proceedings of the American Congress on Laser Neurosurgery II, pp. 31. Chicago.

The Light for the Future:
Excimer and Free-Electron Lasers

T. LETARDI and A. RENIERI

ENEA—Dip. TIB, Divisione Fisica Applicata, C.R.E. Frascati, Rome (Italy)

Contents

I. Introduction 236
II. Excimer Lasers: Introduction 237
    II.1. Pumping Requirements 238
    II.2. Lasing Systems 238
    II.3. Further Developments 241
III. The Free-Electron Laser (FEL) 241
    III.1. The FEL Operating Principles 242
    III.2. FEL Scenario 247
    III.3. The Future of the FEL: Conclusions and Outlooks 247
References 248

I. Introduction

In these last years a great effort has been done in order to develop new tunable, powerful and efficient laser sources operating both in the infrared (IR) and ultraviolet (UV) and vacuum ultraviolet (VUV) spectral regions.

Two different laser schemes appear now as the best candidates for the realization of these sources. Namely, for the short wavelength region (UV and VUV), the "excimer lasers", while, for IR (and hopefully, in the future, UV, VUV and X too), the "free-electron lasers" (FEL).

In this article we briefly describe the operating principles and the state of the art of these sources. Namely Sect. II is devoted to excimer lasers, whose technology is now at a noticeable level of development, while theoretical and experimental aspects of FEL devices (which are at the very first stage of investigation, with only six operating sources in all the world!) are discussed in Sect. III.

Table 1. *List of the Symbols*

c	light velocity
e	electron charge
m	rest electron mass
λ	radiation wavelength
σ	stimulated emission cross-section
IR	infrared
UV	ultraviolet
VUV	vacuum ultraviolet
RGH	rare gas halide
FEL	free-electron laser
UM	undulator magnet
λ_u	undulator magnet period

The list of the symbols more frequently utilized throughout the text is reported in Table 1.

II. Excimer Lasers: Introduction

The existence of molecular systems which are bound in the excited state and dissociated in the ground state was observed for the first time by Lord Rayleigh[1], while Stevens and Hutton[2] suggested the term "excimer" to distinguish them from normal excited states. The importance of these molecular systems as laser media is evident: being the gain $G = \sigma (n_2 - n_1)$ proportional to the difference between the upper state population n_2 and the lower one n_1, in these systems it reaches the maximum value, because it is always $n_1 = 0$.

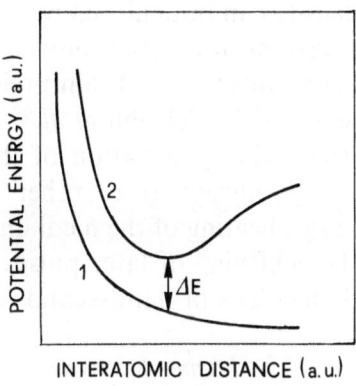

Fig. 1. Potential energy vs interatomic distance, in arbitrary units, for a typical biatomic excimer molecule

In the case of a molecular system formed by two atoms, the curves of potential energy vs interatomic distance will have the general form shown in Fig. 1, where the curve 1 refers to the ground state, and the curve 2 refers to the electronically excited state. The transition energy ΔE, which defines the emission wavelength, is in the region of few e.V. (λ from visible to ultraviolet). Experimental evidence of laser emission from excimer systems was observed for the first time in pure noble gas by Basov et al.[3]. In the following time, other important excimer systems were made to lase, as the Rare Gas Halogen (RGH) excimers (Searles et al.[4]), and the metal vapor lasers (Bazhulin et al.[5], Eden[6]).

In the following, the general working scheme of these systems will be shown, comprising the excitation methods, than the main characteristics (wavelength, efficiency, power and energy per pulse) will be detailed, and finally particular methods to extend the capabilities of excimer lasers (wavelength, peak power, pulse length) will be described.

II.1. Pumping Requirements

In laser systems, very high pumping levels are required as far as the emission wavelength is decreased. Indeed (Hutchinson)[7] the stimulated emission cross-section can be written as (for the symbols see Table 1)

$$\sigma = \frac{\lambda^4}{8\pi\tau\Delta\lambda c},$$

where τ is the lifetime of the excited state and $\Delta\lambda$ is the emission bandwidth. Taking into account that the upper level mean population, in stationary conditions, is linked to the pump power P by

$$n_2 \alpha P\tau,$$

we can conclude that the pumping power density, for gain threshold conditions, scales as λ^{-5}.

High power pump density can be achieved by means of particle beams, usually electrons, but also protons (Baranov et al.[8]), by fast electric discharges, after UV, X-ray or electron beam preionization, and also by means of microwave devices (Mendelsohn et al.[9]).

Even if in these systems the dissociation of the lower level gets the condition $\Delta n = n_2 - n_1 > 0$ always true, other mechanisms, such as instabilities of the discharge, heating of the medium, growing of absorbing species, do not allow the achieving of laser pulses longer than $\sim 1\,\mu\text{sec}$, while in most cases only few tens of nanoseconds are achieved.

II.2. Lasing Systems

Excimer molecules, condidates as laser media, form a very large family (Rhodes[10]) which span in wavelength from VUV to visible, but not all have succeeded to lase, and only the class of RGH excimer lasers has, up to now, reached the stage of commercial development.

Anyway it is worthwhile to mention the class of pure noble gas excimer lasers, which have the shortest wavelength. Laser emission has been observed in Xe (Koehler et al.[11]) ($\lambda = 172$ nm), krypton (Hoff et al.[12]) ($\lambda = 146$ nm), argon (Hughes et al.[13]) ($\lambda = 126$ nm). The very high pumping power needed, due to the very short wavelength, can be achieved only by means of electron beams. Indeed laser pulses of 10 J, 400 MW have been obtained (Ault et al.[14]), using Xe.

Anyway, the complexity of the electron pumping apparatus limits the development of this class of lasers to laboratory systems.

Only recently, in the class of metal vapors excimers, the systems operating with HgBr have reached very attractive performances. The laser wavelength is 502 nm, and fast electric discharge, after UV or X-ray preionization, can be used as pumping system. High energy per pulse (3.2 J) and high overall efficiency (2%) have been obtained (Fisher et al.[15]).

The RGH excimer lasers use, as active medium, an excited molecule (RgH) formed by a noble gas atom Rg (Ar, Kr, Xe) and a halogen atom H (F, Cl, Br). As general scheme, few torrs of the two species Rg and H are mixed together, and some atmospheres of a noble gas (Ar, Ne) are added to absorb the energy from the pumping system and transfer it to the reacting species. Different pumping devices can be used: electron beams, proton beams, discharge sustained by electron beams, self-sustained discharge after UV or X-ray preionization, microwave devices. In Table 2 it is shown the RGH systems in which laser action has been observed, with the corresponding wavelength in nm (Lakoba and Yakovlenko[16]).

Table 2. *RGH Excimer Molecules in which Laser Emission has been Observed, with Corresponding Wavelength in Nanometers*

	Ar	Kr	Xe
F	193	248	350
Cl	175	222	308
Br			282

If we define the intrinsic efficiency as the laser pulse energy divided by the energy deposited in the gas, the highest value (14%) has been obtained with KrF (Salesky and Kimura[17]) while with XeCl it has been obtained 5% (Champagne[18]) in both cases in electron-beam pumped systems. The overall efficiency, it is laser pulse energy divided by the energy furnished by the power supply for the pump system (be it a discharge or an electron beam) is always lower, because it takes into account the transfer efficiency and the coupling to the gas system. Anyway, very recently (Long et al.[19]) discharge systems for XeCl have been developed in which an overall efficiency of 4%, very close to intrinsic efficiency, has been obtained.

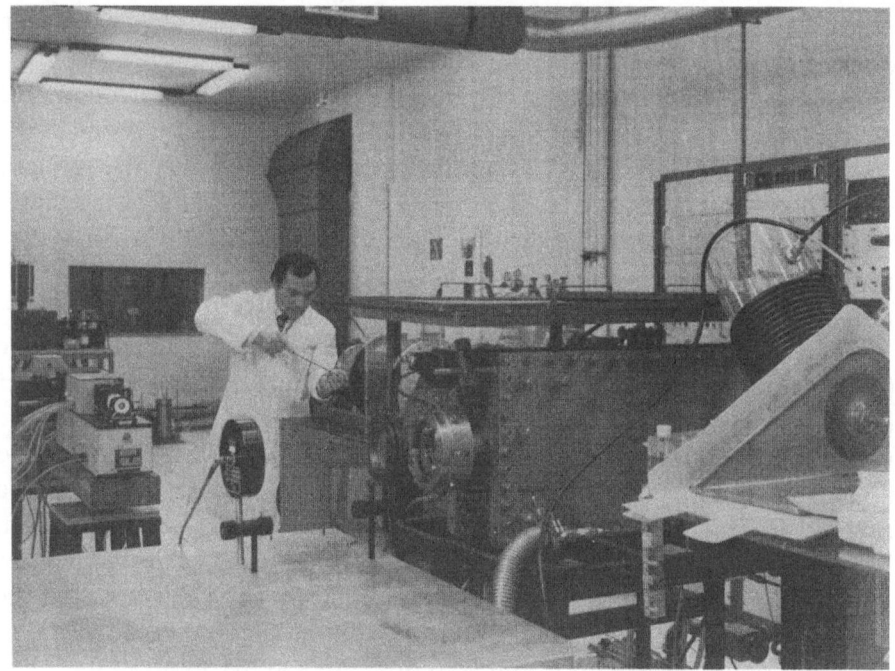

Fig. 2. Excimer laser source developed at the Frascati ENEA Center

The maximum values of energy per pulse have been achieved in electron-beam pumped systems: 850 J for KrF (Goldhar et al.[20]) and 100 J for XeCl (Baranov et al.[21]). The scalability for this configuration has been confirmed.

Self-sustained discharge systems have volume instabilities which limit the scalability. Only for XeCl output energy of 42 J per pulse have been obtained (Giallorenzi and McMahon[22]) in a self-sustained discharge system, while a much lower energy ($\sim$ 5 J/pulse) has been obtained (Watanabe and Endoh[23]) with KrF.

The laser energy which can be extracted from a given active volume (laser energy density) depends, also for a given type of laser, from the pumping method. For electron beam pumping, 40 J/l (Tisone et al.[24]) for KrF and 9 J/l (Tisone and Hoffman[25]) for XeCl have been extracted from the active volume, while in self-sustained discharge systems 4 J/l is the maximum value for XeCl and 5 J/l for KrF (Baranov[26]).

Commercial systems are now available with laser mean power of 200 W, both for KrF and XeCl, typically with pulses of ~ 50 nsec, at a repetition rate ranging from 100 to 500 Hz.

Experimental systems with higher power have been presented (Baranov[26], Fahlen[27]).

As to laser beam angular divergence, typical values for stable oscillators are in the region of few milliradiants, but diffractation limited beams (few tens of microrad) can be obtained (McKee et al.[28]) using unstable cavity configurations. If these techniques are used in oscillator-amplifier systems, low loss of overall efficiency can be obtained. Spectral linewidth of few Å is typical for normal oscillator configurations, but can be enhanced by means of intracavity devices (etalons, etc) to single-mode limit (60 MHz) (Pacala et al.[29]). A pulse length of 1 nsec has been achieved in small systems (Takahashi et al.[30]) or using compression and mode-locked techniques (Takahashi et al.[30], Watanabe et al.[31], Efthimiopoulos[32]).

As example, in Fig. 2 it is shown a laser system, developed at the Frascati ENEA Center, which, operating with a discharge system preionized by electron beam or X-ray, can give laser pulses of 4 J energy (Fiorentino et al.[33]).

II.3. Further Developments

The performances obtained by RGH excimer lasers can be extended in more sophisticated systems.

Raman compression techniques (Murray et al.[34]) permits the achieving of shorter pulses, at higher peak power, starting from conventional systems. With nonlinear optical processes in atoms and molecules (Bischel et al.[35]) higher armonics can be produced. In this way, coherent radiation up to 39.5 nm can be obtained (Egger et al.[36]). Finally, the combination of a dye laser pumped by an excimer laser (Hohla[37]) permits the construction of laser sources with high efficiency, tunability, high optical qualities.

III. The Free-Electron Laser (FEL)

One of the most interesting and promising coherent radiation sources developed in these last years is the free-electron laser, designed and operated the first time by J. M. J. Madey and coworkers of Stanford University at the beginning of 1977 (Deacon et al.[38]).

The more peculiar characteristics of this source is that the active medium is not made of atoms or molecules but it is simply a beam of high energy electrons running in a periodic magnetic structure. The mechanisms which drives the lasing action of this source is not completely new. Indeed it is very similar to that relevant to the "free-electron" microwave devices (Slater[39]) whose development started between the two world wars, like klystrons, magnetrons, travelling wave tubes and, more recently, Giratrons, Ubitrons and Orotrons. The novelty of FEL sources is the possibility of the operation at short wavelength, *i.e.,* in the spectral region where, up to now, coherent radiation was generated only by standard (*i.e.,* atomic or molecular) lasers. This possibility is provided by the high energy of the electrons [many tens of millions of electron volt (MeV) instead of few thousands of electron volt], which generates a very large relativistic Doppler shift and makes possible the operation at short wavelength (*i.e.,* IR and visible instead of microwaves). Indeed the FEL is just the "relativistic version" of the Ubitron (Phillips[40]), which was developed about twenty years before the first successful Stanford experiment.

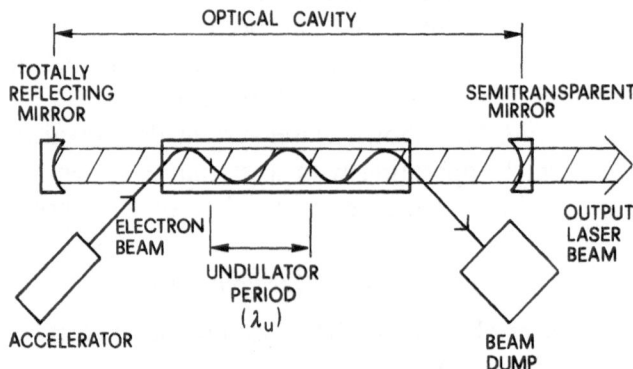

Fig. 3. Layout of a typical FEL source

A detailed and analytical description of the physics involved in the FEL process can be found in many review articles[41] and textbooks[42]. In the next sections we report a very short description of the FEL working principles (section III.1) and we outline the state of art of this source (section III.2). Finally in Sect. III.3 are reported some outlooks for the future.

III.1. The FEL Operating Principles

A sketch of a typical FEL device is reported in Fig. 3. The electrons, generated by an accelerating machine, are injected in a special magnet which creates a spacially periodic magnetic field. As a consequence electrons are forced to oscillate around the magnetic axis [for this reason this item is usually called "undulator magnet" (UM)] and they emit electromagnetic radiation (synchrotron emission) whose wavelength depends on electron energy and magnetic field intensity and period. Moreover, if the radiation is trapped in an optical cavity, it is possible to obtain stimulated emission and, if the gain overcomes the losses, lasing action. The mechanism which drives the stimulated emission is very simple. Namely the electric field of the wave trapped into the optical cavity and running together the electrons, modulates the energy of the electron beam. This energy modulation is transformed, during the passage along the UM, in density modulation at the same wavelength of the radiation itself and the electrons emit coherently just at this wavelength and in phase with the stimulating field. The role of the periodic magnetic field is fundamental. Indeed electrons are forced to oscillate around the UM axis and then they acquire a transverse velocity parallel to the stimulating wave electric field. In this way the electric field can work on the electrons and modulates their energy.

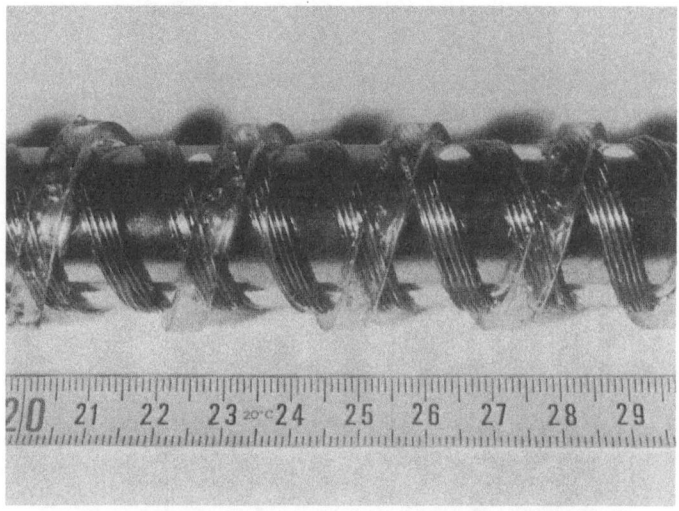

Fig. 4. Helical undulator magnet (electromagnet)

Two kinds of UMs are usually utilized for "undulating" the electrons in FEL devices, namely:

1. Helical UM. The magnetic field is rotating along the UM axis and the electrons follow an helical trajectory. The emitted light is circularly polarized.

2. Linear UM. The magnetic field oscillates in a fixed plane and the electrons follow a sinusoidal trajectory which lies in a plane perpendicular to the magnetic field. The emitted light is linearly polarized.

In Figs. 4 and 5 two examples of helical and linear UMs are shown. Both UMs are presently utilized for the operation of a FEL source tunable in the FIR region ($\lambda = 10$–$30 \, \mu m$) (Bizzarri et al.[43]), under development at the ENEA Frascati Center.

Let us now outline some interesting features of FEL sources. The more impressive one is certainly the very large tunability. Indeed in conventional lasers the radiation wavelength depends on atomic or molecular energy

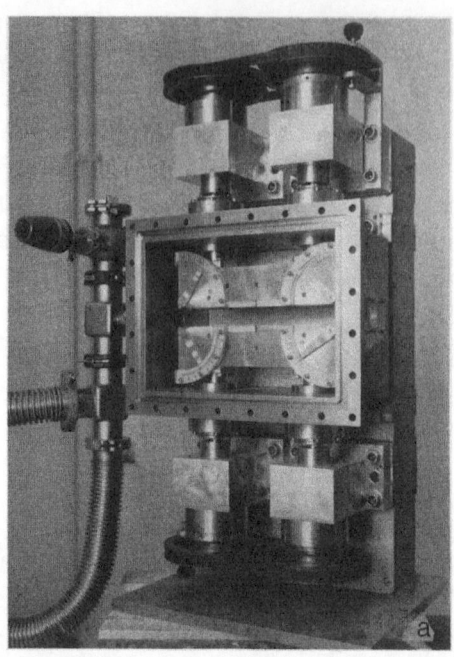

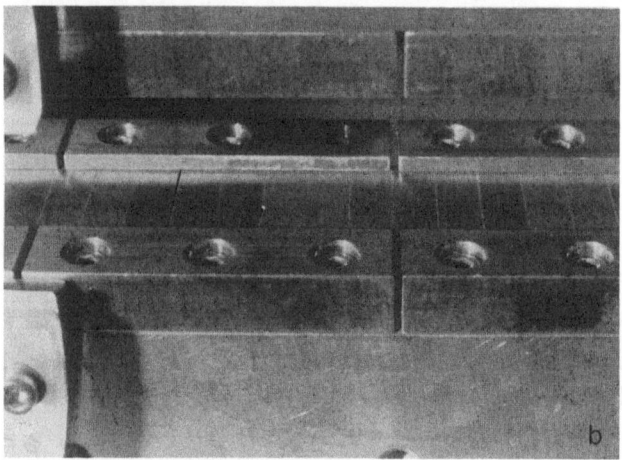

Fig. 5. Linear undulator magnet: (a) general view: (b) permanent magnets

levels of the lasing medium and then it is not possible, in general, to have a large tuning range (apart dye lasers). FEL sources, on the other hand, can be easily tuned simply by changing electron energy or UM parameters. More precisely the relationship between radiation wavelength λ, electron energy E and r.m.s. magnetic field $\bar{B}$ and period λ_u of the UM, reads (for the symbols see Table 1)

$$\lambda = \frac{\lambda_u}{2} \left[1 + \left(\frac{e\bar{B}\lambda_u}{2\pi mc^2} \right)^2 \right] \left(\frac{mc^2}{E} \right)^2. \tag{1}$$

In FEL literature it is usually defined the following "undulator parameter",

$$K = \frac{e\bar{B}\lambda_u}{2\pi mc^2}, \tag{2}$$

so that Eq. (1) can be written in the form

$$\lambda = \frac{\lambda_u}{2} (1 + K^2) \left(\frac{mc^2}{E} \right)^2. \tag{3}$$

Equation (3) holds for both helical and linear UMs. In addition the tunability of linear UMs is greatly enhanced by the fact that they can operate (if the gain is sufficiently high) also at odd harmonics of the fundamental, *i.e.*,

$$\lambda = \frac{1}{n} \frac{\lambda_u}{2} (1 + K^2) \left(\frac{mc^2}{E} \right)^2 \tag{4}$$

$$(n = 1, 3, 5, \ldots).$$

For typical values of λ_u ($\sim$ cm), K ($\sim$ 1) and E ($\sim$ 1/1,000 MeV) the emitted radiation ranges from millimeter to X-rays region. This very impressive operating bandwith is a unique features of FEL sources.

In addition to this wide tunability, FEL sources present the possibility of modulation of the wavelength during the laser pulse, just by changing the electron beam energy, and, with a linear UM, the operation at several wavelengths in the same laser beam at the same time [see Eq. (4)].

Another interesting aspect of FEL sources is the laser beam time structure, which follows the electron beam one. We can distinguish between single pulse devices, like that operating with induction linac (pulse duration $\sim$ 10–100 nsec) on Pelletron (pulse duration $\sim$ 100 μsec), and radio-frequency (r.f.) accelerators (linacs, microtrons, storage rings). In this last case, the electrons are collected in trains of several microbunches, whose duration ranges from few psec to a fraction of nsec. As a consequence of this pulse structure, the laser linewidth is Fourier-transform limited, *i.e.*, it reads

$$\frac{\Delta\lambda}{\lambda} \gtrsim \frac{\lambda}{c\tau}, \tag{5}$$

where τ is the microbunch duration. We stress that the limit given by Eq. (5) can be very severe for some possible applications, in which very high

Table 3. *Operating FEL Sources*

Year	Laboratory	Accelerator	E (MeV)	λ (μm)	τ (psec)	Macropulse duration (μsec)	Peak power (W)
1977	Stanford	LINAC	43	3.3	4	$\sim 10^3$	$\sim 10^6$
1983	Orsay	STORAGE RING	160	0.65	500–1,000	c.w.	1
1983	TRW/Stanford	LINAC	66	1.6	4	$\sim 10^3$	$\sim 10^6$
1983	Los Alamos	LINAC	20	9–11	30	70	10^6
1983	Livermore	INDUCTION LINAC	4.5	8×10^3	3×10^4	—	8×10^7
1984	S. Barbara	PELLETRON	3	400	60×10^6	—	10^3

Table 4. *FEL Scenario*

Laboratory	λ (μm)	Accelerator	E (MeV)	I (A)	Undulator	λ_u (cm)
Livermore	$(2\text{–}10) \cdot 10^3$	Induction Linac	4	10^3	pulsed (tapered)	9.8
S. Barbara 1-stages	400	Pelletron	3–6	2	permanent magnet	3.6
S. Barbara 2-stages	1–10	Pelletron	3	2	FEL laser wave	0.01–0.1
Bell Labs	100–400	Microtron	18–20	5	electromagnet	20
Frascati (ENEA)	10–30	Microtron	20	6.5	permanent magnet	5
UK Project	2–20	Linac	20–100	10	permanent magnet	8
TRW	1.6	Linac	66	2.5	permanent magnet	3.56
Los Alamos	9–11	Linac	20	25	permanent magnet	2.4
MSNW-BAC	10.6	Linac	19	100	permanent magnet	2.54–2.22
Stanford	3.3	Linac	43	1.3	electromagnet	3.23
Novosibirsk	0.6328	Storage ring	370		permanent magnet	10
Orsay	0.65	Storage ring ACO	166		permanent magnet	7.78
Frascati (INFN)	0.5145	Storage ring ADONE	300, 624		electromagnet	11.6
Brookhaven	0.25–0.45	VUV Storage ring	300–500		permanent magnet	6.5

monochromaticity of laser radiation is required. For example, at $\lambda \sim 30\,\mu m$, $\tau \sim 20\,psec$ (ENEA IR source—Bizzarri et al.[43]) we obtain

$$\frac{\Delta\lambda}{\lambda} \geqslant 0.5\%.$$

III.2. FEL Scenario

As pointed out in the introduction, only six FEL devices have been able to lase up to now. In Table 3 the main characteristics of these sources are reported together with the year of realization. It is interesting to point out the large delay between the first device (Stanford 1977) and the second one (Orsay 1983), mainly due to the complexity of FEL sources in which high level accelerator, magnet and optical technologies are required. The FEL scenario is developing very fastly. Indeed there is a lot of experiment under realization (see Table 4). In a near future, the number of operating oscillators will increase very rapidly and certainly their performances will be greatly improved. In particular a great effort is presently done in many laboratories (TRW/Stanford, Livermore, Los Alamos, MSNW) in order to increase efficiency and power output by using UMs of special design (tapered and multicomponent devices).

Namely the maximum efficiency obtained up to now is of the order of few percent with a fraction of watt of average output power (let us stress that these values are in very good agreement with theoretical predictions). For the near future efficiencies up to ten percent together with average output power of the order of many hundreds of watts are foresee in FIR and IR. Finally, as to the bandwidth, the operating wavelength ranges presently from 8 mm (Livermore) to visible (Orsay). It is worth noticing that very promising schemes have been recently proposed[44], which would allow operation up to soft X-rays spectral region.

III.3. The Future of the FEL: Conclusions and Outlooks

It is not a simple task to foresee the future for a source like the FEL, whose development started only few years ago and where very few devices have been able to lase up to now. However it is possible to outline some very general considerations. Namely, the present FEL devices show a number of disadvantages, i.e.,

1. the operation requires radiation shielding,
2. the system dimensions are very large (from few tens to many hundreds of meters),
3. FELs are very expensive devices (some millions of dollars).

It is difficult to overcome completely the drawbacks relevant to point 1., which are due to the operating principle itself of FEL sources (see sections III and III.1). However, it is possible to minimize the problem. Namely there is a noticeable experimental work aimed to reduce the electron energy (which, in any case, remains relativistic) for a given operating wavelength, by utilizing short period magnetic undulators, wave undulators[45] (*i.e.,* in place of UMs it is utilized microwave radiation) and dielectric waveguide systems, in which instead of stimulated synchrotron emission (see section III.1), it is utilized Cerenkov emission[46].

As to the points 2 and 3, we must take into account that the present FEL devices are just experiments. This means that they need a lot of diagnostics, they must be very flexible, in order to operate in many different experimental configurations, and, finally, they are prototypes which utilize, in general, electron accelerators designed for completely different applications (nuclear physics, synchrotron radiation, nuclear weapon simulation, etc.). On the other hand, dedicated FEL sources will be optimized for a given operating regime and they will utilize accelerating systems designed just for FEL operation. In addition compactness and reduction of the cost will be achieved with the integration of many parts of the system, *e.g.,* the electron beam guiding and focusing channel with the UM itself. Finally it is possible to foresee a strong reduction of cost for the fact that these sources would not be prototypes.

All these considerations are very preliminary, however the outlined technological trend (if confirmed by further investigation) will allow FEL devices to have a noticeable impact in many fields[47], like research, industrial and medical applications and energy production (controlled fusion devices).

References

1. Lord Rayleigh, 1966: Proc. R. Soc. London *A 116,* 702.
2. Stevens, B., Hutton, E., 1960: Nature *186,* 1045.
3. Basov, N. G., Danilychev, V. A., Propov, Yu. M., Khodkevich, D. D., 1970: JEPT Lett. *12,* 329.
4. Searles, S. K., Hart, G. A., 1975: Appl. Phys. Lett. *27,* 243.
5. Bazhulin, S. P., Basov, N. G., Zuev, V. S., Leonov, Yu. S., Stoilov, Yu. Yu., 1978: Sov. J. Quantum Electron. *8,* 402.
6. Eden, J. G., 1978: Appl. Phys. Lett. *33,* 495.
7. Hutchinson, M. H. R., 1980: Appl. Phys. *21,* 95.
8. Baranov, S. V., Bystritskii, V. M., Didenko, A. N., Kozhevnikov, A. V., Prokhorov, A. M., Sulakshin, S. S., Usov, Yu. P., 1982: Sov. J. Quantum Electron. *12,* 70.
9. Mendelsohn, A. J., Normandin, R., Harris, S. E., Young, J. F., 1981: Appl. Phys. Lett. *38,* 603.
10. Rhodes, Ch. K., 1983: Excimers Lasers. 2nd ed. Berlin-Heidelberg-New York: Springer.
11. Koehler, H. A., Ferderber, L. J., Rehhead, D. L., Ebert, P. J., 1972: Appl. Phys. Lett. *21,* 198.
12. Hoff, P. W., Wingle, J. C., Rhodes, C. K., 1973: Appl. Phys. Lett. *23,* 245.

13. Hughes, W. M., Shannon, J., Hunter, R., 1974: Appl. Phys. Lett. *24*, 488.
14. Ault, E. R., Bradford, R. S., Jr., Bhaumik, M. L., 1975: Arpa Contract N 00014-72-C-0456.
15. Fisher, C. H., Znotins, T. A., Smilanski, I., Pindroh, A. L., De Hart, T. E., Ewing, J. J.: 1st Conf. on Lasers and Electro-Optics. Cleo '83. Tec. Digest, p. 240.
16. Lakoba, I. S., Yakovlenko, S. I., 1980: Sov. J. Quantum Electron. *10* (4), 389.
17. Salesky, E. T., Kimura, W. D.: Conf. on Lasers and Electro-Optics. Cleo '84, Postdeadline Papers ThR6.
18. Champagne, L. F., 1979: Appl. Phys. Lett. *33*, 523.
19. Long, W. H., Jr., Plummer, M. J., Stappaerts, E. A., 1983: Appl. Phys. Lett. *43*, 735.
20. Goldhar, J., Jancaitis, K. S., Murray, J. R.: Conf. on Laser and Electro-Optics, Cleo '84. Tech. Digest, p. 136.
21. Baranov, V. Yu., Velikhov, E. P., Gaidarenko, D. V., Isakov, I. M., Krasnikov, Yu. G., Malyuta, D. D., Novobrantsev, I. V., Pis'mennyi, V. D., Smakovskii, Yu. B., Strel'tsov, A. P., 1983: Sov. Tech. Phys. Lett. *9*, 88.
22. Giallorenzi, T. G., McMahon, J. M., 1984: Laser Focus/Electro-Optics, May 1984, p. 75.
23. Watanabe, S., Endoh, A., 1982: Appl. Phys. Lett. *41*, 799.
24. Tisone, G. C., Patterson, E. L., Rice, J. K., 1979: Appl. Phys. Lett. *35*, 437.
25. Tisone, G. C., Hoffman, J. M., 1982: IEEE J. of Quant. Elec. *QE-18*, 1008.
26. Baranov, V. Yu., 1983: IEEE J. of Quant. Elec. *QE-19*, 1577.
27. Fahlen, T. S., 1980: IEEE J. of Quant. Elec. *QE-16*, 1260.
28. McKee, T. J., Stoicheff, B. P., Wallace, S. C., 1977: Appl. Phys. Lett. *30*, 278.
29. Pacala, T. J., McDermid, I. S., Laudenslager, J. B., 1984: Appl. Phys. Lett. *45*, 507.
30. Takahashi, A., Maeda, M., Noda, Y., 1984: IEEE J. of Quant. Elec. *QE-20*, 1196.
31. Watanabe, S., Watanabe, M., Endoh, A., 1983: Appl. Phys. Lett. *43*, 533.
32. Efthimiopoulos, T., 1984: Appl. Phys. Lett. *45*, 346.
33. Fiorentino, E., Letardi, T., Marino, A., Sabia, E., Vannini, M.: to be published in "Laser and Particles Beams".
34. Murray, J. R., Goldhar, J., Eimerl, D., Szöke, A., 1979: IEEE J. of Quant. Elec. *QE-15*, 342.
35. Bischel, W. K., Bokor, J., Klinger, D. J., Rhodes, C. K., 1979: IEEE J. of Quant. Elec. *QE-15*, 380.
36. Egger, H., Pummer, H., Rhodes, C. K., 1982: Laser Focus, p. 59.
37. Hohla, K. L., 1982: Laser Focus, p. 67.
38. Deacon, D. A. G., Elias, L. R., Madey, J. M. J., Ramian, G. T., Schwettman, H. A., Smith, T. I., 1977: Phys. Rev. Lett. *38*, 892.
39. See, *e.g.,* Slater, J. C., 1963: Microwave Electronics. Princeton: Van Nostrand.
40. Phillips, R. M., 1960: IRE Trans. Electron Devices, *ED-7*, 231.
41. See, *e.g.,* the special issue devoted to FEL devices, IEEE J. of Quant. Elec. *QE-17* issue no. 8, 1981, and Dattoli, G., Renieri, A.: Experimental and theoretical aspects of the free-electron laser. In: Laser Handbook, Vol. 4 (Stich, M. L., Bass, M. S., eds.). North Holland.

42. On FEL topics have been done many workshops, Conferences and schools. The proceedings of the more recent meetings are: Colloque International sur les Lasers a Electron Libres. Bendor, Sept. 1982, J. de Physique, Colloque C 1, Suppl. 2, *44* (1983).
Free Electron Generation of Coherent Radiation. Orcas Island, 1983, SPIE Vol. 453 (1984).
1984 FEL Conference. Castelgandolfo, 1984, Nucl. Instrum. and Meth. in Phys. Res. Vol. A 237 (1985).

43. Bizzarri, U., Ciocci, F., Dattoli, G., De Angelis, A., Fiorentino, E., Gallerano, G. P., Marino, A., Renieri, A., Vignati, A.: first of references[42], p. 677, second of references[42], p. 313, and last of references[42], p. 213.

44. See, *e.g.,* proceedings of "Topical Meeting on Free Electron Generation of Extreme Ultraviolet Coherent Radiation" AIP 118, Brookhaven (1983) and Murphy J. B., Pellegrini C.: last of references[42], p. 159.

45. Segall, S. B., see the second of references[42], p. 383.

46. Dattoli, G., Walsh, T. E., Johnson, B., Renieri, A., 1984: Phys. Rev. Lett *53*, 779.

47. See, *e.g.,* Scoles, S., ed., 1979: "The Possible Impact of Free-Electron Lasers in Spectroscopy and Chemistry" IRST, Riva del Garda.
Proc. of "Workshop on Application of FEL", Castelgandolfo 1984, to appear on Nucl. Instrum. and Meth. in Phys. Res.

The Role of Laser in Neurosurgery. Conclusions

Victor A. Fasano

Institute of Neurosurgery, University of Turin (Italy)

Rather than a new surgical tool the laser, as a new source of energy, is a new surgical method.

We know at present two different laser techniques: noncontact and contact laser surgery.

1. Conventional noncontact laser surgery.

On the basis of a personal experience in more than 700 cases operated utilizing three lasers (CO_2, Nd: YAG, argon) free-hand with magnification glasses or with the aid of the operating microscope, comes out that lasers, in comparison with the traditional technique, consent a decrease of postoperative morbidity, a more extended removal and a reduction of the blood loss.

Ultrasonic aspirator is currently used to debulk large neoplasms. CO_2 laser is suitable to vaporize layer by layer small deep-seated lesions or tumor remnants and to dissect them from the critical areas.

Nd: YAG laser finds its application to coagulate vascularized lesions (tumors and arteriovenous malformations). Use of this source in the following situations is however risky:

a) Tumors in and around the brain stem because of the possibility of penetration beyond the tumor into normal brain tissue.

b) Radiation of residual tumors because of the risk of hemorrhage from the tissue which had been rendered necrotic by Nd: YAG laser radiation but not excised.

Argon laser is mostly used in vascular pathology.

Computerized CO_2 laser is used in brain stem tumors to improve selectivity.

Preliminary results seem to suggest the usefulness of lasers in other pathologies.

A peculiar effect on the collagen fibers of the wall is produced after CO_2

and argon irradiation; this involves the elastic response to strain, and resistance to overstretching increases subsequently.

Endovascular thrombosis can be obtained after Nd:YAG and argon irradiation in thin wall vessels with low blood flow.

Both effects have made a new method of surgery of arterio-venous malformations and arterial aneurysms possible.

Experimental applications of the laser are in progress in microvascular surgery for anastomizing blood vessels and in endoscopy to remove arterial obstructions.

The use of laser coupled with computerizing imaging devices (CT scan, NMR) and stereotactic technique will allow increasing precision in the treatment of deep-seated lesions of the brain, brain stem and spinal cord.

On the other hand a greater knowledge of the absorption characteristics of pathological tissue will make a more correct use of the various wavelengths possible.

Photoradiation therapy with hematoporphyrin derivative and laser hyperthermia offer great promise especially in intrinsic brain tumors, where infiltration of neoplastic tissue precludes the classical oncologic surgery practice of resection leaving a safe margin. The ability to destroy these cells without affecting adjacent tissue has not been sufficiently tested yet, as extensive clinical trials on the benefit of these therapies do not exist.

2. Contact laser surgery.

The goal of this technique is the progressive transformation of the traditional surgical instruments using radiofrequency into a laser unit which will allow increased rapidity and precision of the surgical maneuver, and a reduction of blood loss and side effects. In comparison with the electrosurgical unit carbonization, smoke and sticking are avoided.

The first instrument of the contact laser surgery is the laser scalpel, available for all sources delivered through optic fibers. This scalpel, useful for cutting and dissecting maneuver, shows considerable advantages in comparison with the conventional technique and noncontact lasers. When Nd:YAG laser is used, scalpel becomes an ideal surgical tool which produces a sharp cut associated to a complete hemostasis.

Such an atomic system, wheter it be gaseous, solid or liquid can lead to a laser.

The opportunity to exploit new wavelength is the key to the future. A more rapid removal and a more complete hemostasis can be expected by the use of new wavelengths. Copper vapor lasers (CVL) are studied in cardiovascular research; heavy metal vapor lasers are still under investigation as rivals of the dye laser in photoradiation therapy.

Other laser sources in advanced study are the Nd:YAG 1.2 nm, the X- and gamma-ray lasers.

The free-electron laser, as a source of high average power of coherent radiation of tunable wavelengths, seems to be applicable in surgery in order to find suitable wavelengths which may provide for both cutting and coagulation; wavelengths between those of CO_2 and Nd : YAG laser seem to be particularly attractive.

The free-electron laser may cover the entire spectrum from millimeter waves to ultraviolet waves. The importance of this type of laser is obvious where tunable sources are not available, for example in the ultraviolet range. The development of centralized laser apparatuses with a fiberoptic delivery system to the operating rooms could reduce the present problems of size and costs.

3. Ultrasonic Aspiration in Neurosurgery

Ultrasonic Aspiration in Neurosurgery

Victor A. Fasano

Institute of Neurosurgery, University of Turin (Italy)

Contents

1. General Principles 257
    1.1. Historical Data 257
    1.2. Technical Characteristics.. 258
2. Surgical Applications 259
    2.1. Tumor Removal 260
        2.1.1. Experimental Data.. 260
        2.1.2. Clinical Data 260
    2.2. Tissue Dissection 266
        2.2.1. Experimental Data.. 266
        2.2.2. Clinical Data 268
3. Surgical Results.. 270
4. Conclusive Considerations 271
References 272

I. General Principles

1.1. Historical Data

Various methods have been proposed for the removal of either normal or pathological tissues.

In 1928, Cushing and Bovie reported the use of radiofrequency electrical currents (loop electrode) to facilitate the removal of intracranial tumors[3]. Successively other methods, including cryogenic probes, coherent infrared radiation and mechanical dissectors, as the Biotome or the House-Urban rotary dissector, have been introduced in surgery[10].

Recently the ultrasonic aspirator (CUSA: Cavitron Ultrasonic Surgical Aspirator), an instrument capable of fragmenting and then aspirating the tissue has become available. This instrument was first applied to the removal of dental plaque (Cavitron Dental Scaler, 1947). Since 1967 a precursor of the CUSA, the Kelman Phacoemulsifier, has been used in more than 1,000,000 cataract procedures, and this application prompted attempts to adapt ultrasonic emulsification and aspiration to neurosurgical procedures[9]. After the original equipment proved to be inadequate to fragment the firm tissue encountered in intracranial tumors, a new design was introduced in 1976[5, 6]. Over 7,000 cases have been reported especially meningiomas, low grade gliomas, acoustic neuromas and intramedullary spinal cord tumors. Exploration of general surgical applications of the CUSA began in 1977, and its use in hepatic resection, partial nephrectomy, and mucosa proctectomy have facilitated these complex procedures[2, 8, 9, 11].

1.2. Technical Characteristics

The ultrasonic aspirator consists of a control and power console and a gas-sterilizable surgical handpiece. It is a self-contained unit requiring only standard operating room electrical connections, with all controls and indicators located on the control panel. Three major systems operate simultaneously to provide fragmentation, irrigation and aspiration of tissue coming into contact with the vibrating surgical tip.

The handpiece can be assembled in three configurations: regular handpiece, straight or curved 4 inch extender for deep-access tumors or sites where surgical microscope will be used. It can be held directly by the surgeon or by means of a supporting pistol grip. A vibrating suction device oscillates longitudinally along its axis, thereby fragmenting and aspirating tissue within a 1 to 2 mm radius of the tip. The vibration is imperceptible, with a magnitude in the range of 100 microns, and is produced at the ultrasonic frequency of 23 kHz.

The console contains a system of aspiration and irrigation (to facilitate suction of the fragmented tissue and guarantee the cooling of the tip) and provides the energy source for the vibration. Electric energy activates a magneto-structure transducer in the handpiece. The longitudinal contractions of this acoustic vibrator cause the tip to impact tissue resulting in fragmentation at the tip/tissue interface. Power emitted by the vibration can be taken up to a maximum of 70 watts; the aspiration pressure can be varied from 0 to 600 mm Hg and the flow rate of the irrigating physiological solution from 3 to 10 ml/minute (Fig. 1).

Onboard computer logic directs and monitors setup and surgical procedure to assure that:

a) The unit is properly primed.

b) The vibration/irrigation is set and checked.

c) The console control is inactive while the surgeon has handpiece control.

On-off controls of both the irrigation and vibration are provided by switches in the handpiece.

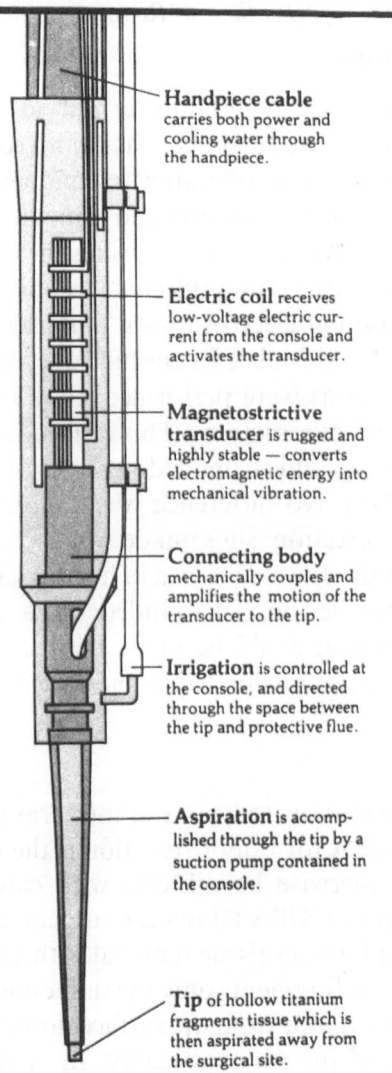

Fig. 1. Ultrasonic aspiration handpiece

Tip suction is automatically inoperative when applying flush irrigation and momentarily interrupted whenever tip vibration is terminated.

2. Surgical Applications

The focused energy of the CUSA is concentrated in the ultrasonically vibrating tip of the device which is used mostly in two groups of procedures:
   a) Dissection.
   b) High-volume debulking of large tumor.

2.1. Tumor Removal

2.1.1. Experimental Data

Studies were undertaken by Flamm et al.[6] to compare the damage produced in the cat brain when tissue was removed using the ultrasonic aspirator and various standard operative techniques. On each side of the brain of twelve cats a cortical resection and removal of about $2 cm^3$ of the underlying white matter was carried out using the ultrasonic aspirator at maximal power for 10 seconds and different techniques (standard suction and cautery, cutting loop of electrosurgical unit and bone rongeur). After surgery all animals received 3 ml of Evans blue dye. After sacrifice 72 hours later brain coronal sections were performed: they showed a zone of blue staining around all types of resections. This ranged from 3 to 5 mm around the edge of the lesion and extended in a rostral caudal direction approximately 2 to 3 cm. No difference was seen in the amount of blue staining around the resection sites made with the various techniques. Histological examination showed an area of hemorrhage and necrosis in the immediate area of the lesion, surrounded by a zone of edema. No quantitative differentiation could be made between lesions produced by ultrasonic aspirator and lesions created by the other types of brain removal.

2.1.2. Clinical Data

Observations are based on 153 cases of intracranial tumors. The major advantage in using CUSA for tumor resection is the rapid removal of firm tumors that would otherwise be difficult with cautery and suction. In comparison with cautery, CUSA allows the surgeon to achieve a rapid and highly controlled layer by layer tissue removal with a limited depth of tissue damage, since the CUSA fragments only the tissue contacted by the tip. It is possible to extirpate the tumor from the surface downwards thus constantly controlling the limits of the surgical cavity. In comparison with normal suction, which is effective only on very soft tissues, the aspiration occurs without significant pressure, minimizing damage, pulling and distortion of surrounding tissue.

The selective fragmentation of highly acqueous tissues relative to those of greater collagenous and elastic character allows the sparing of vessels and nerves of a certain caliber; the lower the power used in fragmentation, the greater the vascular salvage. Cerebral vessels within lesions are easily skeletonized and hemostasis is achieved with bipolar coagulation; nerves adherent to tumoral tissue however, cannot to be spared in the same way. At the capillary level the sheer limited thermal effect produced by the vibration of the tip often permits satisfactory hemostasis, the heat bonding effect on small vessels occurring more rapidly by reducing the flow of irrigation. Continuous irrigation and aspiration enhance the surgeon's ability to work quickly and precisely in a relatively dry field. The surgical procedure may be modulated by changing power of vibration; slow or fast maneuvers may influence the removal: the former is used when operating near high functional structures, the latter to debulk tumoral mass.

Our series of tumors operated with CUSA is presented in Table 1. The rapidity of action of the CUSA is conditioned by the consistency of the tissue encountered. Soft tumors (gliomas, medulloblastomas, degenerated

Table 1. *Tumors Operated with CUSA*

SOFT   TUMORS   :   76   CASES
‾‾‾‾‾‾‾‾‾‾‾‾‾‾‾‾‾‾‾‾‾‾‾‾‾‾‾‾‾
- 35 GLIOMAS (14 DEEP - SEATED AND 2 SUBCORTICAL)
- 13 CEREBELLAR TUMORS (6 MEDULLOBLASTOMAS , 5 SPONGIOBLASTOMAS , 2 EPENDYMOMAS)
- 12 ACOUSTIC NEUROMAS
- 2 INTRAMEDULLARY GLIOMAS
- 4 PYNEALOMAS
- 5 BRAIN - STEM TUMORS (3 INTRINSIC GLIOMAS AND 2 MEDULLOBLASTOMAS WITH EXTRA - AXIAL
                         EXTENSION)
- 5 PITUITARY ADENOMAS

FIRM   TUMORS   :   77   CASES
‾‾‾‾‾‾‾‾‾‾‾‾‾‾‾‾‾‾‾‾‾‾‾‾‾‾‾‾‾
- 35 BASAL MENINGIOMAS (15 ADJOINING VESSELS , 20 ADJOINING VASCULAR AND NERVE STRUCTURES)
- 35 SUPERFICIAL MENINGIOMAS (15 PARASAGITTAL MENINGIOMAS , 13 CONVEXITY MENINGIOMAS,
                             7 MENINGIOMAS OF THE FALX)
- 6 MENINGIOMAS OF THE PONTO - CEREBELLAR REGION
- 1 INTRADURAL SPINAL CORD MENINGIOMA

meningiomas, neurinomas, adenomas and pynealomas) are easily and rapidly fragmented and aspirated. In gliomas and meningiomas the elective preservation of large caliber vasculature facilitated hemostasis, while in adenomas and pynealomas the effective hemostasis from CUSA is largely sufficient for dealing with these poorly vascularized tumors. In very soft tumors, as necrotic glioblastomas, surrounded by edema, the rapidity of removal requires great attention because of the risk of extending the fragmentation to surrounding tissues. Firm tumors are also rapidly removed, while hard tumors are not readily handled and fragmentation is very slow and difficult; in these cases CUSA is used as a scalpel to resect, step by step, parts of the tumor.

In gliomas, cerebellar and mid-line tumors the non-traumatic removal is very useful to respect highly functional structures (especially in deep-seated astrocytomas and pinealomas).

In capsular tumors (acoustic neurinomas, meningiomas) the CUSA is used to perforate the capsule and reduce the tumor bulk. The capsule

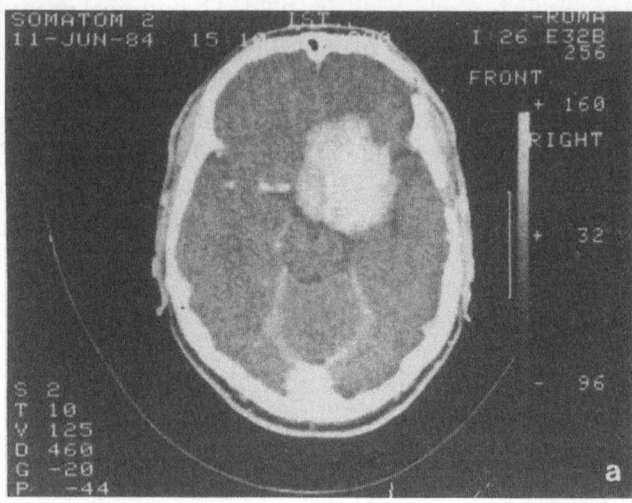

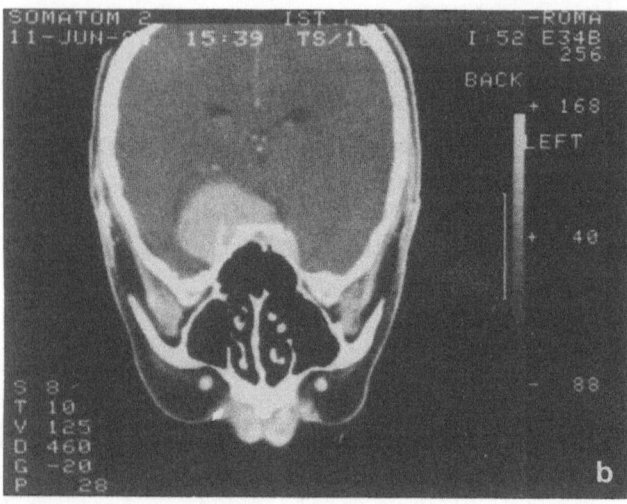

Fig. 2. Medial sphenoid ridge meningioma extending to the anterior and medial cranial fossa bilaterally to sellar region and third ventricle. After removal with CUSA the visual function was preserved and there were no neurological deficits. a)–b) preoperative CT scan, c)–d) preoperative angiography, e) postoperative CT scan, f)–g) postoperative angiography

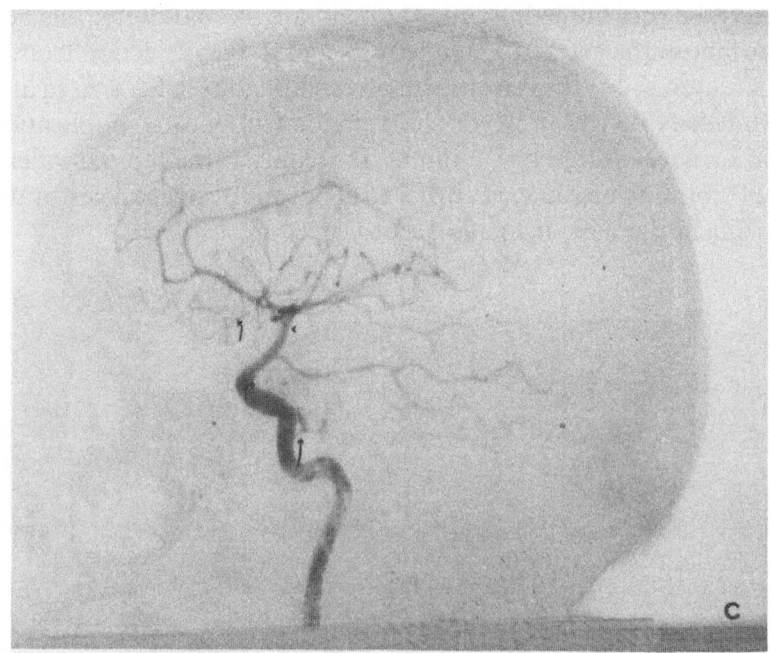

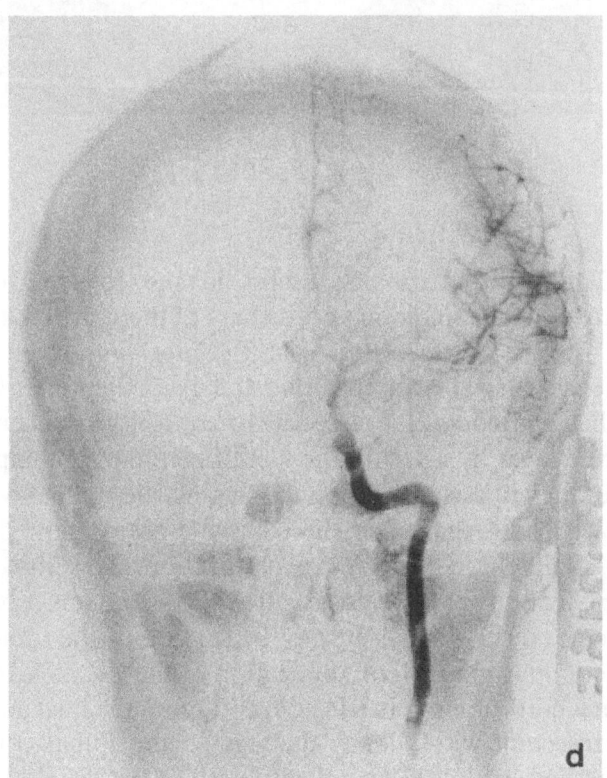

Figs. 2 c and d

incision must be very limited in order to maintain its continuity, this being very important in the extraction maneuvers and in the dissection from the adjacent structures. For the intracapsular resection the CUSA is used at the maximal intensity of vibration for short periods in repeated applications, total duration never exceeding 7 minutes. In vicinity of the capsule walls the intensity of vibration is reduced in order to avoid any accidental perforation with consequent damage of the adjacent tissue.

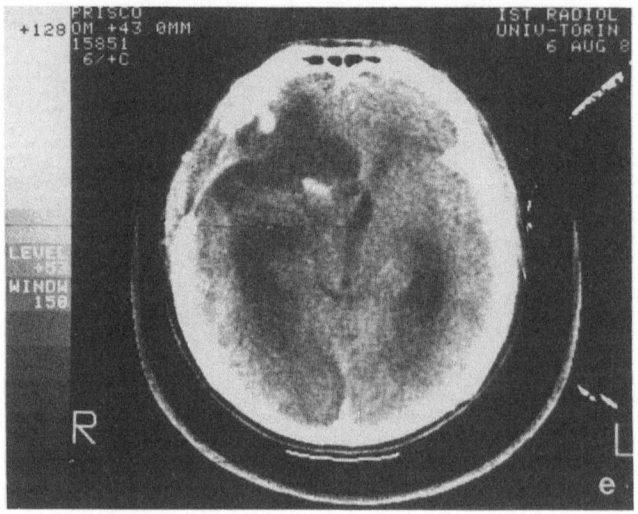

Fig. 2 e

The CUSA is particularly useful in the removal of parasagittal meningiomas and meningiomas of the base of the skull, mostly in sellar and parasellar regions. In the latter case the most important problem is to respect the vascular structures within the mass. Tumor is first reduced in volume, then shifted with a dissector to control vascular adherences and then resected layer by layer till the identification of the important arteries which are then dissected from the neoplastic tissue with traditional instruments. In this maneuver the CUSA is used at low power and very slowly to avoid the risk of vessel perforation. This risk should not be underestimated since rupture can easily occur aside from any contact owing to the traction on the vessel during the suction of the tumor (Fig. 2).

Another important field of application of the CUSA is in the treatment of the spinal cord tumors. In intradural tumors the instrument consents a complete resection without any damage to the spinal cord. In intrinsic tumors after incision of the spinal cord with CO_2 laser, the surgeon has the great advantage of a tactile feedback which allows him to distinguish

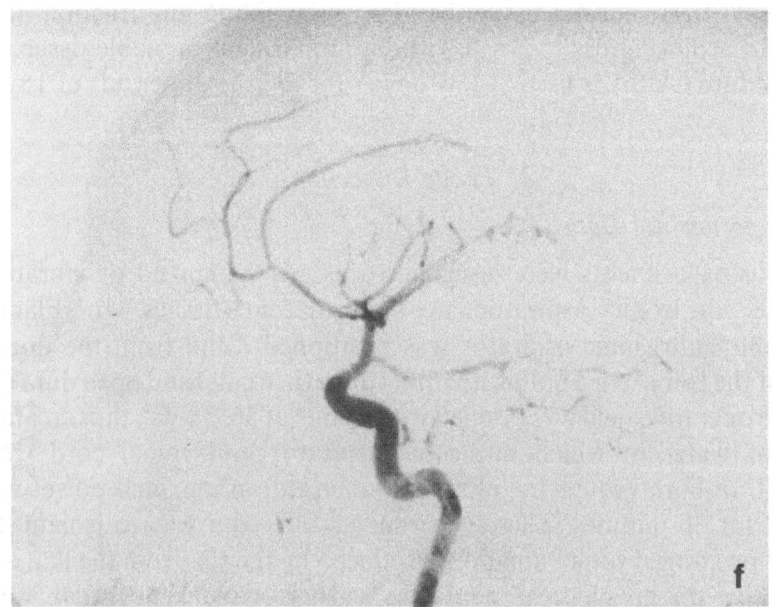

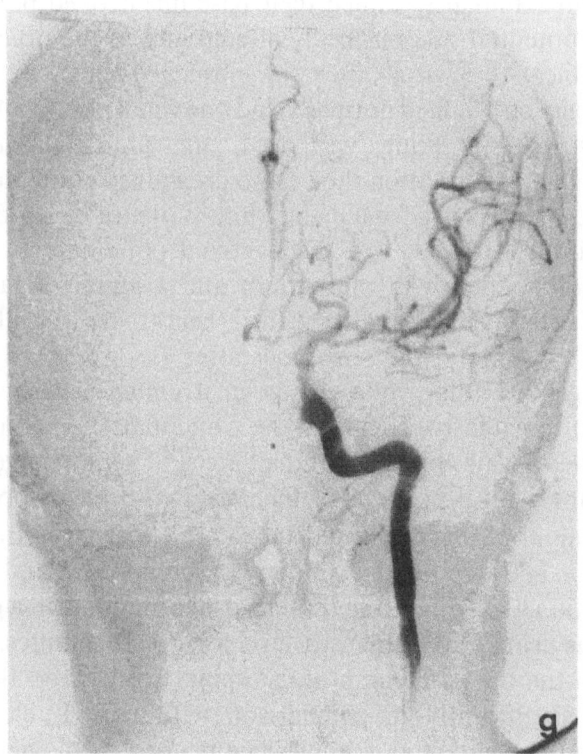

Figs. 2 f and g

pathological from normal tissue; besides, by avoiding any traction, it is possible to achieve gross removal without impairment of viable tissue. In this procedure CUSA is used at low power for 2–3 short periods of 15–30 seconds.

2.2. Tissue Dissection

2.2.1. Experimental Data

Various experiments were designed to assess the spread of vibration from the ultrasonic aspirator to the adjacent tissues. In Flamm experiments[6] ultrasonic aspirator was positioned 3 mm from the dorsal surface of the spinal cord both with intact dura (in 6 cats) and open dura (10 cats). The operative field was flooded with saline (at 36–38 °C), thus creating a pool of water in which ultrasonic aspirator and spinal cord were immersed. In both groups the ultrasonic aspirator at maximal power was activated for 30 minutes. These experiments offered a way to isolate the effects of prolonged sonic radiation, produced by the tip, from the damage incurred by direct physical contact. Sensory evoked potential were monitored before and after the exposure interval. In the group with intact dura, three animals retained their base line evoked potentials, in two the evoked potential was markedly altered and in the other it was no longer obtainable. At 1 week after the surgical exposure, four animals were paraplegic, one walked normally and one was a poor walker. By 6 weeks five animals were walking well and one animal remained paraplegic. Histological examination showed no gross disruption but did show, even at 6 weeks, evidence of edema in the white matter of the cord. In the group with open dura, 6 animals lost their evoked potentials, 3 animals showed a considerable change in the pattern and 1 animal retained the base line evoked potential. 8 animals regained their ability to walk (2 within the first week after surgery; the remainder after 7–8 weeks). 2 animals remained paraplegic. In this group histological changes were more marked. In addition to extensive edema in the white matter, even in the animals that were able to walk, there were small areas of hemorrhage and glial scarring within the central portions of the spinal cord at the operating site.

Young et al.[14] investigated the acute effects of ultrasonically induced lesions on action potential conduction, blood flow, and nerve conduction. The suction was adjusted so that the probe maintained a gentle contact with the tissue using a 20% intensity level for 1 to 10 minutes. After a lesion was made in the dorsal column of cat spinal cord blood flow values did not change significantly in comparison with the H_2 clearance flow rates measured in the lateral column. The neurophysiological responses of the spinal tracts surrounding the lesion also remained intact. Examination of the spinal cord with the light microscope revealed normal tissue at the borders of the lesion. There was little evidence of edema or neuronal loss as

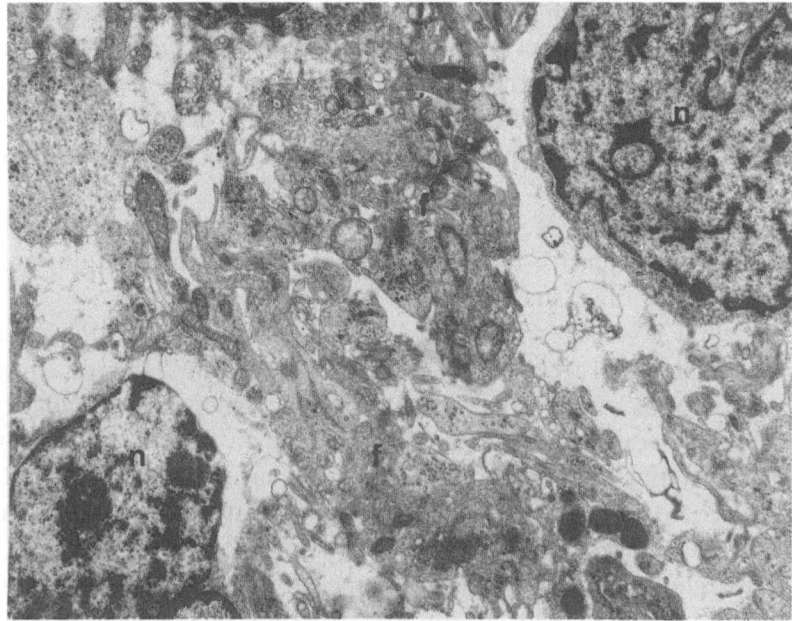

Fig. 3. Transmission electron microscope of a cerebral astrocytoma after CUSA application. × 7,500. Effects on the outer periphery of the lesion. (*n* nucleus; *f* fragments of cytoplasm with organules partly disgregated)

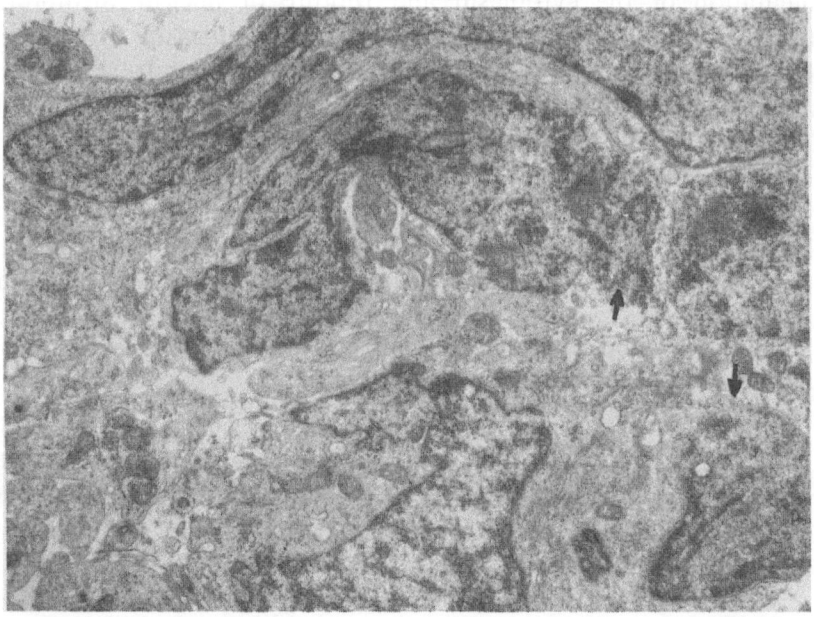

Fig. 4. Transmission electron micrograph of a cerebral astrocytoma after CUSA application. × 7,500. Effects on the outer periphery of the lesion. Arrows indicate the site of rupture of the nuclear membrane

close as 50 microns. Capillary structures appeared patent. The study of the effects of direct and indirect contact of the CUSA probe on rat sciatic nerve conduction showed that if the tip did not touch the nerve, regardless of the intensity or duration of ultrasonic vibration the action potential was conducted normally, but if the tip touched the nerve the action potential was abolished quickly.

The discrepancy between Flamm's and Young's studies may be related to the different intensity of vibration and time of application causing different damage on tissues.

Brock and co-workers[1] studied at electron microscope the changes occurring in perifocal area. This zone appears intact under the conventional light microscope. Two days after ultrasonic aspiration of a circumscribed area of rat cortex, electron microscope reveals a marked dilatation of endoplasmic reticulum of neurones. Both neuronal and glial cells have large vacuoles. There is swelling in myelinated and unmyelinated axons. At 72 hours axonal changes persist. There is a prominent cortical and subcortical edema. Phagocytes are increased in number in the perivascular spaces but vessels appear to be intact. These ultrastructural changes correspond to those observed following mechanical lesions of nervous tissue.

These changes have been studied by Fasano et al. (unpublished data) in meningiomas and gliomas. The effects of the ultrasonic vibration on cerebral gliomas consist in a breaking up of the tissue. The hit cells show fragmentation of the cytoplasm and rupture of nuclear membranes. Cellular debris showing damaged cytoplasmic organules are evident (Fig. 3). Tight junctions are rarely affected. A distinct boundary line exists between the area of impact of the vibration and the healthy tissue. At this level cells can show slight damages often limited to portions of nucleus or nuclear membrane (Fig. 4). The effects of the ultrasonic vibration on meningiomas consist in the widening of the intercellular spaces by exfoliation. Cellular debris are never detectable (Fig. 5). Cells and cytoplasmic organules are spared. Nuclear lesions are rare. Tight junctions are often damaged showing a total or partial disgregation (Fig. 6). In the areas strictly adjacent to the CUSA impact cells are fragmented and the boundary line with the adjacent tissue is not always clearly detectable.

These different responses to vibration seem to be correlated to the compactness of the tissue. The effects on fibrous meningiomas are characterized by a prevalent damage of tight junctions without a significant cellular damage whereas in soft astrocytomas the effects of fragmentation prevail.

2.2.2. Clinical Data

The tactile feedback provided by the CUSA in distinguishing various types of tissue as brain, collagenous structures (vessels, tumor capsule wall)

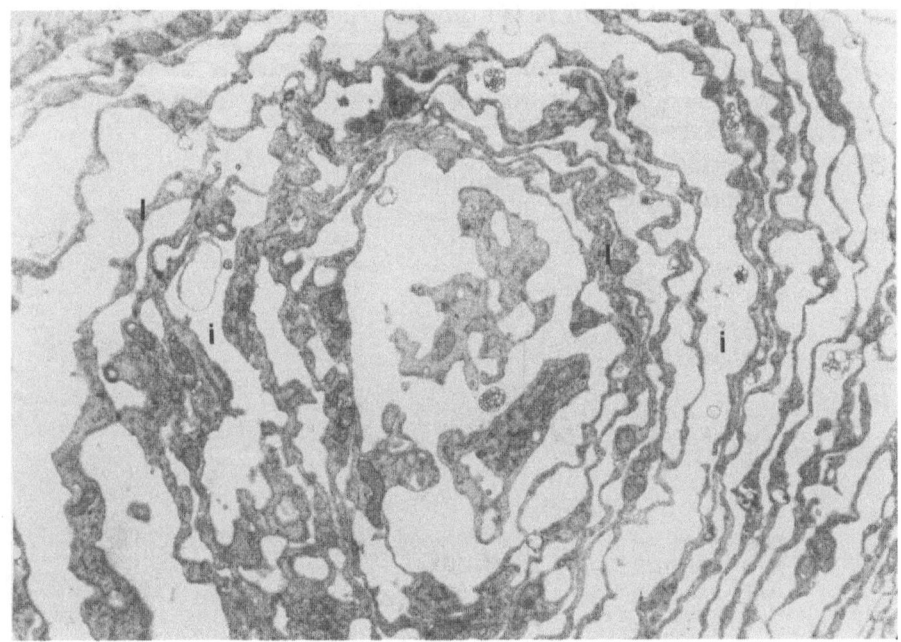

Fig. 5. Transmission electron micrograph of a meningioma after CUSA application. × 3,000. Effects on the outer periphery of the lesion. (*i* intercellular spaces; *l* exfoliated cytoplasmic laminae)

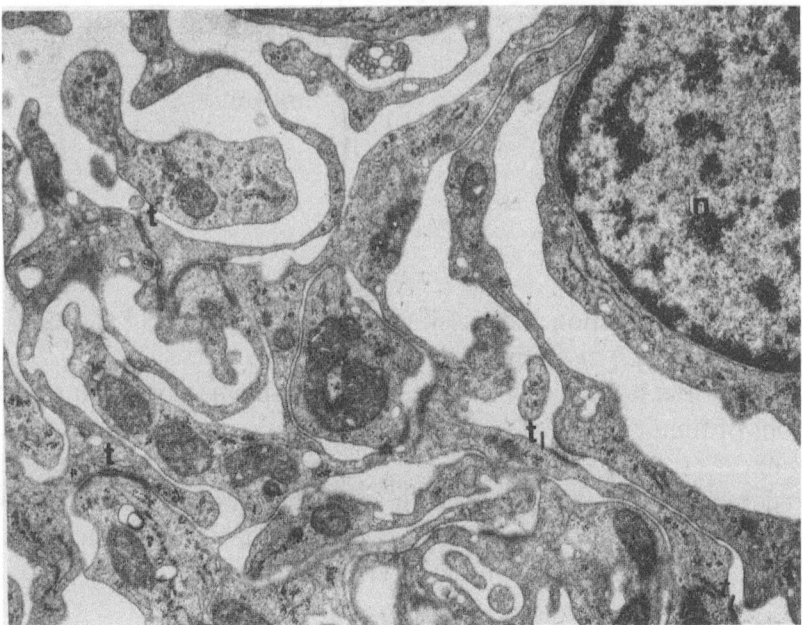

Fig. 6. Transmission electron micrograph of a meningioma after CUSA application. × 13,000. Effects on the outer periphery of the lesion. (*n* nucleus; *t* tight junctions; t_1 partial gap of a damaged tight junction)

Table 2. *Surgical Results in 153 Cases of Tumor Operated with CUSA*

	POST – OPERATIVE MORBIDITY	TUMOR VOLUME ON CT – SCAN		
		FROM	TO	AVERAGE
DEEP – SEATED AND SUBCORTICAL GLIOMAS	NO MORBIDITY	2,25 x 2,25 cm	4,5 x 6,3 cm	3,6 x 4 cm
MENINGIOMAS OF THE BASE OF THE SKULL a) ADJOINING VESSELS b) ADJOINING NERVES	IN 12% OF CASES NO MORBIDITY	4,95 x 4 cm	5,85 x 6,75 cm	5,4 x 5,4 cm
SUPERFICIAL MENINGIOMAS	IN 11% OF CASES	3,15 x 3,6 cm	4,5 x 5,85 cm	3,8 x 4,7 cm
TUMOR OF THE PONTO – CEREBELLAR ANGLE	NO MORBIDITY	3,6 x 4 cm	5,85 x 6,75 cm	4 x 4,9 cm
CEREBELLAR TUMORS	NO MORBIDITY	2,25 x 2,7 cm	3,6 x 4 cm	2,7 x 3,15 cm
BRAIN – STEM TUMORS	NO MORBIDITY			
INTRAMEDULLARY TUMORS	NO MORBIDITY	DETERMINATION NOT POSSIBLE		
TUMORS OF THE PINEAL REGION	NO MORBIDITY			
INTRADURAL SPINAL CORD TUMORS	NO MORBIDITY			

allows delicate dissection and incisions which are more rapid and safer than with the traditional dissecting tools.

Dissection is particularly important in falx meningiomas to resect the portions of tumor adherent to the falx cerebri after reduction in volume of the bulk.

In convexity endotheliomas which are often very large and fibrous, we also use CUSA as a dissecting tool to resect the tumor from adjacent cortex. To dissect, CUSA is used at low vibration intensity.

3. Surgical Results

The advantages of the CUSA depend on the rapidity of the maneuver and the reduced manipulation of the adjacent tissue. Table 2 shows the postoperative morbidity. In all cases the cortical incision was 3–4 cm. The extent of removal and the edema were evaluated on the CT scan. Resection was macroscopically complete in 90% of cases of deep seated gliomas, in 85% of meningiomas of the skull base, in 100% of superficial meningiomas, acoustic tumors and meningiomas of the ponto-cerebellar region, in 90% of cerebellar tumors. Removal was also complete in all tumors of the pineal region. Concerning the rate of edema formation a slight increase of shift of the median structures was noted in 40% of cases, a discrete increase in 20% of cases. A slight reduction was noted in 40% of cases. Blood transfused never exceeded 500 ml.

In agreement with Flamm, who operated 38 patients at New York University Medical Center[5], our results confirm the precision and the accuracy of the CUSA when operating on a bulk mass (no operative morbidity in deep-seated gliomas, tumors of the ponto-cerebellar angle, cerebellar tumors).

The resection of brain stem tumors, intramedullary tumors and tumors of the pineal region has been also performed without deficits and in all patients with intramedullary tumors an effective improvement of the neurologic status was noticed. This is in accordance with Epstein who operated at the New York University Medical Center 4 patients with intramedullary tumors and noticed postoperative neurological improvements[4]. Postoperative morbidity noticed in superficial meningiomas and basal meningiomas depends on the vascular perturbation following the tumor removal and cannot therefore be modified by CUSA or other instruments.

4. Conclusive Considerations

The advantages and disadvantages of the CUSA can be summarized as follows:

I. Advantages

1. Improvement of visibility of the operative field resulting from:

a) The characteristics of the tip that performs as three instruments in one: scalpel, aspirator, irrigator.

b) The layer by layer extirpation from the surface downwards.

c) The lack of charring, smoke and reduced blood loss because of the continuous aspiration.

2. The reduction of bleeding because of the vessel skeletonizing effect and coagulation of the smaller vessels by frictional heat at the tip/tissue interface.

3. Rapid debulking of soft and firm mass.

4. Delicate resection without traction and important thermal effects on the surrounding tissue.

5. Discriminatory capability in removing the tissue through tactile feedback.

6. Minimal damage to adjacent tissues under conditions of clinical use making possible resection in important areas (brain stem tumors, intramedullary tumors).

II. Disadvantages

   1. Ineffectiveness in the fragmentation of very hard tumors.

   2. Risk of perforation of main cerebral arteries and venous sinuses.

   3. Easy laceration of nerves stretched and compressed by tumor growth.

   4. Although it was thought that tissue fragmentation did not allow histological examination, recent researches [12, 13] show that tissue obtained by ultrasonic aspiration is suitable for histological examination and cell culture. Examination of pooled tissue fragments from tumor aspiration would permit a relatively large proportion of the tumor to be surveyed in contrast to the limited sample obtained by conventional biopsy procedures. Williams and Hodgson [13] compared the microscopic features of CUSA fragments of dog liver with tissue obtained by sharp dissection. The ultrasonically aspirated liver fragments revealed a recognizable sinusoidal pattern of hepatocytes with erythrocytes adherent to the fragments. More recently, in order to evaluate the usefulness of the CUSA-aspirated fragments of intracranial tumors as possible source of material for histopathological study and tissue culture, Richmond and Hawksley [2] compared the microscopic features and viability in tissue culture of CUSA tissue fragments and biopsies obtained by conventional methods. The authors reported two cases (a meningioma and a subependymal astrocytoma) treated with CUSA and confirm the good preservation of histological details.

At present we use the CUSA directly on the tumor bulk to achieve a rapid removal or a reduction in volume of the mass thus facilitating the dissection from the surrounding tissues. When used in this way the CUSA offers effective advantages on the traditional instruments. The dissection of remaining tumor tissue from high functional structures is better performed by the laser because of its greater selectivity and the predictability of the maneuver.

References

1. Brock, M., Ingwersen, I., Roggendorf, W., 1984: Ultrasonic aspiration in neurosurgery. Neurosurg. Rev. 7, 173–177.
2. Chopp, R. T., Shah, B. B., Addonizio, J. C., 1983: Use of ultrasonic surgical aspirator in renal surgery. Urology XXII, 157–159.
3. Cushing, H., Bovie, W. T., 1928: Electrosurgery as an aid to the removal of intracranial tumors. Surg. Gynec. Obstet. 47, 751–784.
4. Epstein, F., Epstein, N., 1982: Surgical management of extensive intramedullary spinal cord astrocytoma in children. In: Concepts in Pediatric Neurosurgery II (American Society for Pediatric Neurosurgery), pp. 29–44. Basel: S. Karger.

5. Fasano, V. A., Zeme, S., Frego, L., Gunetti, R., 1981: Ultrasonic aspiration in the surgical treatment of intracranial tumors. J. Neurosurg. Sci. *25*, 35–40.

6. Flamm, E. S., Ransohoff, J., Wuchinich, D., Broadwin, A., 1978: Preliminary experience with ultrasonic aspiration in neurosurgery. Neurosurg. *2*, 240–245.

7. Heimann, T. M., Kurtz, R. J., Schwarz, S. S., Aufses, A. H., Jr., 1983: Mucosal proctectomy and endorectal pullthrough using ultrasonic tissue fragmentation. Surgical Forum *34*, 202–203.

8. Hodgson, W. J. B., McElhinney, A. J., 1982: Ultrasonic partial splenectomy. Surgery *91*, 346–348.

9. Kelman, C. D., 1973: Phaco-emulsification and aspiration: a report of 500 consecutive cases. Am. J. Ophthalmol. *75*, 764–768.

10. Link, W. J., Incropera, F. P., Glover, J. L., 1976: A plasma scalpel: comparison of tissue damage and wound healing with electrosurgical and steel scalpels. Arch. Surg. *111*, 392–397.

11. Putnam, C. W., Techniques of ultrasonic dissection in resection of the liver. Surg. Gynec. Obstet. *157*, 474–478.

12. Richmond, I. L., Hawksley, C. A., 1983: Evaluation of the histopathology of brain tumor tissue obtained by ultrasonic aspiration. Neurosurg. *13*, 415–419.

13. Williams, J. W., Hodgson, W. J. B., 1979: Histologic evaluation of tissues sectioned by ultrasonically powered instruments (a preliminary report). Mt. Sinai J. Med. NY *46*, 105–106.

14. Young, W., Cohen, A. R., Hunt, C. D., Ransohoff, J., 1981: Acute physiological effects of ultrasonic vibrations on nervous tissue. Neurosurg. *8*, 689–694.

4. Localized Hyperthermia for the Treatment of Cerebral Tumors

Localized Hyperthermia for the Treatment of Cerebral Tumors

ALLAN W. SILBERMAN and ROBERT W. RAND

Division of Surgical Oncology, John Wayne Cancer Clinic,
Division of Neurosurgery, Department of Surgery,
UCLA School of Medicine,
Los Angeles, California (U.S.A.)

Contents

I. Introduction 277
II. Hyperthermia 278
III. Localized Hyperthermia Techniques 279
IV. Malignant Brain Tumors 279
V. UCLA Experience with Localized Radiofrequency Hyperthermia by
    Magnetic-Loop Induction 279
    A. Animal Studies 280
    B. Human Studies 285
VI. Discussion 291
VII. Literature Review 297
References 300

I. Introduction

Hyperthermia is a cancer-treatment modality that can cause tumor necrosis by concentrated heating of tumor tissue. The treatment of human tumors by the application of heat is an idea rooted in antiquity. Both Hippocrates (400 BC) and Galen (200 AD) described the palliative effects of red-hot irons applied to superficial tumors. A more recent rationale for hyperthermia in cancer therapy was based on the observation that patients with high fevers had spontaneous remissions of their tumor. In 1893, Coley described tumor responses to bacterial toxin therapy associated with fevers of 39–40 °C of several days duration[1]. Although hyperthermia has been of historical interest for some time, in the last two decades it has reemerged as an investigational therapy. The renewed interest is due, in part, to the crucial observation by Cavaliere *et al.* (1967), that tumor cells are selectively thermosensitive compared to normal cells at temperatures between 42–45 °C[2]. In addition, data from in vitro, animal, and human studies have shown an additive or synergistic response between heat and chemotherapy, and heat and radiation therapy, at 41–43 °C. Furthermore, today's hyperthermia technology, although still in its infancy, has the capability of producing therapeutic temperatures with minimal morbidity to the host. Thus, a new modality has emerged coincident with the realization that standard cancer therapy—surgery, radiation, chemotherapy—can cure only one of three afflicted patients.

Nowhere is the frustration with standard therapy more evident than in patients with malignant brain tumors. Patients with glioblastoma multiforme, the most common primary brain tumor in adults, have a median survival time of 3–8 months regardless of therapy[7]. The median survival time following the diagnosis of intracerebral metastases is less than 4 months[8]. Although standard therapy provides palliation for these unfortunate patients, their long-term survival is not markedly improved.

In this chapter, we hope to provide the reader with some insight into the rationale for, and the use of, localized or regional hyperthermia for the treatment of solid cancers in general, and to discuss its applicability, feasibility, and safety for the treatment of human cerebral tumors.

II. Hyperthermia

The biological rationale for hyperthermia as a cancer therapy is based on the observation that tumor cells are more thermosensitive than normal cells between 42 and 45 °C. Muckle and Dickson (1972) showed that at 42 °C there was a marked and progressive decrease in the viability of tumor cells with time[9]. The mechanism of thermal kill is not clearly understood; however, the effect of heat at ≥ 42 °C appears to alter the function of vital enzyme systems[10, 11]. In addition, there is a reduction in both DNA and RNA synthesis, an increase in permeability of both the cell membrane and the lysosomal membrane[12, 13], and liberation of lysozymes[14]. These effects appear to be more pronounced in hypoxic cells[15]. The efficiency of thermocytotoxicity increases rapidly as temperatures are increased from 42–45 °C, the threshold of thermal pain in man. At temperatures ≥ 45 °C, the differential thermosensitivity between malignant and normal cells is reduced and is replaced by a linear cell kill from progressive protein denaturation[16]. Thus, host tissue tolerance becomes a limiting factor at temperatures ≥ 45 °C.

Westermark, in 1927, when heating tumor-bearing rat limbs with high-frequency currents, found that tumor temperatures from 44–48 °C could be obtained without injury to normal surrounding tissues. He postulated that differences in vascularity might account for the heat variations observed[17]. In 1962, Crile observed that the heat generated in human-hepatic metastases was retained, while the remaining normal liver was cooled by portal blood flow[18]. Mantyla, in 1979, confirmed that ambient tumor blood flow was generally less than that of normal host tissues[19]. These findings have led to the exciting conclusion that tumor tissue can be "selectively" heated while the normal surrounding tissue remains cool. After extensive temperature measurements during hyperthermia therapy of spontaneous animal and human neoplasms, Storm *et al.* (1979) suggested that many tumors selectively retain more heat than normal tissues because tumor neovascularity is incapable of augmenting blood flow in response to thermal stress[20]. Thus, *nonfocused* microwaves and capacitive, inductive, and magnetic-loop radiofrequency applicators can heat a region of the host containing a tumor, and provide selective tumor heating. This phenomenon of "selective tumor heating" after regional energy deposition suggests that potentially effective independent tumor heating might be possible within the body, even without the ability to focus such energy.

III. Localized Hyperthermia Techniques

Many ingenious techniques have been used to produce localized or regional hyperthermia. These include isolated limb perfusion[4], low-frequency current fields[21, 22] ferromagnetic coupling[23], ultrasound[24, 25], microwaves[26], and radiofrequency waves[27]. The interested reader is referred to several excellent reviews[28–30].

IV. Malignant Brain Tumors

Primary malignant brain tumors occur at an annual rate of approximately 4.5 cases per 100,000 population. Forty-three percent of these cases are designated as malignant gliomas and include glioblastoma multiforme, malignant astrocytoma, and anaplastic astrocytoma. These tumors are inevitably fatal, with a historical median survival of 6 months[31]. A randomized study by the Brain Tumor Study Group comparing postsurgical radiation vs postsurgical radiation and a nitrosourea showed no statistical differences in survival by the addition of a chemotherapeutic agent[31]. It has been become apparent that standard therapy has not effectively altered the outcome of this dreaded disease. This failure has encouraged the development of experimental therapies, with hyperthermia therapy recently coming to the forefront.

V. UCLA Experience with Localized Radiofrequency Hyperthermia by Magnetic-Loop Induction

In 1977, radiofrequency hyperthermia by magnetic-loop induction (Magnetrode™) was introduced as an investigational cancer therapy by

Storm *et al.* (1979–1982) at UCLA[20, 32-35]. This device employs a non-invasive circumferential electrode, operating at a radiofrequency of 13.56 MHz, to produce hyperthermia at depth without preferential surface tissue heating[20, 32-38]. The design, engineering, and heat distribution principles of the Magnetrode™ have been reported elsewhere[36, 37]. Results to date suggest that this type of localized hyperthermia can be applied safely to most types of solid human tumors independent of their histology or size[32]. In addition to the safety of the methodology, the UCLA group has also demonstrated the potential efficacy of combining localized hyperthermia with chemotherapy[39]. Patients with advanced cancer who had documented disease progression while receiving chemotherapy alone were subsequently treated with the same drug, by the same dose and route, but combined with localized hyperthermia. Thirty-four patients whose diseases included metastatic colon carcinoma, melanoma, sarcoma and hepatoma were treated with combination thermochemotherapy for 1 hour daily for 5 days/month. Effective heating from 41–45 °C was possible in $^{17}/_{19}$ (89%) tumors in which temperatures could be measured safely. There were 5 (15%) tumor regressions for 1–5 months (median, 2 months), and 19 (56%) tumor stabilizations (arrest of previously progressive disease) for 1–9 months (median, 4 months). Subjective improvement in activity and/or pain control was achieved in 6 (18%) patients and 20 (59%) had no progression of symptoms during treatment. Moreover, there was no detectable morbidity from localized hyperthermia, and no evidence of increased chemotherapy toxicity. Thus, while the mechanism(s) of response was poorly understood, the documented disease regression and stabilization of previously progressive disease in 24 (71%) patients during secondary combination thermochemotherapy provided some evidence that the addition of hyperthermia may have had useful anticancer activity.

Because both the safety and potential therapeutic value of non-invasive thermochemotherapy for advanced extracranial disease could be demonstrated, it was not long before our group began to study the effects of this technique on the brain and surrounding tissues. Our principle concern in undertaking brain hyperthermia was related to the possible detrimental effect of localized heat on intracranial pressure, particularly in the face of an intracranial tumor with its attendant secondary edema. A second intriguing question was whether normal brain tissue could tolerate temperatures in the tumoricidal range (42–44 °C).

A. Animal Studies

In our initial study[40], we examined the effect of localized hyperthermia on the brain of normal rabbits in an effort to shed light on these two concerns.

New Zealand white rabbits weighing approximately 2 kg were

anesthetized with 5% Surital intravenously and 1% Xylocaine locally. A 2 cm incision was made through the skin and subcutaneous tissue overlying the midportion of the skull. Using a high-speed dental drill, two 2 mm twist-drill holes were created in the skull, exposing both the right and left hemispheres of the brain. The twist-drill holes provided access to the brain for both temperature measurements and intracranial pressure monitoring.

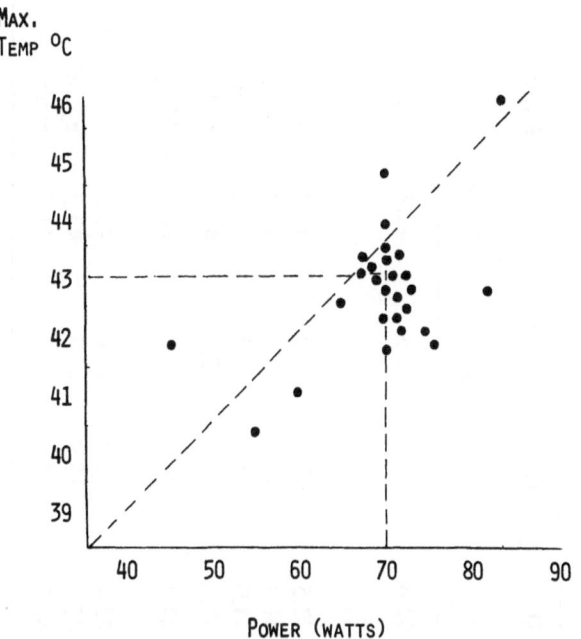

Fig. 1. Effect of power (watts) on resultant brain temperature. Relationship between amount of power applied from a 5-inch Magnetrode™ applicator and brain temperature. Seventy watts of power consistently achieved the desired brain temperature of 42–44 °C (N = 26)

The animal then was placed within a 5-inch Magnetrode™ applicator and heat was applied for 1 hour. The rabbit's head was air-cooled at 25 °C throughout the heating period. At 15-minute intervals, the temperatures of the skin, subcutaneous tissue, skull, external eye, and brain were measured during a brief period of wave cessation by the introduction of a 26-gauge thermocouple probe (Bailey Instruments, Inc., Saddlebrook, N.J.; Model BAT-12). Brain temperature was recorded in each hemisphere at various depths (2–15 mm) to ascertain the temperature variation throughout the cerebrum.

Intracranial pressure was monitored by placing an 18-gauge plastic tube into a 2 mm twist-drill hole, sealing it with Permabond® cement, and connecting it to a standard water manometer. Continuous pressure

Table 1. *Effect of Hyperthermia on the Skin, Subcutaneous Tissue, External Eye, Skull, and Brain in Rabbits*

Experiment	Animal group	Temperature °C at 1 hour					Outcome at 1 week
		Skin/Sq	Bone	Brain Superf.	Deep	External eye	
A. Effect of hyperthermia on brain and surrounding tissues at temperatures < 45 °C (N = 26)[a]	N = 26 average T°C	42.6	39.0	42.3	42.4	39.6	alive
B. Experiments at brain temperatures ≥ 45 °C (N = 4)[b]	1.	42.5	39.5	45.2	45.2	39.8	died
	2.	41.8	43.7	45.1	45.0	42.0	died
	3.	44.9	35.9	44.5	45.1	38.9	died
	4.	47.0		45.7	44.4	50.0	died
C. Experiments at superficial temperatures ≥ 45 °C (N = 4)[c]	1.	48.9	46.8	44.3	44.0	44.9	scal burn, corneal burn
	2.	45.4	41.9	43.0	43.0	eyelid closed	scalp burn
	3.	45.0	37.8	43.3	43.2	eyelid closed	alive
	4.	45.7	43.5	43.2	41.8	eyelid closed	alive

[a] Animals were alive and neurologically intact at 1-week posthyperthermia with no evidence of burn injury to the superficial tissues. There was no statistical difference between the superficial (2–3 mm) and deep (10–15 mm) brain temperatures.

[b] All animals died within minutes of reaching brain temperatures ≥ 45 °C.

[c] Although all animals survived, burn injury occurred in 2 out of 4 rabbits with superficial tissue temperatures ≥ 45 °C.

measurements were obtained in the closed system as increasing incident power was applied.

To study the effect of tumoricidal temperatures (42–44 °C) on normal brain tissue, rabbits were subjected to radiofrequency hyperthermia at 70 w of power for 1 hour and were sacrificed at 2 days, 3 days, and 5 months posthyperthermia. Previous work had demonstrated that 70 w of power produced a brain temperature between 42 and 44 °C. The brains were prepared for examination by intravital perfusion with 10% formalin while in situ, and then were fixed in 10% formalin for 7 days. The brains were sectioned in the coronal plane, embedded in epon, and subsequently cut, mounted, and stained with hematoxylin and eosin (H & E). Rabbit brains from both treated and control animals were examined microscopically by a neuropathologist who had no knowledge of the treatment regimen.

Figure 1 illustrates the relationship between the amount of power applied from a 5-inch Magnetrode™ applicator and the resultant brain temperature. Seventy watts of power consistently produced a brain temperature of between 42 and 44 °C. Furthermore, when power at 70 w was applied without a twist-drill hole, there was no increase in morbidity or mortality. This finding suggested that the presence of a twist-drill hole did not confer a protective effect; however, without it, brain temperatures obviously could not be measured.

Table 1 shows the effect of localized radiofrequency hyperthermia on the superficial brain (2–3 mm), deep brain (10–15 mm), and surrounding tissues. A comparison of the superficial and deep brain temperatures in 26 animals showed that there was little variation in temperature at various depths or locations within the brain and that temperatures between 42 and 44 °C were well tolerated by the brain, skin, subcutaneous tissue, bone, and external eye. Temperatures of 45 °C or greater were not tolerated by the brain. Rabbits rapidly succumbed within several minutes of reaching a brain temperature of 45 °C. Although the animals survived brain temperatures of less than 45 °C, the results in four animals (Table 1 C) indicated that the external tissue must also remain less than 45 °C to avoid burn injury.

The effect of hyperthermia on intracranial pressure is shown in Fig. 2. As power was increased, only a minimal rise (less than 2 cm of water) was observed in the intracranial pressure. This lack of significant pressure elevation was apparent even when the animal was agonal at brain temperatures greater than 45 °C. Animals that survived the heating period (42–43 °C) demonstrated similar intracranial pressure curves.

The animals appeared to be neurologically intact within 24 hours of the hyperthermia treatment; i.e., their eating habits, behavior, and response to handling appeared normal. Light microscopy revealed occasional "glial knots," possibly attributable to encephalitis, common in rabbits, or to fixation artifacts. The cerebellum was examined with particular care, because hyperthermia, or "heat stroke," is known to cause more extensive pathologic changes in this area than in the forebrain of mammals[41]. There were no definite pathologic changes seen in the brains of any of the rabbits subjected to localized radiofrequency hyperthermia compared to nontreated animals.

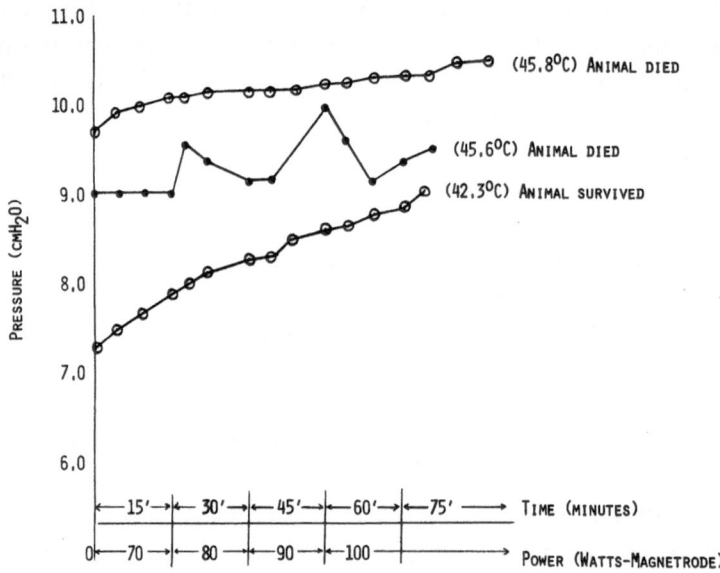

Fig. 2. Effect of localized magnetic-loop hyperthermia on intracranial pressure. Intracranial pressure was monitored by placing an 18-gauge plastic tube into a 2-mm twist-drill hole and sealing it with Permabond® cement. The tube was connected to a standard water manometer and its proper function confirmed by a fluctuating water column. Continuous pressure measurements in cm H_2O were obtained in the closed system as increasing incident power was applied from the Magnetrode™. The reported temperature of the brain was measured at the conclusion of the experiment

To test whether radiofrequency hyperthermia could be safely applied to the head in the presence of a solid brain tumor, we developed an experimental brain tumor model in rabbits using transplanted VX-2 carcinoma[42]. These tumor-bearing animals were then treated with combination thermochemotherapy[43]. Tumor implantation was accomplished by injecting 0.125 ml (5×10^6 cells) of viable VX-2 carcinoma suspension through the right-sided twist-drill hole 8–10 mm into the right hemisphere of the rabbit's brain. The scalp was closed with a single layer of running nylon suture. The animals were returned to their cages and allowed to recover. On Day 3, 4, or 5 following tumor implantation, the rabbits were anesthetized with 5% Surital® intravenously. The scalp incision was reopened to expose the two twist-drill holes. Baseline temperatures of the skin, subcutaneous tissue, external eye, skull, superficial brain (2–3 mm), and deep brain (10–15 mm) were recorded with the thermocouple probe. Each animal under study was placed within the magnetic-loop applicator and heat was applied for 1 hour. Temperatures of the brain and surrounding tissue were measured at 15-minute intervals. During the second 15-minute heating period, Carmustine (BCNU) was given over 5–10 minutes as a one-time intravenous injection at a dose of 14 mg/kg. Following the thermochemotherapy treatment, the animals were returned to their cages, inspected each day and followed until spontaneous death occurred. The number of days subsequent to the implantation of VX-2 carcinoma was recorded, and this record formed the basis for the evaluation of survival time. Upon death, rabbit brains were removed and fixed in standard 10% formalin solution for 48 hours. The brains were serially sectioned in the coronal plane and examined grossly for evidence of tumor formation. When tumor was visible, the greatest tumor dimensions were measured. Thirty animals with transplanted intracerebral VX-2 carcinoma not treated by either hyperthermia or chemotherapy served as a comparison group.

The results of localized radiofrequency hyperthermia combined with intravenous BCNU in rabbits with transplanted intracerebral VX-2 carcinoma are shown in Table 2. All 16 animals were alive 24 hours after the thermochemotherapy regimen. Fifteen of 16 animals were neurologically intact at 24 hours, *i.e.,* their eating habits, behavior and response to handling appeared normal; however, Animal no. 2, although alive, was not neurologically intact, most likely the result of a scalp burn suffered when the skin-subcutaneous tissue temperature reached 45.4 °C. This animal died on Day 3 following thermochemotherapy. Because no tumor was noted at autopsy, the animal's death was probably secondary to the burn. The average maximum brain temperature achieved during treatment was 43.1 °C (range 41.8–44.7 °C), compared to an average brain temperature of 39.8 °C in 43 nonheated animals (range 38.1–41.3 °C). The mean survival from the time of tumor implantation was 18.6 days. This finding compared very favorably to the survival of a group of 30 animals used in the development of our rabbit brain tumor model ($p < 0.0001$). The survival time for rabbits with untreated transplanted intracerebral VX-2 carcinoma was 9.3 days. Fourteen of 16 treated animals had gross tumor visible at autopsy with an average tumor area of 30.3 mm². The untreated group had a tumor take of 90% [27, 30] with an average tumor area of 42.6 mm².

B. Human Studies

Because of the apparent safety of brain hyperthermia in our animal model and because earlier studies had shown that thermochemotherapy in

Table 2. *Effect of Thermochemotherapy on Rabbits with Transplanted Intracerebral VX-2 Carcinoma (N = 16)*

Animal	Temperature °C at 1 hour						Outcome 24 hours p. hyperth.	Survival from tumor implantation (days)	Tumor dimensions (mm)	Area (mm²)
	Skin/Sq	Bone	Brain (a, b)			External eye (c)				
			Superf.	Deep	Maximum					
1	44.2	—	42.7	42.4	42.7	42.2	alive	13	2 × 3	6
2	45.4	41.9	43.0	43.0	43.0	eyelid closed	scalp/burn	7	0	0
3	42.6	37.0	41.4	41.8	41.8	eyelid closed	alive	21	6 × 3	18
4	43.6	38.2	43.2	43.3	43.3	eyelid closed	alive	39	9 × 9	81
5	43.4	41.2	43.1	43.2	43.2	eyelid closed	alive	16	12 × 5	60
6	44.2	38.6	43.0	43.2	43.2	eyelid closed	alive	26	5 × 6	30
7	44.3	41.4	43.9	43.7	43.9	eyelid closed	alive	22	5 × 4	20
8	44.0	41.1	43.4	43.1	43.4	eyelid closed	alive	6	3 × 2	6
9	43.3	37.1	43.1	43.0	43.1	eyelid closed	alive	14	2 × 5	10
10	45.0	37.8	43.3	43.1	43.3	eyelid closed	alive	16	2 × 3	6
11	45.7	43.5	43.2	41.8	43.2	eyelid closed	alive	23	1 × 2	2
12	42.3	39.3	43.0	42.9	43.0	eyelid closed	alive	29	5 × 9	45
13	43.4	39.7	42.6	42.5	42.6	eyelid closed	alive	13	10 × 10	100
14	42.4	40.6	42.3	42.1	42.3	eyelid closed	alive	13	7 × 3	21
15	42.3	40.9	42.3	42.2	42.3	eyelid closed	alive	21	10 × 8	80
16	43.8	39.1	44.4	44.7	44.7	eyelid closed	alive	18	0	0
Average					43.1 °C			18.6 days		30.3 mm²

(a) Brain temperatures in 43 animals prior to heating averaged 39.8 °C (range 38.1–41.3 °C). (b) There was no statistical difference between the superficial (2–3 mm) and deep (10–15 mm) brain temperatures. (c) Previous experience has shown that the eyelid can be safely closed during hyperthermia.

Table 3. *Patient/Tumor Profile*

Patient*	Age, Sex	Primary tumor	Previous therapy for brain tumor	Brain tumor location	Number of tumors
A	60, f	chordoma	surgery, XRT	clivus	single
B	46, f	cystic glioblastoma	surgery, XRT	L frontal lobe	single
C	43, m	melanoma	XRT, chemo	throughout cerebrum	multiple
D	37, f	lung	XRT	R temporal lobe	single
E	63, m	nasopharyngeal carcinoma	XRT, chemo	brain stem	single
F	29, m	glioma	surgery, XRT, chemo	R fronto/parietal lobes	single
G	46, m	adenocarcinoma ? primary	surgery, XRT, chemo	L fronto/parietal lobes	multiple
H	53, f	lung	XRT, chemo	R frontal lobe	multiple
I	45, m	lung	XRT, chemo	R frontal lobe	single
J	46, m	lung	XRT, chemo	L frontal lobe	multiple
K	58, f	glioma	surgery, XRT, chemo	R fronto/parietal lobes	single
L	33, m	glioma	surgery, XRT, chemo	thalamus	single
M	41, m	glioma	surgery, XRT, chemo	R parietal lobe	single

* All patients received BCNU (80–120 mg/m² IV) over 1 hour during hyperthermia except Patient G, who received 5-FU (600 mg/m² IV) and Adriamycin (30 mg/m² IV).

Table 4. Intracranial Pressure (ICP) Profile

Treatment session	Patient	Opening ICP (cm H_2O)	Maximum ICP (cm H_2O)	Closing ICP (cm H_2O)	ΔP (C—O)
1	A	20.0	25.0	25.0	+5.0
2	A	13.0	26.0	26.0	+13.0
3	B	15.0	35.0	25.0	+10.0
4	B	19.0	42.0	34.0	+15.0
5	B	—	27.4	22.8	—
6	B	—	26.6	21.6	—
7	B	17.4	20.0	19.6	+2.2
8	B	15.8	15.8	15.0	−0.8
9	C	45.0	45.0	30.0	−15.0
10	B	28.0	28.0	21.2	−6.8
11	B	19.7	25.7	21.2	+1.5
12	D	40.0	46.8	43.9	+3.9
13	D	38.3	38.6	38.6	+0.3
14	E	15.9	15.9	12.2	−3.7
15	E	12.0	12.0	11.0	−1.0
16	F	19.0	22.3	22.3	+3.3
17	F	—	—	—	—

18	G	19.0	19.0	15.5	−3.5
19	G	12.1	19.2	17.6	+5.5
20	H	16.5	18.5	13.2	−3.3
21	I	30.0	47.5	37.2	+7.2
22	H	13.0	19.5	17.0	+4.0
23	J	27.0	48.6	44.0	+17.0
24	H	7.5	14.5	11.5	+4.0
25	H	6.0	11.0	9.3	+3.3
26	K	22.0	22.0	8.0	−14.0
27	K	22.0	22.0	13.0	−9.0
28	L	7.6	8.2	8.0	+0.4
29	L	5.0	7.5	6.0	+1.0
30	K	29.0	29.0	16.6	−12.4
31	K	21.2	21.2	19.3	−1.9
32	M	18.2	18.2	9.6	−8.6
33	M	26.6	26.6	22.0	−4.6
34	L	8.2	9.0	7.4	+0.8
35	L	7.2	7.5	7.4	+0.3

cancer patients with noncerebral malignancy caused both disease regression and disease stabilization, we began a Phase I investigation of combination radiofrequency hyperthermia and intravenous chemotherapy in patients with both primary and metastatic brain tumors[44].

To date, 13 patients have undergone 35 thermochemotherapy sessions using the Magnetrode™ experimental hyperthermia device (Table 3). There have been 5 female and 8 male patients, ranging in age from 29–63. Tumor histology varied, and included 6 primary brain tumors and 7 metastatic tumors. For our first 4 patients, a 10-inch diameter applicator was used to deliver the heat. Since then, an oblique 16-inch diameter applicator has been used. Both applicators function at the ISM frequency of 13.56 MHz; consequently, no screen room, Faraday cage, or other shielding device is necessary. The newly designed oblique applicator can treat a larger surface of the patient's head without including the patient's eyes in the heat field; in addition, it can be reversed to heat the lower face and neck.

Normal-brain and brain-tumor temperatures were constantly monitored during the hyperthermia treatment using a tissue-implantable thermocouple microprobe (Bailey Type IT-18) connected to the Bailey Clinical Thermometer TM-10 (Bailey Instruments, Inc. Saddlebrook, N.J.). Temperatures were confirmed during brief periods of wave cessation.

Oral temperature was measured every 15 minutes during the hyperthermia treatment using disposable Tempa-Dot® oral thermometers. The skin (forehead) was constantly monitored with Stik-Temp™ disks. The range of maximum normal brain temperatures after 1 hour of hyperthermia was 38.6–43.4 °C, with a median temperature of 41.3 °C and an average of 41.1 °C. The range of maximum tumor temperatures was 38.8–46.3 °C, with a median temperature of 42.5 °C and an average of 42.6 °C ($p < 0.01$). In 73% of the treatments, the measured tumor temperature was at least 42.0 °C, whereas normal brain temperature reached $\geqslant 42$ °C in only 23% of the treatments.

The opening, maximum, and closing intracranial pressures (ICP) are listed in Table 4 for each treatment session. The change in pressure (ΔP) between the closing and opening pressure is also shown.

Vital signs were monitored throughout the heating period. Minimal, transient elevations in blood pressure, pulse, and respiratory rate were often observed during the hyperthermia sessions; however, these changes were not clinically significant and no therapy was required. Bradycardia consistent with elevated intracranial pressure was not observed in any patient. There were no treatment-related deaths, permanent neurologic deficits, or local complications. There were three transient neurologic complications.

VI. Discussion

Hyperthermia, which can be delivered by various ingenious techniques, has been reintroduced over the last 10–15 years as an experimental cancer therapy by many groups around the world. Theoretically, if a tumor can be heated to a high enough temperature for a long enough time, it can be destroyed. The problem encountered in hyperthermia therapy has been to protect the normal surrounding tissue, *i.e.,* host tolerance, during the heating period. The various hyperthermic devices differ in their ability to provide this necessary safety factor. Our group has used a magnetic-loop induction device that seems to be applicable to most types of advanced solid human malignancy, including intracranial neoplasms. Its exciting potential is enhanced by the fact that toxicity has been minimal in the internal organs tested to date. This type of hyperthermia appears to be effective against both small tumors and the larger tumors that have the poorest response to traditional therapy. When combined with one or more of the standard treatments, such as radiation therapy or chemotherapy, relatively low-dose hyperthermia (42–43 °C) appears to induce a synergistic or additive effect [3-6].

Until recently, the effects of localized radiofrequency hyperthermia on the brain have not been adequately studied because of the potential hazards involved in applying effective heat to this organ while preserving surface tissues. However, the combined presence of a devastating disease and a new modality stimulated us to study the effects of hyperthermia on the brain. In our initial animal study [40], we found that normal rabbits could tolerate localized radiofrequency hyperthermia to the head with tumoricidal temperatures (42–43 °C) achieved in the brain without apparent histopathologic or clinical damage to the brain or surrounding tissues. We were somewhat surprised that the intracranial pressure remained stable even as the brain temperature reached 45 °C. However, the animal may have succumbed before significant cerebral edema developed. It appeared that the cause of death was primarily a respiratory one and not due to increased intracranial pressure. The animals did develop hyperpnea during the treatment, which may counter any rise in intracranial pressure that would otherwise be detectable. More importantly, in animals subjected to the Magnetrode™ for 1 hour at 70 w of power, a power output which consistently yielded a tumoricidal temperature (42–43 °C), there was no histopathologic evidence of cerebral edema at 24 or 48 hours. Furthermore, there was no evidence of pathological change in brains at 5 months posthyperthermia.

In our second study using intravenous chemotherapy in addition to hyperthermia, equivalent brain temperatures were achieved with the same degree of safety in a group of rabbits with solid brain tumors [43]. The brain tumor-bearing animals that were simultaneously treated with one dose of intravenous BCNU achieved a statistically significant survival advantage over an untreated control group. The differences in tumor size between the treated (30.3 mm^2) and untreated animals (48.5 mm^2), although favoring the thermochemotherapy group, were not statistically significant. Because the safety of the Magnetrode™ has been well established for treatment of extracranial disease in over 14,000 treatments in 1,170 patients in a multiinstitutional national cooperative trial[45], together with our animal data indicating the safety of brain hyperthermia in our rabbit model, we began a Phase I trial of thermochemotherapy in patients with both primary and metastatic brain tumors who had failed standard therapy.

All patients but one received BCNU chemotherapy during the 1-hour hyperthermia treatment. BCNU was chosen as the chemotherapeutic drug because of its established ability to cross the blood-brain barrier (BBB), its relatively low toxicity, and because the nitrosoureas have been shown both in vitro and in vivo to be synergistic with hyperthermia[46]. Whether it is important to use drugs that cross the BBB is controversial, since evidence exists that the BBB is broken in part, if not entirely, in the presence of neoplastic involvement. Rosner et al. (1983) from Roswell Park recently demonstrated a 52% objective response in 66 patients with breast cancer metastatic to the brain using standard "breast" drugs without the addition of radiation[47]. As our study evolves, the use of more tumor-specific chemotherapeutic agents will be tested.

Of the 26 brain-tumor temperatures measured, the median was 42.5 °C (average 42.6 °C; range 38.8–46.3 °C), whereas 35 normal-brain temperatures had a median of 41.3 °C (average 41.1 °C; range 38.6–43.4 °C) ($p < 0.01$). In 21 of 26 treatments in which both the normal-brain and brain-tumor temperatures were measured, the tumor temperature was greater than the corresponding normal-brain temperature. This finding demonstrates the "selective inability" of brain-tumor tissue to dissipate heat. In 73% of the treatments, the brain tumor reached 42 °C, whereas the normal brain reached 42 °C in only 23% of the treatments. The "selective inability" of brain-tumor tissue to dissipate heat is probably caused by its poor blood supply compared to normal-brain tissue. As in extracranial tumors, the neovascularity of the brain tumor may be incapable of augmenting blood flow in response to the heat; hence, the tumor becomes hotter than the surrounding normal tissue. We have found that some tumors have a normal or near-normal blood supply and may increase blood flow to dissipate the heat[48]. Thus, some tumors are incapable of reaching tumoricidal temperatures during hyperthermia therapy.

We felt it was important to know the toxicity of the *maximum* temperature achieved in both the normal brain and the brain tumor to establish the *safety* of the methodology, because excess heat contributes to local complications. However, the *minimum* tumor temperature achieved is probably of more importance for determining the efficacy of the therapy, since the maximum tumor temperature may be achieved in the necrotic center of the tumor. Tumor temperature mapping will be the object of future studies. We are currently developing a calibrated microprobe to be placed under CT guidance that will allow us to perform temperature mapping at various locations within the tumor.

Vital signs were monitored throughout the heating sessions. Although mild elevations in blood pressure, pulse, and respiratory rate were noted, these transient cardiovascular changes were clinically insignificant and required no therapy. Bradycardia secondary to elevated intracranial pressure was never observed, even in patients with intracranial pressures > 40 cm H_2O.

Intracranial pressure was measured continuously in every patient during the hyperthermia treatment by a standarded H_2O manometer (Table 4). The closing pressure (ICP at the completion of the hyperthermia treatment) was elevated compared to the opening pressure (ICP immediately prior to the hyperthermia treatment) in 19 treatments and lower in 13 treatments. The largest observed change in pressure (ΔP) was 17 cm H_2O; however, it caused no adverse sequelae. Three of our patients had opening pressures of 30 cm H_2O or greater, and in two of these patients adverse effects possibly related to the hyperthermia occurred. As more experience is gained, it may be that an opening ICP of 30 cm H_2O will be a contraindication to hyperthermia therapy. The maximum ICP observed was rarely the closing pressure; it was usually observed about 30 minutes into the treatment. The fall-off in pressure may have been due to the slow continued loss of cerebrospinal fluid through the teflon screws used for insertion of the microprobes. These screws, then, may act as a vent for elevated pressure, and they, or an equivalent device, may be a necessary safety factor during hyperthermia therapy delivered to the head.

No mortality or increase in chemotherapeutic toxicity could be attributed to the thermochemotherapy. There were no skin, bone, or local complications noted in the 35 treatments. Three patients, A, C, and I, suffered transient neurologic complications that may have been caused by the hyperthermia. Patient A, a 60-year-old female with a recurrent clivus chordoma, tolerated the thermochemotherapy procedure quite well in terms of intracranial pressure and cardiovascular parameters. As expected, her heart rate and respiratory rate steadily increased throughout the heating period. A sinus tachycardia and tachypnea have been consistently observed during localized hyperthermia to other parts of the body (chest and abdomen). Her systolic and diastolic blood pressure presented no special problems and there were no cardiac arrhythmias noted. Swan-Ganz monitoring was performed: the mean pulmonary artery pressure and cardiac index were stable; however, the central venous pressure, pulmonary artery diastolic pressure and pulmonary capillary wedge pressure showed some mild fluctuations probably secondary to the patient's volume status. Although there was no worsening of the patient's neurologic deficits during the procedure, she was disoriented to time and place at the conclusion of the first treatment session. The maximum and closing ICP reached during this session was 25 cm H_2O, with a ΔP of 5 cm H_2O. Her normal-brain temperature was 39.8 °C; tumor temperature was not measured due to its difficult location. The change in mental status cleared within 24 hours. A CT scan taken during the period of disorientation offered no explanation and was unchanged from her pretherapy scan. The disorientation did not occur during Treatment no. 2, in which the ICP reached 26 cm H_2O with a ΔP of 13 cm H_2O. The normal-brain temperature reached 40.0 °C. Because this was our first patient to undergo brain hyperthermia, and safety was our main concern, the procedure was performed in the operating room with stereotaxic placement of the temperature probe. The length of the session, including the 1-hour hyperthermia treatment, lasted 5 hours. We feel that the patient's anxiety, coupled with her neurologic deficits (double vision, lack of coordination), the newness of the procedure, and the length of the first heating session, probably accounted for her change in mental status. With future patients who require temperature-probe placement under stereotaxic control, we plan to perform the procedure the day before the first heating session. Currently, neither the twist-drill hole placement nor the hyperthermia is performed in the operating room.

The second complication occurred in Patient C, a 43-year-old male who was suffering from multiple melanoma metastases throughout his cerebrum. He developed a 30-second grand mal seizure immediately following hyperthermia Treatment no. 9. The patient's opening ICP was 45 cm H_2O and fell to 30 cm H_2O by the conclusion of the hyperthermia session. His normal-brain temperature reached 41.3 °C. This patient had not been on anti-convulsant therapy because there was no prior seizure history; however, from this experience we have routinely placed all patients on Dilantin (300 mg/day) several weeks prior to therapy. No additional seizures have occurred in any patient. Due to his elevated ICP and seizure, Patient C was not treated again.

The last complication occurred in Patient I, a 45-year-old male with a right frontal lobe metastasis secondary to lung carcinoma. He tolerated Treatment no. 21 without difficulty, despite an elevated opening ICP of 30 cm H_2O, a maximum pressure of 47.5 cm H_2O, and a closing ICP of 37.2 cm H_2O. His normal-brain temperature reached 40.5 °C, and his tumor temperature reached 43.6 °C. However, 24 hours following the treatment, he became totally disoriented and developed left lower extremity paralysis. Prior to therapy, this limb had been paretic and demonstrated ankle clonus. An emergency CT scan demonstrated increased edema. His daily steroid

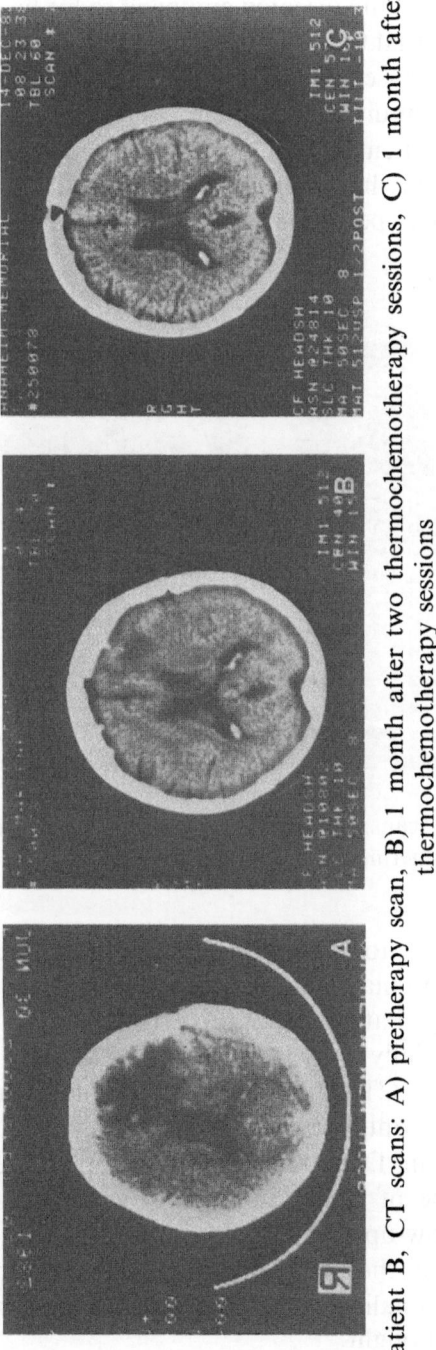

Fig. 3. Patient **B**, CT scans: A) pretherapy scan, B) 1 month after two thermochemotherapy sessions, C) 1 month after four thermochemotherapy sessions

dose was increased from 16 to 32 mg Decadron, and by the following day both the disorientation and paralysis were much improved. At his 1-week outpatient visit, he was totally oriented and back to his baseline neurologic status. We do not think that the complication in Patient A was attributable to the hyperthermia, because her maximum normal-brain temperature was only 39.8 °C, with a maximum ICP of 25 cm H_2O. However, the second and third complications in Patients C and I may have been, in some way, caused by the heat. Both patients had markedly elevated ICP pressures (45 and 30 cm H_2O) prior to the hyperthermia that may have been exacerbated by the heat.

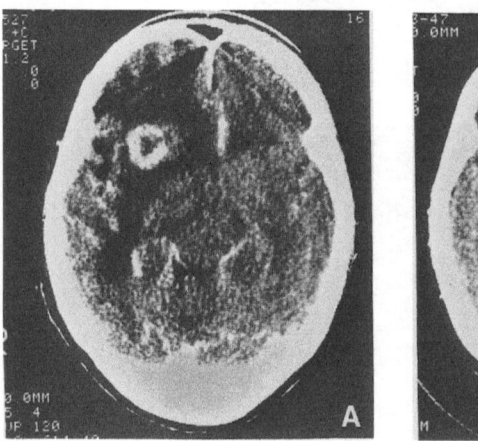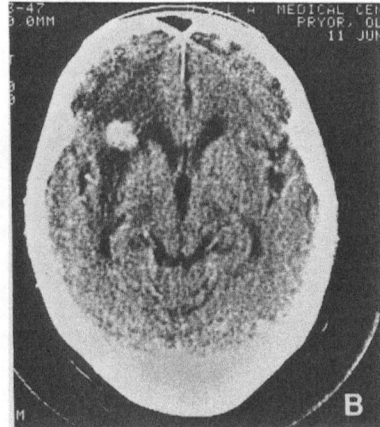

Fig. 4. Patient H, CT scans: A) pretherapy scan, B) 1 month after four thermochemotherapy sessions

Although it is too early to discuss the efficacy of thermochemotherapy for the treatment of brain malignancy, two patients, B and H, have had a response to the therapy. Patient B, a 46-year-old female with recurrent cystic glioblastoma, initially presented in late 1981 with complaints of headache and vomiting. A CT scan of her head revealed a large mass in the left frontal lobe. A left frontal craniotomy with complete excision of the tumor was performed in December 1981. Postoperatively the patient underwent a full course of radiation therapy which was completed in February 1982. A follow-up CT scan in June 1982 (Fig. 3 A) showed recurrence of the lesion in the left frontal area. Her symptoms at the time consisted of subtle personality changes, overall weakness without focal signs, and slowness in thought.

The patient was entered into our brain hyperthermia protocol in September 1982 and subsequently underwent a total of eight hyperthermia treatments. Each treatment was given simultaneously with an intravenous dose of BCNU (80 mg/m²). Her follow-up CT scans are shown in Fig. 3 B and 3 C demonstrating improvement. This patient, however, received BCNU for the first time during her initial course of thermochemotherapy, and it may be that her dramatic response was completely due to the BCNU. The response rate for BCNU in patients with recurrent gliomas is 46%, with an average survival of 3.25 mos[49]. However, applying the response criteria of Levin et al. (1977)[40], Egan and Scott (1983)[51], obtained regression rates of 13.3–33.3% for single-agent nitrosoureas. Because of the possible response to BCNU alone, all subsequent patients have received at least one course of IV BCNU before the combined therapy so the effect of chemotherapy alone can be assessed. After six treatments, Patient B stopped therapy, and unfortunately her disease recurred again after 9 months. She was treated two more times without benefit and died 8 months later.

Patient H is a 53-year-old female with recurrent metastatic lung carcinoma to the right frontal lobe following radiation therapy. She received an initial course of IV BCNU without success; however, a partial response was obtained with thermochemotherapy (Fig. 4). She remains alive with disease 11 months from the time of the diagnosis of her disease recurrence.

VII. Literature Review

The field of brain hyperthermia is in its early stages; however, a number of important in vitro, animal and human studies have already been done. Thuning et al. (1980) from the Goodwin Institute in Florida, demonstrated a synergism between hyperthermia and a nitrosourea (CCNU) in the treatment of a murine ependymoblastoma[46]. Using whole-body hyperthermia at 40 °C in combination with intraperitoneal CCNU, they found a statistically significant survival advantage for combined therapy over heat or drug therapy alone. This study is important because it demonstrates the synergism between heat and a chemotherapeutic agent active against human brain tumors. In addition, the tumor model was a primary brain tumor.

Lin and Lin (1982, 1984) from the University of Illinois studied the effects of microwaves on cerebrovascular permeability in rats[52, 53]. They used the extent of Evan's blue dye penetration into brain tissue as a measure of blood-brain barrier permeability. Their results demonstrated that BBB changes induced by microwave hyperthermia occurred only when the brain temperature reached 44 °C for at least 5 minutes. This study has important clinical implications, because if hyperthermia causes an increase in blood-brain barrier permeability, it may allow drugs to enter the brain that do not ordinarily cross the blood-brain barrier.

Britt et al. (1983) from Stanford, studied the feasibility of using ultrasound-generated hyperthermia in cats[54]. Bilateral craniotomies were performed to expose the dural surface, then ultrasonic radiation was applied for 50 minutes to generate temperatures up to 48 °C. At temperatures of less than 42 °C for 50 minutes, no evidence of damage could be detected histologically in either gray or white matter; however, at temperatures of 44–45 °C there was definite loss both of neurons in the gray matter and of myelin tracts in the white matter. This study demonstrated that ultrasound could effectively heat the brain in a controlled manner. These investigators also showed that the normal brain could withstand temperatures to 42 °C, the temperature at which neoplastic cells begin to show cytotoxic effects, without showing histologic evidence of damage. Furthermore, this study emphasizes the importance of monitoring maximum normal-brain temperature to avoid damage to normal-brain tissue.

Salcman et al. (1982) from the University of Maryland have conducted extensive animal studies with an implantable miniature microwave antenna for invasive heating of restricted tumor volumes. In normal cat brains, they found no evidence of alteration in vital functions, intracranial pressure, or tissue morphology[55]. This same group recently reported on six patients in whom the miniature microwave antenna was implanted[56, 57]. The antenna was inserted into the center of the residual tumor at the time of surgery. Each patient received two 1-hour treatments with the center of the field at 45 °C. No changes in vital signs, intracranial pressure or neurologic status were observed. In addition, the authors also noted that the tumor tissue was incapable of dissipating heat, presumably because of decreased blood flow. They concluded that hyperthermia may be applied safely to the human brain.

At the recent 4th International Symposium on Hyperthermic Oncology held in Aarhus, Denmark, several interesting papers were presented in the field of brain hyperthermia. The group from Niigata University in Japan studied the influence of hyperthermia on cerebral blood flow (CBF), cerebral metabolism as measured by tissue PO_2 and pH, and electroencephalography (EEG) in a rabbit model[58]. They found that CBF increased gradually as the cortical temperature increased to 40 °C but increased markedly at temperatures ≥ 43 °C. Tissue PO_2 and pH in the cerebral cortex increased as cortical temperature increased, and the peak frequency of the power spectrum of EEG also increased as the temperature was raised. High-amplitude rhythmic slow wave bursts appeared at 44 °C and soon changed to a flat pattern. It was noted that if the core aortic temperature of the animals remained under 43.5 °C, cerebral functions were preserved until the brain temperature reached 44 °C.

The same group also reported on the effects of radiofrequency hyperthermia on an experimental brain tumor in animals[59], and on human malignant brain tumors[60]. They found that localized hyperthermia at a radiofrequency of 13.56 MHz provided selective hyperthermia between tumor and normal-brain tissue in a monkey model. Temperatures as high as 50 °C were obtained in the tumor with virtually no injury to normal brain. This study supports the notion that normal brain, due to its excellent blood supply, is particularly difficult to heat and, as a result, normal-brain tissue can remain relatively cool during effective brain tumor heating. In their human study, four patients received "intracranial heating", *i.e.,* invasive heating, at the time of craniotomy. Radiofrequency electrodes were placed on the cerebral convexity and medial surface with the tumor between the electrodes. Each patient was heated for approximately 1 hour. "Extracranial heating" was performed in four additional patients. Following a bilateral craniectomy, a pair of radiofrequency electrodes were placed on the scalp bilaterally in order to put the tumor between the electrodes. These tumors were heated for approximately 1 hour, 2 times/week for 4 weeks. During this time the patients also received postoperative radiochemotherapy. As in their animal study, selective tumor heating was accomplished; however, complications (edema, bleeding) occurred in all patients receiving intracranial heating. Although responses were noted in several of their patients, a statement regarding the efficacy of hyperthermia per se cannot be made because of the uncontrolled use of multimodality therapy.

Sutton (1984) from the University of South Florida, reported on a regimen combining invasive hyperthermia with an immersion heater and parenteral chemotherapy[61]. To date, 18 patients with malignant gliomas have been treated. Tumor specimens removed en bloc from the 18 patients after 40 hours of invasive hyperthermia revealed four zones of histological change: 1. coagulation necrosis around the heater surface; 2. vasodilatation extending for 1–1.5 cm beyond the surface; 3. a zone of degenerating tumor cells; and 4. a peripheral zone of healthy unheated tumor. The authors conclude that moderate hyperthermia (42 °C) can kill glial tumor cells in man and that safe delivery of local hyperthermia to neoplasms within the human brain is feasible.

Thus, several groups around the world have some preliminary data in human patients that seem to indicate that brain hyperthermia is feasible and can be accomplished with a minimum of morbidity. The safety of brain hyperthermia is most likely the result of the normal brain's ability to dissipate incident heat by augmenting blood flow. We believe that noninvasive hyperthermia has definite advantages over the invasive techniques such as the microwave antenna or the immersion heater. First, of course, surgery is not required to provide the heat, and second, patients with multiple tumors and tumors in eloquent areas of the brain may be treated. In addition, the treatment can be repeated on a regular basis. It is our opinion that the ultimate role of hyperthermia in the treatment of malignant brain tumors will be in combination with radiation and/or chemotherapy. Furthermore, the *preoperative* use of combined thermoradiotherapy and/or thermochemotherapy may provide the maximum benefit by destroying the active tumor cells at the periphery of the tumor. The neurosurgeon and radiation therapist could then treat the remainder of the tumor and achieve local control, which in primary brain tumors is tantamount to cure. It is ironic that for most solid human cancers local control of the tumor can usually be accomplished, although the patient succumbs to distant disease. However, for patients with primary brain tumors, tumors which rarely metastasize, the patient succumbs to local disease because the exquisite nature of the brain does not allow the performance of radical surgery.

References

1. Coley, W. B., 1893: The treatment of malignant tumors by repeated innoculations of erysipelas: with a report of 10 original cases. Amer. J. Med. Sci. *105*, 487–511.
2. Cavaliere, R., Ciocatto, E. C., Giovanella, B. C., Heidelberger, C., Johnson, R. O., Margottini, M., Mondovi, B., Moricca, G., Rossi-Fanelli, A., 1967: Selective heat sensitivity of cancer cells: Biochemical and clinical studies. Cancer *20*, 1351–1381.
3. Hahn, G. M., Li, G. C., 1982: Interactions of hyperthermia and drugs: Treatments and probes. J. Nat. Cancer. Inst. Monogr. *61*, 317–323.
4. Stehlin, J. S., Giovanella, B. C., Ipolyi, P. D., Mueg, L. R., Anderson, R. F., 1975: Results of hyperthermic perfusion for melanoma of the extremities. Surg. Gynec. Obstet. *140*, 339–348.
5. Kim, J. H., Hahn, E. W., Tokita, N., Nisce, L. Z., 1977: Local tumor hyperthermia in combination with radiation therapy. Cancer *40*, 161–169.
6. Hornbeck, N. B., Shupe, R. E., Shidnia, H., Joe, B. T., Sayoc, E., Marshall, C., 1977: Preliminary clinical results of combined 433 MHz microwave therapy and radiation therapy on patients with advanced cancer. Cancer *40*, 2854–2863.
7. Salcman, M., 1980: Glioblastoma multiforme. Amer. J. Med. Sci. *279*, 84–94.
8. Zimm, S., Wampler, G. L., Stablein, D., Hazra, T., Young, H. F., 1981: Intracerebral metastases in solid-tumor patients: Natural history and results of treatment. Cancer *48*, 384–394.
9. Muckle, D. S., Dickson, J. A., 1972: The selective inhibitory effect of hyperthermia on the metabolism and growth of malignant cells. Br. J. Cancer *5*, 771–778.
10. Mondovi, B., Finazzi-Agro, A., Rotilio, G., Strom, R., Moricca, G., Rossi-Fanelli, A., 1969: The biochemical mechanism of selective heat sensitivity of cancer cells. II. Studies on nucleic acids and protein synthesis. Eur. J. Cancer *5*, 137–147.
11. Strom, R., Santoro, A. S., Crifo, C., Bozzi, A., Mondovi, B., Rossi-Fanelli, A., 1973: The biochemical mechanism of selective heat sensitivity of cancer cells. IV. Inhibition of RNA synthesis. Eur. J. Cancer *9*, 103–112.

12. Hahn, G. M., 1975: Thermochemotherapy: Interactions between hyperthermia and chemotherapeutic agents. In: Proc. Int. Symp. on Cancer Therapy by Hyperthermia and Rad. Washington, D.C. Amer. Coll. Rad. Press, pp. 61–65.
13. Strom, R., 1970: Ricerche sul meccanismo d'azione del calore sui tumori. Atti. Soc. Ital. Cancer. V. Nat. Congr. Vol. 7, Part 2, 49–60.
14. Turano, C., Ferraro, A., Strom, R., Cavaliere, R., Rossi-Fanelli, A., 1970: The biochemical mechanism of selective heat sensitivity of cancer cells. III. Studies on lysosomes. Eur. J. Cancer 6, 67–72.
15. Dickson, J. A., Calderwood, S. K., 1983: Thermosensitivity of neoplastic tissues in vivo. In: Hyperthermia in Cancer Therapy (Storm, F. K., ed.), pp. 63–140. Boston: G. K. Hall.
16. Hardy, J. D., Stolwijk, J. A. J., Hammel, H. T., 1965: Skin temperature and cutaneous pain during warm water immersion. J. Appl. Physiol. 20, 1014–1021.
17. Westermark, N., 1927: The effect of heat upon rat tumors. Skand. Arch. Physiol. 52, 257–322.
18. Crile, G., 1962: Selective destruction of cancers after exposure to heat. Ann. Surg. 156, 404–407.
19. Mantyla, M. J., 1979: Regional blood flow in human tumors. Cancer Res. 39, 2304–2306.
20. Storm, F. K., Elliott, R. S., Harrison, W. H., Morton, D. L., 1979: Normal tissue and solid tumor effects of hyperthermia in animal models and clinical trials. Cancer Res. 39, 2245–2251.
21. Doss, J. D., 1975: Use of RF fields to produce hyperthermia in animal tumors. Proc. Int. Symp. on Cancer Therapy by Hyperthermia and Rad, pp. 226–227. Washington, D.C.: Amer. Coll. Rad. Press.
22. Sternhagen, C. J., Doss, J. D., Day, P. W., Edwards, W. S., Doberneck, R. C., Herzon, F. S., Powell, T. D., O'Brien, G. F., Larkin, J. M., 1978: Clinical use of radiofrequency current in oral cavity carcinomas and metastatic malignancies with continuous temperature control and monitoring. In: Cancer Therapy by Hyperthermia and Rad. (Streffer, C., ed.), pp. 331–334. Baltimore: Urban & Schwarzenberg.
23. Rand, R. W., Snow, H. D., Brown, W. J., 1982: Thermomagnetic surgery for cancer. J. Surg. Res. 33, 177–183.
24. Lele, P. P., 1975: Hyperthermia by ultrasound. In: Proc. Int. Symp. on Cancer Therapy by Hyperthermia and Rad., pp. 168–178. Washington, D.C.: Amer. Coll. Rad. Press.
25. Schwan, H. P., 1980: Electromagnetic and ultrasonic induction of hyperthermia in tissue-like substances. Radiat. Environ. Biophys. 17, 189–203.
26. Guy, A. W., Chou, C. K., 1983: Physical aspects of localized heating by radiowaves and microwaves. In: Hyperthermia in Cancer Therapy (Storm, F. K., ed.), pp. 279–304. Boston: G. K. Hall.
27. Le Veen H. H., Wapnick, S., Piccone, V., Falk, G., Ahmed, N., 1976: Tumor eradication by radiofrequency therapy. Response in 21 patients. J.A.M.A. 235, 2198–2200.
28. Storm, F. K., 1983: Hyperthermia in Cancer Therapy. Boston: G. K. Hall, Medical Publ.

29. Lehmann, F. J., 1982: Therapeutic Heat and Cold, 3rd ed. Baltimore: Williams and Wilkins.

30. Third Int. Symposium: Cancer therapy by hyperthermia, drugs, and radiation. NCI Monograph 61, 1982.

31. Walker, M. D., Green, S. B., Byar, D. P., et al., 1980: Randomized comparisons of radiotherapy and nitrosoureas for the treatment of malignant glioma after surgery. NEJM 303, 1323–1329.

32. Storm, F. K., Harrison, W. H., Elliott, R. S., Hatzitheofilou, C., Morton, D. L., 1979: Human hyperthermic therapy: Relationship between tumor type and capacity to induce hyperthermia by radiofrequency. Amer. J. Surg. 138, 170–174.

33. Storm, F. K., Harrison, W. H., Elliott, R. S., Morton, D. L., 1980: Hyperthermic therapy for human neoplasms: Thermal death time. Cancer 46, 1849–1854.

34. Storm, F. K., Harrison, W. H., Elliott, R. S., Kaiser, L. R., Silberman, A. W., Morton, D. L., 1981: Clinical radiofrequency hyperthermia by magnetic-loop induction. J. Microwave Power 16, 179–184.

35. Storm, F. K., Morton, D. L., Kaiser, L. R., Harrison, W. H., Elliott, R. S., Weisenburger, T. H., Parker, R. G., Haskell, C. M., 1982: Clinical radiofrequency hyperthermia: A review. J. Natl. Cancer. Inst. Monogr. 61, 343–350.

36. Elliott, R. S., Harrison, W. H., Storm, F. K., 1982: Electromagnetic heating of deep-seated tumors. IEEE. Trans. Biomed. Engin. 29, 61–64.

37. Storm, F. K., Harrison, W. H., Elliott, R. S., Silberman, A. W., Morton, D. L., 1982: Thermal distribution of magnetic-loop induction hyperthermia in phantoms and animals: Effect of the living state and velocity of heating. Int. J. Rad. Oncol. Biol. Phys. 8, 865–871.

38. Baker, H. W., Snedecor, P. A., Goss, J. C., Galen, W. P., Gallucci, P., Horowitz, I. J., Dugan, K., 1982: Regional hyperthermia for cancer. Amer. J. Surg. 143, 586–590.

39. Storm, F. K., Silberman, A. W., Ramming, K. P., Kaiser, L. R., Harrison, W. H., Elliott, R. S., Haskell, C. M., Sarna, G., Morton, D. L., 1984: Clinical thermochemotherapy: A controlled trial in advanced cancer patients. Cancer 53, 863–868.

40. Silberman, A. W., Morgan, D. F., Storm, F. K., Rand, R. W., Bubbers, J. E., Brown, W. J., Morton, D. L., 1982: Localized magnetic-loop induction hyperthermia of the rabbit brain. J. Surg. Oncol. 20, 174–178.

41. Krainer, L., 1949: Lamellar atrophy of the purkinje cells following heat stroke. Arch. Neuro. Psychiat. 51, 441–444.

42. Morgan, D. F., Silberman, A. W., Bubbers, J. E., Rand, R. W., Storm, F. K., Morton, D. L., 1982: An experimental brain tumor model in rabbits. J. Surg. Oncol. 20, 218–220.

43. Silberman, A. W., Morgan, D. F., Storm, F. K., Rand, R. W., Benz, M., Drury, B., Morton, D. L., 1984: Combination radiofrequency hyperthermia and chemotherapy (BCNU) for brain malignancy: Animal experience and two case reports. J. Neuro-Oncol. 2, 19–28.

44. Silberman, A. W., Rand, R. W., Storm, F. K., Drury, B., Benz, M. L., Morton,

D. L., 1985: Phase I trial of thermochemotherapy for brain malignancy. Cancer *56*, 48–56.

45. Storm, F. K., Baker, H. W., Scanlon, E. F., *et al.*, 1985: Magnetic-induction hyperthermia: Results of a 5-year multi-institutional national cooperative trial in advanced cancer patients. Cancer *55*, 2677–2687.

46. Thuning, C. A., Bakir, N. A., Warren, J., 1980: Synergistic effect of combined hyperthermia and a nitrosourea in treatment of a murine ependymoblastoma. Cancer Res. *40*, 2726–2729.

47. Rosner, D., Nemoto, T., Pickren, J., Lane, W., 1983: Management of brain metastases from breast cancer by combination chemotherapy. J. Neuro-Oncol. *1*, 131–137.

48. Olch, A. J., Kaiser, L. R., Silberman, A. W., Storm, F. K., Graham, L. S., Morton, D. L., 1983: Blood flow in human tumors during hyperthermia therapy: Demonstration of vasoregulation and an applicable physiological model. J. Surg. Oncol. *23*, 125–132.

49. Goldsmith, M. A., Carter, K. S., 1974: Glioblastoma multiforme—A review of therapy. Cancer. Treat. Rev. *1*, 153–165.

50. Levin, V. A., Crafts, D. C., Norman, D. M., Hoffer, P. B., Spire, J. P., Wilson, C. B., 1977: Criteria for evaluating patients undergoing chemotherapy for malignant brain tumors. J. Neurosurg. *47*, 329–335.

51. Egan, R. T., Scott, M., 1983: Evaluation of prognostic factors in chemotherapy of recurrent brain tumors. J. Clin. Oncol. *1*, 38–44.

52. Lin, J. C., Lin, M. F., 1982: Microwave hyperthermia-induced blood-brain barrier alterations. Rad. Res. *89*, 77–87.

53. Lin, J. C., Lin, M. F., 1984: Blood-brain barrier changes under microwave hyperthermia. Hyperthermic. Oncol. *1*, 737–738. Abstract.

54. Britt, R. H., Lyons, B. E., Pounds, D. W., Prionas, S. D., 1983: Feasibility of ultrasound hyperthermia in the treatment of malignant brain tumors. Med. Instrum. *17*, 172–177.

55. Samaras, G. M., Salcman, M., Chung, A. Y., Abdo, H. S., Schepp, R. S., 1982: Microwave-induced hyperthermia: An experimental adjunct for brain tumor therapy. Natl. Cancer. Inst. Monogr. *61*, 477–482.

56. Salcman, M., Kaplan, R. S., Samaras, G. M., Ducker, T. B., Broadwell, R. D., 1982: Aggressive multimodality therapy based on a multicompartmental model of glioblastoma. Surg. *92*, 250–259.

57. Salcman, M., Samaras, G. M., 1983: Interstitial microwave hyperthermia for brain tumors. J. Neuro-Oncol. *1*, 225–236.

58. Yamada, N., Tanaka, R., Kanayama, T., Suzuki, Y., Takeda, N., Sekiguchi, K., Saito, Y., 1984: The influence of hyperthermia on cerebral functions— blood flow, metabolism and electroencephalography. Hyperthermic. Oncol. *4*, T_1. Abstract.

59. Tanaka, R., Kim, C. H., Yamada, M., Saito, Y., 1984: RF hyperthermia of experimental brain tumor. Hyperthermic. Oncol. *4*, T_5. Abstract.

60. Tanaka, R., Yamada, N., Kim, C. H., Saito, Y., 1984: RF hyperthermia of human malignant brain tumor. Hyperthermic. Onco. *4*, T_6. Abstract.

61. Sutton, C. H., 1984: Invasive hyperthermia and chemotherapy for the treatment of malignant gliomas of the brain. Hyperthermic. Oncol. *4*, T_7. Abstract.

Subject Index

Acoustic tumors 118, 121, 261–264, 271
A-mode echoencephalography 20–25
Anesthesiological technique 228–234
Argon laser 56, 59, 62, 64, 65, 67, 68, 85,
  86, 88–91, 95, 98, 99, 121, 126, 127, 132,
  142, 143, 145–152, 196, 251, 252
Arterial aneurysms 10, 33, 39, 40–44, 127–
  135
Arterio-venous malformations 10, 42, 43,
  44, 124–127
Atherosclerotic disease 35, 56, 195, 196,
  197

Bipolar coagulation 99, 100, 120
Bipolar cutting 124
Bonding mechanisms 185
Brain stem tumors 119, 123, 271

Carotid endoarterectomy, ultrasound control 18
Cerebellar tumors 119, 122, 261, 271
Computerized-assisted stereotactic laser
  procedures 162–174
Computerized laser 56
Contact laser 140–144, 252
Copper vapor laser 252
CO_2 laser 56, 59, 62, 63, 64, 65, 72–83, 85,
  87, 88–91, 93, 94, 95, 98, 99, 108, 110,
  116, 117, 118, 119, 120, 121, 124, 126,
  127, 135, 136, 143, 155, 163, 175, 178,
  196, 251
Craniopharyngiomas 117, 118, 148
Cutting 98

Discectomy 16, 136
Doppler sonography
  anastomosis 36–39
  aneurysms 33, 39, 40, 44
  arterio-venous malformations 42, 43,
    44
  extracranial-intracranial by pass proce-
    dures 37–39
  instrumentation 31–33
  normal cerebral arteries 33, 34
  stenosis 35
  techniques 28–31

Dorsal Root Entry Zone Lesions (DREZ)
  136, 150, 151
Dye laser 57, 211–223

Excimer laser 58, 201, 202, 237–241
Extraaxial cerebral tumors 116–118, 147–
  149, 154–160
Eyes damage by laser 104, 105, 229, 230

Free-electron laser 241–248, 252, 253

Gamma ray laser 57, 58, 252
Gliomas 24, 25, 110, 121, 122, 142, 149,
  212, 219, 222, 261, 271

Heavy metal vapor laser 252
Hematoporphyrine derivative (HpD)
  concentration of HpD in tumors 66,
    213–215
  HpD tumor cell killing efficiency 66,
    215–218
  phototoxicity of HpD 215
Hemostasis 99, 100
He-Neon laser 56, 57, 59, 64, 65, 67
High frequency jet ventilation (HFJV) 232,
  233
High-peak pulsed irradiation CO_2 laser 63,
  97, 110
Historical review 20, 21, 27, 28, 51, 52, 211,
  212, 257, 258, 277
Hyperthermia 277–300
  animal studies 116, 281–285, 291, 292,
    297, 298
  combination of hyperthermia and che-
    motherapy 284, 285, 290, 291, 292,
    296, 297, 299, 300
  complications of hyperthermia 293–296
  effects on intracranial pressure 283,
    290, 293, 297, 298
  human studies 116, 285–290, 293–296,
    299, 300
  localized hyperthermia techniques 279,
    297, 298, 299
  tumoricidal temperatures 66, 278, 279,
    283, 290, 292

Intraaxial cerebral tumors   118, 119, 149, 150
Intramedullary tumors   15, 120, 150, 264–266, 271

Laser
  l. absorption   54, 97
  absorption coefficients in tissues   59, 108, 218, 219
  active medium   54, 55, 56, 57, 238–241
  characteristics of l.   57
  l. emission   54
  functional studies on l. effects   94, 95, 127, 128, 135, 229
  generation of l.   53–55
  interaction of l. with matter
    qualitative   57
    quantitative   58, 108, 146
  l. lesion
    brain tissue damage in the target area
      acute 72–74, 93, 94
      chronic   82
    brain tissue damage in the outer periphery of the lesion   74, 82
    defect of the blood-brain barrier   74, 78, 80, 94
    effect on atherosclerotic obstruction 198–202, 203, 204
    effect on thrombotic obstruction   204
    histochemical data   82, 83
    nerves damage   83
    vessels damage
      acute   85–91, 99, 124, 125, 127
      chronic   91, 92, 124, 127
  optical cavity   55
  pumping   55, 238
  l. recanalization   206
    risk of l. recanalization   204–206
  l. risks   229–232
    carcinogenic effects   106
    electrical risk   104
    inhalation of toxic vapour   105
    mechanical r.   104
    r. of fire   106
    r. of microbiological contamination 105
  l. scalpel   140–144
  l. terminology   60
  l. tissue effects   61
    biologic effects   67, 68
    effects related to electromagnetic field 67
    mechanical effects   67
    photochemical reaction   65, 66
    thermal effects on tissue   62, 63
    thermal effects on vessels and blood 64, 125
    thermal recording in tissue   64, 65

M-CO$_2$ laser   186, 116–118
Meningiomas   24, 25, 111, 121, 122, 142, 148, 261–264, 271
  basal meningiomas   33, 117, 120, 264, 271
  convexity meningiomas   116, 270
  parasagittal meningiomas   177–182
Microscope   88

Nd:YAG laser   57, 59, 62, 67, 68, 72–83, 86, 87, 88–91, 95, 98, 99, 108, 115, 117, 118, 119, 121, 124, 125, 126, 127, 142, 143, 157, 159, 196, 251, 252
Nerves coaption   176, 179
Nerves repair
  current microsurgical techniques   176
  laser repair   177–182
Neurinomas   25, 118, 121, 148, 261

Operative technique
  arterial aneurysms   131–135
  AVMs   125–127, 149, 171
  nervous system tumors   116–123, 147–150, 154–160, 167–173

Pain procedures   136, 150, 151
Photofrin   213
Photoradiation therapy   (P.R.T.)   211–223
  application of HpD P.R.T. by irradiation of tumor bed after resection 220–222
  clinical studies on HpD P.R.T.   219–222
  stereotactic application of HpD P.R.T. 66, 219, 220
Pinealomas   117, 118, 261, 271
Pituitary adenomas   117, 118, 148, 261

Radiofrequency hyperthermia by Magnetrode 279–280
Real-time sonography
  abscesses   10
  angiomas   10
  aneurysms   10
  AVMs   10
  cerebral tumors   10
  disc fragments   16
  extradural extramedullary tumors   16
  instrumentation   4–6, 10, 11, 12, 14, 18
  intracerebral hematomas   10
  intradural extramedullary tumors   16
  intramedullary tumors   15
  localization/characterization   8–10
  metastatic tumors   8, 9
  spondylosis   17, 18
  syringomyelia   15, 16
  technique   6–8, 14, 15
  trauma   10, 18

Safety procedures   103–106
Skin damage by laser   105
Spinal cord tumors   15, 16, 119, 150, 264–
  266
Stereotactic CO_2 laser approach of
  deep-seated AVMs   171
  deep-seated tumors   162–174
Syringohydromyelia   15, 16, 135, 136, 151

Thermochemotherapy   284, 285, 290, 300
Transconjunctival oxygen monitoring system
  233, 234

Ultrasonic aspirator (CUSA)   251, 257–
  272
  dissection procedures   266–270
  functional studies on CUSA effects   266
  histology of CUSA lesion   260, 266,
    267, 268, 269, 272

technical characteristics of CUSA   258,
  259
tumor removal with CUSA   123, 124,
  260–266
Ultrasound   3–18, 20–25, 27–45
Ultrasound guidance of
  biopsy cannula   11, 12, 14
  drainage of cysts or abscesses   13, 14, 18
  ventricular catheter   14

Vaporization   98, 99
Vascular repair by laser
  arterial anastomoses   187–190
  growing anastomoses   191, 192
  venous anastomoses   190

Welding   100, 127, 130, 191, 192

X-ray lasers   57, 252

Differential Approaches in Microsurgery of the Brain

By Professor **Wolfgang Seeger,** M. D.,
Medical Director of the Department of General Neurosurgery and Chairman of
Neurosurgery of the Neurosurgical Clinic, University of Freiburg i. Br., FRG

In Collaboration with **W. Mann**

1985. 201 figures. VII, 414 pages.
Format: 23,7 cm × 32 cm. ISBN 3-211-81857-X

In this book the various possible approaches to the same target are presented with
their advantages and disadvantages for the first time. The normal anatomical variations seen preoperatively and the specific processes which are similar but never
identical may require different operative procedures even for the same target area.
This problem concerns almost exclusively the deep lying processes in the area of the
brainstem and ventricular system. In most routine interventions in the cerebrum and
cerebellum this problem is not present, so that one can limit the operative approaches
according to this cisterns. The dorsal cisternal area of the brainstem is especially
important and has only in recent years been increasingly operated on. Here the
danger of psychological disturbances due to damage of the limbic system is
particularly great. Until now a systematic review of this area from the microsurgical
aspect has been absent.

As in his previous volumes Professor Seeger proves once again to be not only an
extremely experienced and gifted specialist in his field but also a man with rare
artistic talents. The book presents highly valuable information to specialists working
in the fields of neurosurgery, neurorhinootology, neurology, neuroradiology, neuro-
pathology, anatomy, pathology, ophthalmology, microvascular surgery, oral surgery,
and plastic surgery.

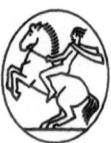

Springer-Verlag Wien New York